全国高等中医药院校中药学类专业双语规划教材
Bilingual Planned Textbooks for Chinese Materia Medica Majors in TCM Colleges and Universities

药理学

Pharmacology

（供中药学类、药学类及相关专业使用）

(For Chinese Materia Medica, Pharmacy and other related majors)

主　编　周玖瑶

副主编　殷玉婷　彭　芙　徐志立　王芙蓉　董世芬

编　者　（以姓氏笔画为序）

马秉亮	上海中医药大学	王　平	成都中医药大学
王志琪	湖南中医药大学	王芙蓉	山东中医药大学
王宏婷	皖南医学院	乌仁图雅	内蒙古民族大学蒙医药学院
白　莉	河南中医药大学	吕　莹	长春中医药大学
朱星枚	陕西中医药大学	辛晓明	上海健康医学院
张　峰	南京中医药大学	张海宁	广州医科大学
周　园	广州中医药大学	周玖瑶	广州中医药大学
徐志立	辽宁中医药大学	殷玉婷	江西中医药大学
陶小军	辽宁中医药大学	彭　芙	四川大学华西药学院
董世芬	北京中医药大学	程媛媛	广州中医药大学

秘书（兼）周　园

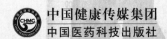

中国健康传媒集团

中国医药科技出版社

内 容 提 要

本教材是"全国高等中医药院校中药学类专业双语规划教材"之一，教材内容经典、精简适用、格式新颖，强调药理学基本知识、基本理论，注重科学性与系统性。全书共 43 章，内容包括：药理学总论、作用于外周神经系统药理、作用于中枢神经系统药理、作用于心血管系统及肾脏药理、作用于内分泌系统药理、作用于消化系统和呼吸系统及子宫药理、抗组胺药、抗贫血药、化学治疗药、免疫调节药。本教材为书网融合教材，即纸质教材有机融合电子教材、教学配套资源（PPT、微课、视频、图片等）、题库系统、数字化教学服务（在线教学、在线作业、在线考试），使教学资源更加多样化、立体化。

本教材供高等中医药院校中药学类各专业双语教学使用，也可供从事药物研究、生产、销售工作的人员参考。

图书在版编目（CIP）数据

药理学：汉英对照 / 周玖瑶主编 . —北京：中国医药科技出版社，2020.8

全国高等中医药院校中药学类专业双语规划教材

ISBN 978 - 7 - 5214 - 1880 - 4

Ⅰ . ①药… Ⅱ . ①周… Ⅲ . ①药理学 – 双语教学 – 中医学院 – 教材 – 汉、英 Ⅳ . ①R96

中国版本图书馆 CIP 数据核字（2020）第 101857 号

美术编辑 陈君杞

版式设计 辰轩文化

出版 **中国健康传媒集团** | 中国医药科技出版社

地址 北京市海淀区文慧园北路甲 22 号

邮编 100082

电话 发行：010 - 62227427 邮购：010 - 62236938

网址 www.cmstp.com

规格 889 × 1194 mm $\frac{1}{16}$

印张 22 ½

字数 572 千字

版次 2020 年 8 月第 1 版

印次 2020 年 8 月第 1 次印刷

印刷 三河市万龙印装有限公司

经销 全国各地新华书店

书号 ISBN 978 - 7 - 5214 - 1880 - 4

定价 **69.00** 元

获取新书信息、投稿、为图书纠错，请扫码联系我们。

近些年随着世界范围的中医药热潮的涌动，来中国学习中医药学的留学生逐年增多，走出国门的中医药学人才也在增加。为了适应中医药国际交流与合作的需要，加快中医药国际化进程，提高来中国留学生和国际班学生的教学质量，满足双语教学的需要和中医药对外交流需求，培养优秀的国际化中医药人才，进一步推动中医药国际化进程，根据教育部、国家中医药管理局、国家药品监督管理局等部门的有关精神，在本套教材建设指导委员会主任委员成都中医药大学彭成教授等专家的指导和顶层设计下，中国医药科技出版社组织全国 50 余所高等中医药院校及附属医疗机构约 420 名专家、教师精心编撰了全国高等中医药院校中药学类专业双语规划教材，该套教材即将付梓出版。

本套教材共计 23 门，主要供全国高等中医药院校中药学类专业教学使用。本套教材定位清晰、特色鲜明，主要体现在以下方面。

一、立足双语教学实际，培养复合应用型人才

本套教材以高校双语教学课程建设要求为依据，以满足国内医药院校开展留学生教学和双语教学的需求为目标，突出中医药文化特色鲜明、中医药专业术语规范的特点，注重培养中医药技能、反映中医药传承和现代研究成果，旨在优化教育质量，培养优秀的国际化中医药人才，推进中医药对外交流。

本套教材建设围绕目前中医药院校本科教育教学改革方向对教材体系进行科学规划、合理设计，坚持以培养创新型和复合型人才为宗旨，以社会需求为导向，以培养适应中药开发、利用、管理、服务等各个领域需求的高素质应用型人才为目标的教材建设思路与原则。

二、遵循教材编写规律，整体优化，紧跟学科发展步伐

本套教材的编写遵循"三基、五性、三特定"的教材编写规律；以"必需、够用"为度；坚持与时俱进，注意吸收新技术和新方法，适当拓展知识面，为学生后续发展奠定必要的基础。实验教材密切结合主干教材内容，体现理实一体，注重培养学生实践技能训练的同时，按照教育部相关精神，增加设计性实验部分，以现实问题作为驱动力来培养学生自主获取和应用新知识的能力，从而培养学生独立思考能力、实验设计能力、实践操作能力和可持续发展能力，满足培养应用型和复合型人才的要求。强调全套教材内容的整体优化，并注重不同教材内容的联系与衔接，避免遗漏和不必要的交叉重复。

三、对接职业资格考试，"教考""理实"密切融合

本套教材的内容和结构设计紧密对接国家执业中药师职业资格考试大纲要求，实现教学与考试、理论与实践的密切融合，并且在教材编写过程中，吸收具有丰富实践经验的企业人员参与教材的编写，确保教材的内容密切结合应用，更加体现高等教育的实践性和开放性，为学生参加考试和实践工作打下坚实基础。

四、创新教材呈现形式，书网融合，使教与学更便捷更轻松

全套教材为书网融合教材，即纸质教材与数字教材、配套教学资源、题库系统、数字化教学服务有机融合。通过"一书一码"的强关联，为读者提供全免费增值服务。按教材封底的提示激活教材后，读者可通过 PC、手机阅读电子教材和配套课程资源（PPT、微课、视频等），并可在线进行同步练习，实时收到答案反馈和解析。同时，读者也可以直接扫描书中二维码，阅读与教材内容关联的课程资源，从而丰富学习体验，使学习更便捷。教师可通过 PC 在线创建课程，与学生互动，开展在线课程内容定制、布置和批改作业、在线组织考试、讨论与答疑等教学活动，学生通过 PC、手机均可实现在线作业、在线考试，提升学习效率，使教与学更轻松。此外，平台尚有数据分析、教学诊断等功能，可为教学研究与管理提供技术和数据支撑。需要特殊说明的是，有些专业基础课程，例如《药理学》等 9 种教材，起源于西方医学，因篇幅所限，在本次双语教材建设中纸质教材以英语为主，仅将专业词汇对照了中文翻译，同时在中国医药科技出版社数字平台"医药大学堂"上配套了中文电子教材供学生学习参考。

编写出版本套高质量教材，得到了全国知名专家的精心指导和各有关院校领导与编者的大力支持，在此一并表示衷心感谢。希望广大师生在教学中积极使用本套教材和提出宝贵意见，以便修订完善，共同打造精品教材，为促进我国高等中医药院校中药学类专业教育教学改革和人才培养做出积极贡献。

全国高等中医药院校中药学类专业双语规划教材
建设指导委员会

数字化教材编委会

主　编　周玖瑶

副主编　殷玉婷　彭　芙　徐志立　王芙蓉　董世芬

编　者（以姓氏笔画为序）

马秉亮	上海中医药大学	王　平	成都中医药大学
王志琪	湖南中医药大学	王芙蓉	山东中医药大学
王宏婷	皖南医学院	乌仁图雅	内蒙古民族大学蒙医药学院
白　莉	河南中医药大学	吕　莹	长春中医药大学
朱星枚	陕西中医药大学	辛晓明	上海健康医学院
张　峰	南京中医药大学	张海宁	广州医科大学
周　园	广州中医药大学	周玖瑶	广州中医药大学
徐志立	辽宁中医药大学	殷玉婷	江西中医药大学
陶小军	辽宁中医药大学	彭　芙	四川大学华西药学院
董世芬	北京中医药大学	程媛媛	广州中医药大学

秘书（兼）周　园

　　药理学是中药学专业的主干课程之一，本教材本着内容经典、精简适用、格式新颖的编写原则，在编写上强调药理学基本知识与理论特色，注重科学性、系统性、可读性及准确性，便于教与学，更好地适应新形势下全国高等中医药院校中药学类专业教育教学改革和发展的需要，培养传承中医药文明、创新型高等中药学类专业人才。

　　1. **内容经典**　参考了多部国外、国内药理学经典教材的内容。

　　2. **精简适用**　针对中医院校中药学类本科生教学，注重把握教材的深度和广度，基于药理学属英文主体的西医学与药学的桥梁学科的特点，采用以英文为主、中英结合的编写方式，通过专业词汇的中英文对照，清除学生学习的语言障碍，力求做到学生好学、教师好教。

　　3. **格式新颖**　①参考药理学英语版经典专著重新创作插图，在保证全书图片清晰美观的基础上有所创新。②引入中文学习目标、重点小结及目标检测等模块，使学习目标明确，重点突出并可检验学习效果。③建设与纸质教材配套的数字化教学资源，即纸质教材有机融合电子教材（含中文电子教材）、教学配套资源（PPT、微课、视频、图片等）、题库系统、数字化教学服务（在线教学、在线作业、在线考试），使教学资源更加多样化、产体化。

　　全书共43章，内容包括：药理学总论（1~3章）；作用于外周神经系统药理（4~9章）；作用于中枢神经系统药理（10~15章）；作用于心血管系统及肾脏药理（16~22章）；作用于内分泌系统药理（23~26章）；作用于消化系统、呼吸系统及子宫药理（27~29章）；抗组胺药（30章）；抗贫血药（31章）；化学治疗药（32~42章）；免疫调节药（43章）。各章节重点介绍代表药物，深入浅出，举一反三。

　　本教材主要供高等中医药院校中药学类各专业双语教学使用，也可供从事药物研究、生产、销售工作的人员参考。

　　本教材在编写过程中得到了各参编单位的大力支持，各位编委各尽其责，确保教材如期出版，在此一并致以真挚的谢意！本教材虽力臻完美，但还有需要不断完善和修订之处，希望广大专家、教师、同学能多提宝贵意见和批评指导，不胜感激！

编　者

2020 年 4 月

Preface

Pharmacology is one of the main courses for Chinese medicine major. Based on the principles of classic content, simplicity, practicality, and novel format, this bilingual textbook emphasizes the basic knowledge and theory, as well as the scientific nature and systematicness, which is convenient for teaching and learning, and better adapt to the teaching reform and development needs of Chinese medicine in universities under the new situation, and trains and inherits Chinese medicine civilization and innovative talents of Chinese medicine specialty.

1. The classic content   It refers to many classic textbooks of pharmacology at home and abroad.

2. Concise and applicative   The textbook mainly aims at the teaching of undergraduates majoring in Chinese Medicine and puts emphasis on grasping the depth and breadth of the teaching materials. Moreover, based on the characteristics of pharmacology as a bridge between modern medicine and pharmacy, the book was written in Chinese and English. Through the comparison of specialized words in Chinese and English, students can break language barrier and better grasp the classical contents and the progress of pharmacology. The ultimate goal is to ensure that students easy to learn and teachers easy to teach.

3. Novel format   ① With reference to the English version of the classic monograph of pharmacology, the illustrations are recreated with innovation to ensure the clarity and beauty of the pictures in the whole book. ② The introduction of learning goal, key summary and target detection module make the learning goal oriented, the key points highlighted, and the learning effect assessable. ③ The construction of digital teaching resources matched with paper-based teaching materials, such as electronic teaching materials, teaching supporting resources (PPT, micro courses, video, pictures, etc.), question bank system, digital teaching services (online teaching, online homework, online examination), which makes teaching resources more diversified and productive.

The textbook consists of 43 chapters, including: general introduction to Pharmacology (chapter 1-3); peripheral neuropharmacology (chapter 4-9); central nervous system pharmacology (chapter 10-15); cardiovascular and renal pharmacology (chapter 16-22); endocrine system pharmacology (chapter 23-26); digestive, respiratory and uterine pharmacology (chapter 27-29); antihistamines (chapter 30); antianemic (chapter 31); chemotherapy drugs (chapter 32-42); immunomodulatory drugs (chapter 43). The contents of pharmacodynamics and pharmacokinetics of representative drugs in each chapter are highlighted, explaining the profound knowledge in a straightforward way and making students draw inferences about other cases from one instance.

This textbook is mainly used by undergraduates majoring in Chinese Medicine in colleges and universities of Chinese medicine. It can also be utilized as a reference for staff engaged in drug research, production and sales.

In the compilation process, this textbook has been greatly supported by all participating organizations. Each editorial committee has its own responsibility to make sure that the textbook is published as scheduled. I would like to place on record my sincere thanks to them. As a teaching material, the textbook still needs to be continuously improved and revised. We are in the hope that experts, teachers and students can provide more valuable comments and critical guidance.

Editor

April,2020

Contents

Chapter 1 Introduction to Pharmacology

 学习目标

1. **掌握** 药理学的概念与研究内容。
2. **熟悉** 药理学的发展简史。
3. **了解** 药理学与药物研发的关系。

1. Drug and Pharmacology

A drug is any natural or synthetic substance which (when taken into a living body) affects its functioning or structure, and is used in the diagnosis, mitigation (缓解), treatment, or prevention of a disease or relief of discomfort. It is also called legal drug or medicine.

Pharmacology (药理学) can be defined as the study of substances that interact with living systems through chemical processes, especially by binding to regulatory molecules and activating or inhibiting normal body processes. These substances may be chemicals administered to achieve a beneficial therapeutic effect on some process within the patient or for their toxic effects on regulatory processes in parasites (寄生虫) infecting the patient. Such deliberate therapeutic applications may be considered the proper role of medical pharmacology, which is often defined as the science of substances used to prevent, diagnose and treat disease. Toxicology is one branch of pharmacology which deals with the undesirable effects of chemicals on living systems, from individual cells to complex ecosystems (复杂的生态系统).

In addition to the known pharmacological action by binding to a particular receptor in a specific tissue, numerous factors contribute to the successful drug therapy. When a drug enters the body, the body begins immediately to work on the drug: absorption (吸收), distribution (分布), metabolism (biotransformation) [代谢(生物转化)], and elimination (排泄). These are the processes of pharmacokinetics (药物代谢动力学). On the other side, the drugs also act on the body mainly by interacting with the specific receptor, which is responsible for the selectivity of drug action and for the quantitative relationship between drugs and effects. The actions and mechanisms of drug action are the processes of pharmacodynamics (药物效应动力学). The time course of therapeutic drug action in the body can be understood in terms of pharmacokinetics and pharmacodynamics.

医药大学堂
WWW.YIYAODXT.COM

2. History of Pharmacology

Since time immemorial time, medicaments have been used for treating disease in humans and animals. The herbal preparations of antiquity describe the therapeutic powers of certain plants and minerals. Belief in the curative powers of plants and certain substances rested exclusively upon traditional knowledge, that is, empirical information (经验信息) not subjected to critical examination.

In the 1500 years or so preceding the present, there were sporadic attempts to introduce rational methods into medicine, but none was successful owing to the dominance of systems of thought that purported to explain all of biology and disease without the need for experimentation and observation. Around the end of the 17th century, reliance on observation and experimentation (观察和实验) began to replace theorizing in medicine, following the example of the physical sciences. As the value of these methods in the study of disease became clear, physicians in Great Britain and on the Continent began to apply them to the effects of traditional drugs used in their own practices.

In the late 18th and early 19th centuries, Francois Magendie, and later his student Claude Bernard, began to develop the methods of experimental animal physiology and pharmacology.

Beginning in the 20th century, the fresh wind of synthetic chemistry began to revolutionise the pharmaceutical industry. New synthetic drugs began to appear, and the era of antimicrobial chemotherapy began with the discovery by Paul Ehrlich in 1909 of arsenical compounds for treating syphilis. Further breakthroughs came when the sulfonamides, the first antibacterial drugs, were discovered by Gerhard Domagk in 1935, and with the development of penicillin by Chain and Florey during the Second World War, based on the earlier work of Fleming. These few well-known examples show how the growth of synthetic chemistry, and the resurgence of natural product chemistry, caused a dramatic revitalisation of therapeutics in the first half of the 20th century. Each new drug class that emerged gave pharmacologists a new challenge, and it was then that pharmacology really established its identity and its status among the biomedical sciences.

The picture of pharmacology that emerges from this brief glance at history (Figure 1-1) is of a subject evolved from ancient prescientific therapeutics (古老的前科学疗法).

Not until the concepts of rational therapeutics, especially that of the controlled clinical trial, were reintroduced into medicine only about 50 years ago, did it become possible to accurately evaluate therapeutic claims. Around the same time, a major expansion of research efforts in all areas of biology began. As new concepts and new techniques were introduced, information was accumulated about drug action and the biologic substrate of that action, the drug receptor. During the last half century, many fundamentally new drug groups and new members of old groups were introduced.

The last three decades have seen an even more rapid growth of information and understanding of the molecular basis for drug action. The molecular mechanisms of action of many drugs have now been identified, and numerous receptors have been isolated, structurally characterized, and cloned. In fact, the use of receptor identification methods has led to the discovery of many orphan receptors which has no ligand being discovered and whose function can only be surmised. Studies of the local molecular environment of receptors have shown that receptors and effectors do not function in isolation; they are

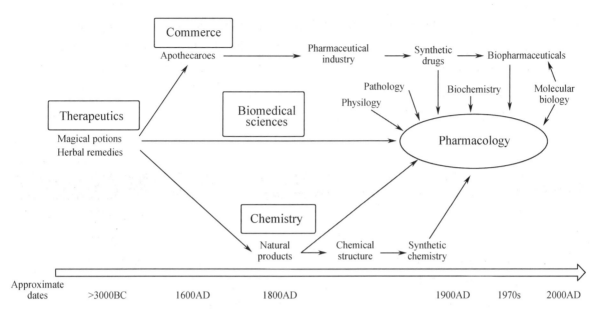

Figure 1-1　The development of pharmacology

strongly influenced by companion regulatory proteins.

As with other biomedical disciplines, the boundaries of pharmacology are not sharply defined, nor are they constant. If it ever had a conceptual and technical core that it could really call its own, the subject is defined by its purpose, that is, understanding what drugs do to living organisms, and more particularly how their effects can be applied to therapeutics, rather than by its scientific coherence.

Figure 1-2 shows the structure of pharmacology as it appears today. Within the main subject fall a number of compartments [Neuropharmacology (神经药理学), Immunopharmacology (免疫药理学),

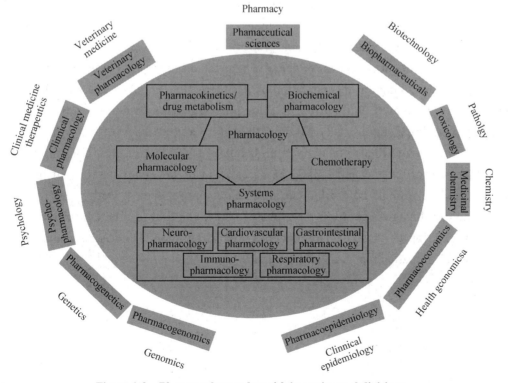

Figure 1-2　Pharmacology today with its various subdivisions

Pharmacokinetics, etc.], which are convenient, if not watertight, subdivisions. Around the edges are several interface disciplines, which form important two-way bridges between pharmacology and other fields of biomedicine. Pharmacology tends to have more of these than other disciplines. Recent arrivals on the fringe are subjects such as Pharmacogenomics (药物基因组学), Pharmacoepidemiology (药物流行病学) and Pharmacoeconomics (药物经济学).

3. Pharmacology and drugs discovered

Most new drugs or drug products are discovered or developed through one or more of six pharmacological approaches (药理学方法).

(1) Identification or elucidation (鉴定或阐明) of a new drug target.

(2) Rational drug design of a new drug based on an understanding of biologic mechanisms, drug receptor structure, and drug structure.

(3) Chemical modification (化学修饰) of a known molecule.

(4) Screening (筛查) for biologic activity of large numbers of natural products, banks of previously discovered chemical entities, and large libraries of peptides, nucleic acids, and other organic molecules.

(5) Biotechnology and cloning using genes to produce peptides and proteins. Efforts continue to focus on the discovery of new targets and approaches, from studies with genomics, proteomics, nucleic acids and molecular pharmacology for drug therapy. Significantly increasing the number of useful disease targets should be a positive driver for new and improved drugs.

(6) Combinations of known drugs to obtain additive or synergistic effects or a repositioning of a known drug for a new therapeutic use. These studies may provide scientific basis for obtaining more desirable pharmacokinetic or pharmacodynamic properties.

The first steps in the development of a new drug is the discovery or synthesis of a potential new drug molecule and seeking an understanding of its interaction (mechanism) with the appropriate biologic targets. Repeated application of this approach leads to compounds with increased potency and selectivity (Figure 1-3). By law, the safety and efficacy of drugs must be defined before marketing. In addition to *in vitro* studies, relevant biologic effects, drug metabolism, and pharmacokinetic profiles and particularly an assessment of the relative safety of the drug must be characterized in animals before human drug trials can be started. With regulatory approval, human testing can then go forward in three phases before the drug can be considered for approval for general use. A fourth phase of data gathering and safety monitoring is becoming increasingly important and follows after approval for general use.

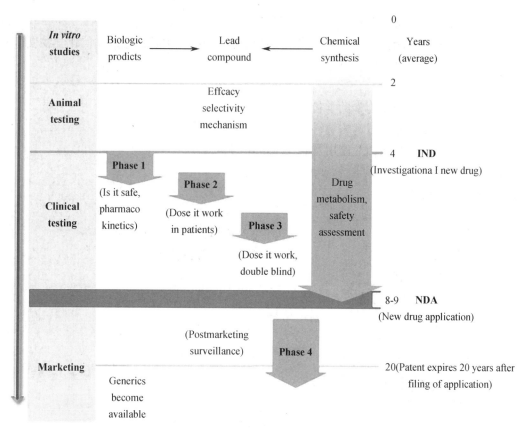

Figure 1-3　The development and testing process required to bring a drug to market

重 点 小 结

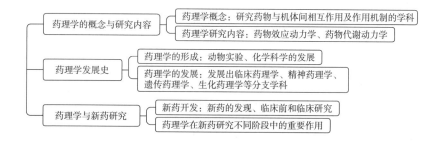

目 标 检 测

题库

一、单项选择题

1. 药物（　　）

　A. 是能干扰细胞代谢活动的化学物质

　B. 是具有滋补营养、保健康复作用的物质

C. 是一种化学物质

D. 是可改变或查明机体的生理功能及病理状态，用以防治及诊断疾病的化学物质

E. 是能影响机体生理功能的物质

2. 药理学（　　　）

    A. 是研究药物代谢动力学的学科

    B. 是研究药物效应动力学的学科

    C. 是研究药物与机体相互作用及其作用规律的学科

    D. 是与药物有关的生理学科

    E. 是研究药物的学科

3. 药物效应动力学研究的是（　　　）

    A. 药物的临床效果　　　　　　　　B. 药物对机体的作用及作用机制

    C. 药物在体内的过程　　　　　　　D. 影响药物疗效的因素

    E. 药物的作用机制

4. 药物代谢动力学研究的是（　　　）

    A. 药物在体内的变化

    B. 药物作用的动态规律

    C. 药物作用的动能来源

    D. 药物作用强度随时间、剂量变化消除规律

    E. 药物在机体影响下所发生的变化及其规律

二、思考题

1. 如何理解药物效应动力学和药物代谢动力学为临床合理用药提供了理论依据？

2. 试述药理学在新药开发研究中的作用。

（周玖瑶）

Chapter 2　Pharmacokinetics

 学习目标

　　1. 掌握　药物的体内过程（吸收、分布、代谢及排泄）及其影响因素。

　　2. 熟悉　生物利用度、表观分布容积、一级动力学消除、零级动力学消除等概念；多次给药的时量曲线和稳态血药浓度；不同给药方式、间隔、剂量对达到稳态血药浓度的时间和水平的影响。

　　3. 了解　药物的转运及转运形式；房室概念及房室模型。

Pharmacokinetics is the study of the variables that affect drug delivery , and removal from, its site of action. Pharmacokinetics includes the study of absorption, distribution, storage, and elimination of drugs. Metabolism and excretion commonly make up the elimination.

Pharmacokinetics is applied to multidisciplinary fields, such as biopharmaceutics, pharmaceutical engineering, clinical pharmacy, etc. It can allow the clinician to design and optimize treatment regimens, including decisions as to the route of administration for a specific drug, the amount and frequency of each dose, and the duration of treatment.

1. Drug transport

In order to play a role, drugs must reach its intended molecular target. Drugs must traverse a number of barriers to be absorbed, distributed, and eliminated. Those barriers are called bio-membrane that consists of a cell membrane and organelle membrane (细胞器膜). Lipid bilayer (脂质双分子层) is the basic structure of bio-membrane, in which proteins (蛋白质) are embedded to form receptors, enzymes, ion channels and carriers of bio-membrane. An understanding of drug transfer is helpful in the determination of drug concentration in systemic circulation and cell. Modes of drug transport across a membrane are described in the following paragraphs.

1.1　Passive transport (被动转运)

This mode is proportional to the concentration gradient (the driving force) of drug between two adjacent compartments. The vast majority of drugs gain access to the body by this mode. Its characters

7

are as follows. ① Transport rate is proportional to lipid solubility. ② The drug moves from a region of high concentration to one of lower concentration without requiring any expenditure of energy. ③ Transport rate is proportional to concentration difference. ④ Transport rate relates to the pKa of the drug and the pH of the solution in which the drug is dissolved. Most drugs are weak acids or bases and, as such, in solution show varying degrees of dissociation into their ionized and nonionized forms. The relationship between the pH of the drug's environment and the degree of its ionization is determined by the Henderson-Hasselbalch equation:

$$\text{Acidic drugs: } 10^{\text{pH}-\text{p}Ka} = \frac{ionization}{nonionization} = \frac{[A^-]}{[HA]}$$

$$\text{Alkaline drugs: } 10^{\text{pH}-\text{p}Ka} = \frac{ionization}{nonionization} = \frac{[BH^+]}{[B]}$$

pKa is the minus log of the dissociation constant K_a which is the pH of the solution at 50% dissociation of drug. Under basic conditions, weak acids are ionized to a greater extent. Under acidic conditions, weak acids are nonionized to a greater extent. The greater the difference between the pH and the pKa, the greater the degree of ionization or nonionization.

Water-soluble (水溶性) drugs penetrate the cell membrane through aqueous channels or pores, whereas lipid-soluble (脂溶性) drugs readily move across most biologic membranes due to their solubility in the membrane lipid bilayers.

1.2   Active transport (主动转运)

This mode is mediated by a very large family of transporters collectively referred to as ATP binding cassette transporters (or ABC transporters). Energy-dependent active transport is driven by the hydrolysis of adenosine triphosphate (ATP). Active transport is different to passive transport that it is capable of moving drugs against a concentration gradient, from a region of low drug concentration to one of higher drug concentration. There are several important features of this mechanism, including saturability, structural selectivity, and ATP dependence.

1.3   Facilitated diffusion (易化扩散)

This mode is a carrier-mediated (载体介导) transport from higher to lower concentration without needing energy and translocating the substrate in the direction of electrochemical gradient (电化学梯度). It can be saturated and may be inhibited by compounds that compete for the carrier. Example of this type of transporter includes glucose transporter-4 (GLUT-4，葡萄糖转运因子-4) enhances the permeation of glucose across a muscle cell membrane.

1.4   Endocytosis and exocytosis (胞吞和胞吐)

A transport mechanism for the movement of large quantities of molecules into and out of cells.

It includes three main types: endocytosis, exocytosis and transcytosis. Vitamin B_{12} is transported across the gut wall by endocytosis, whereas certain neurotransmitter (for example, nor-epinephrine) are stored in intracellular (胞内) membrane-bound vesicles in the nerve terminal and are released by exocytosis.

2.　Drug disposition

2.1　Absorption

Absorption refers to the process of drug from the site of administration into the systemic circulation (体循环). According to the different ways of absorption, it can be divided into gastrointestinal absorption (oral administration, sublingual administration, rectal administration), percutaneous absorption, injection absorption and gastrointestinal absorption. Intravascular administration (血管内给药) such as intravenous injection (静脉注射) hasn't an absorption process. The rate and efficiency of absorption depend on both factors in the environment where the drug is absorbed and the drug's chemical characteristics and route of administration. Absorption pathway is the most important factor. The order of the speed of drug absorption is intraperitoneal injection (腹腔注射) > air-mist-inhalation > sublingual administration (舌下给药) > intramuscular injection (肌内注射) > subcutaneous injection (皮下注射) > oral administration > rectal administration > percutaneous administration.

2.1.1　Oral administration

Oral administration (per os, PO) is the most common route of drug administration. It is the safest and the most convenient method. Oral administration usually requires 30 to 60minutes before significant absorption from the gastrointestinal (GI) tract occurs; therefore, the onset of drug action is delayed. Factors influencing absorption of orally administered drugs include the followings.

(1) Drug formulations and drug chemistry　The general chemical properties of a drug can greatly influence its absorption.

(2) Gastric emptying time and intestinal motility (肠蠕动)　Owing to its large surface, the small intestine is the most important absorption site for most drugs. More rapid gastric emptying facilitates their absorption because the drug is delivered to the small intestine more quickly. Conversely, factors that slow gastric emptying (e.g., food, anticholinergic drugs) generally slow absorption. Increases in intestinal motility (e.g., diarrhea) may move drugs through the intestine too rapidly to permit effective absorption.

(3) Food　In addition to affecting gastric emptying time, food may reduce the absorption of some drugs owing to physical interactions with the drug (e.g., chelation). Alternatively, absorption of some drugs (e.g., clarithromycin) is improved by administration with food.

(4) The pH of gastrointestinal tract　The pH of gastric contents is from 1.0 to 3.0 whereas the pH of intestinal contents is from 4.8 to 8.2. The degree of ionization drug is determined by the pH of gastrointestinal tract. Acidic drugs are apt to be absorbed in the stomach while basic drugs are easier to be absorbed in the intestine.

(5) First-pass hepatic metabolism (首关效应)　When a drug is absorbed across the GI tract, it first enters the portal circulation (门静脉循环) before entering the systemic circulation. If the drug is rapidly metabolized in the liver or gut wall during this initial passage, the amount of unchanged drug that gains access to the systemic circulation is decreased.

2.1.2　Sublimation administration

Placement under the tongue allows a drug to diffuse into the capillary (毛细血管) network, therefore, to enter the systemic circulation directly. This administration has many advantages including rapid absorption, convenience, low incidence of infection, bypass of the harsh gastrointestinal environment, and avoidance of first-pass metabolism, also known as first-pass effect (e.g., nitroglycerin).

2.1.3　Injection administration

The most common routes of injection administration include intramuscular (IM) injection, subcutaneous (SC) injection and intravenous (IV) injection. IM injections are usually delivered into the gluteal or deltoid muscles. The onset of action with IM administration is relatively short, usually within several minutes. SC injections are shots given into the fat layer between the skin and muscle. They are used to give small amounts and certain kinds of medicine (e.g., insulin). IV injections is usually restricted to use in the hospital. IV injection offers the fastest means of drug absorption because the drug is delivered directly into the circulation; therefore, the onset of drug action is almost immediate.

2.1.4　Inhalation administration (吸入给药)

Inhalational administration provides rapid delivery of a drug across the large surface area of the mucous membranes of the respiratory tract (呼吸道) and pulmonary epithelium. The lungs serve as an effective route of administration of drugs. The pulmonary alveoli (肺泡) represent a large surface and a minimal barrier to diffusion. The lungs also receive the total cardiac output as blood flow. Thus, absorption from the lungs can produce an effect almost as rapidly as does IV injection. Drugs must be nonirritating and gaseous or very fine aerosols. The intended effects may be systemic (e.g., inhaled general anesthetics) or local [e.g., bronchodilators (支气管扩张剂) in the treatment of asthma].

2.1.5　Other administrations

(1) Topical administration　Topical application of creams and ointments is used for local effects in the skin and in certain conditions for systemic effects, as with nitroglycerin ointment (硝酸甘油软膏) for the treatment of angina pectoris.

(2) Transdermal administration　It achieves systemic effects by application of drugs to the skin, usually via a transdermal patch depending on the physical characteristics of the skin at the site of application as well as the lipid solubility of the drug.

(3) Rectal administration (直肠给药)　It prevents the destruction of the drug by intestinal enzymes or by low pH in the stomach. This route is useful if the drug induces vomiting when given orally, if the patient is already vomiting, or if the patient is unconscious. However, this rout is also erratic and incomplete, and many drugs irritate the rectal mucosa (黏膜).

2.2　Distribution

After absorption into the bloodstream, drugs are distributed to the tissues via blood flow and diffusion and(or) filtration across the capillary membranes of various tissues. Drug distribution has obvious regularity, most of the drug distribution in the body is uneven and dynamic. Because the circulatory system is the main distribution mechanism and it is a readily accessible body compartment, plasma concentrations are used as an index of tissue concentrations in determining pharmacokinetics of drugs and in clinical management of drug therapy. There are many factors affecting the distribution of drugs, mainly in the following aspects.

2.2.1　Plasma protein binding (血浆蛋白结合率)

The vast majority of drugs would be bound with different proteins (albumin and globulins) in the plasma in varying degrees after absorption. Binding to plasma protein is generally reversible and determined by the concentration of drug, the affinity of the protein for the drug, and the number of binding sites available. Only free drug in the plasma is able to diffuse to its molecular site of action and can exert a pharmacological effect.

$$\text{Drug} + \text{Protein} \longrightarrow \text{Drug-protein complex}$$
$$\text{(Active, free)} \qquad \text{(Inactive, bound)}$$

For highly protein-bound drugs, a small change in plasma protein binding can lead to a large change in the proportion of free drug in the plasma and may lead to toxicity. For dicoumarol (双香豆素) that is 99% bound to plasma protein, only 1% is free in the plasma. Reduction of plasma protein binding to 98% results in a doubling of free drug and drug effect.

A decrease in the concentration of albumin (in liver disease, poor general condition) leads to altered pharmacokinetics of drugs that are highly bound to albumin.

2.2.2　Blood flow

The greater the blood supply in a body organ, the faster the medication is distributed. The various organs of the body receive different amounts of blood. Organs such as the liver, kidneys, and brain have the largest blood supply. Consequently, these organs are usually exposed to the largest amount of drug. Some tissues, such as adipose tissue, receive a relatively poor blood supply and, as a result, do not accumulate large amounts of drug. However, highly lipid-soluble drugs can enter adipose tissue easily, where they can accumulate and remain for an extended period of time.

2.2.3　pH of body fluid

Under physiological conditions, the pH of intracellular fluid is about 7.0, and that of extracellular fluid is about 7.4. Weak acid drugs in the more acidic intracellular solution are more non dissociated and easy to transport from the cell to the extracellular; weak alkaline drugs, on the contrary, have a higher concentration in the cell. For example, oral sodium bicarbonate (碳酸氢钠) can alkalize plasma and urine, not only promote the transport of barbiturates from brain tissue to plasma, but also reduce the reabsorption of renal tubules, accelerate the excretion of drugs from urine, so as to rescue barbiturates poisoning.

2.2.4　Blood-tissue barriers

Drugs are transported in the blood to different tissues of the body. In order to reach their sites of action, they must leave the bloodstream to cross some barriers, such as blood-brain barrier, placental barrier and blood-eye barrier.

(1) Blood-brain barrier　The blood-brain barrier (BBB) is formed by endothelial cells of the capillary wall, astrocyte end-feet ensheathing the capillary, and pericytes embedded in the capillary basement membrane. BBB is a highly selective semipermeable border that separates the circulating blood from the brain and extracellular fluid in the central nervous system (CNS). This barrier is an additional lipid barrier that protects the brain by restricting the passage of electrolytes and other water-soluble substances. Since the brain is composed of a large amount of lipid (nerve membranes and myelin), lipid-soluble drugs pass readily into the brain. As a general rule, then, a drug must have a certain degree of lipid solubility if it is to penetrate this barrier and gain access to the brain.

(2) Placental barrier (胎盘屏障)　The placental barrier is a semipermeable membrane made up of placental tissues and limiting the kind and amount of material exchanged between mother and fetus thiazides (噻嗪类) cross the placental barrier and appear in cord blood. Some drugs can pass through the placenta and then lead toxicity, even teratogenesis to the fetus. Therefore, pregnant women should be especially careful in the use of drugs.

(3) Blood-ocular barrier   The blood-ocular barrier is a barrier created by endothelium of capillaries of the retina and iris (视网膜和虹膜), ciliary epithelium and retinal pigment epithelium. It is a physical barrier between the local blood vessels and most parts of the eye itself and stops many substances including drugs from traveling across it. Because of the blood-ocular barrier, topical application is preferred for eye drugs.

2.2.5 Drug transporters

Drug transporters are membrane proteins involved in the uptake or efflux (外排) of drugs by several tissues such as the intestine, liver, kidney and brain. They can have a significant impact on the pharmacokinetics of endogenous (内源性的) and exogenous (外源性的) compounds. Also, co-administered drugs can influence the transporter activity which may lead to changes in the pharmacokinetics of drugs and, as a result, possibly to reduced efficacy or increased toxicity.

2.3 Biotransformation (metabolism)

Drug biotransformation (metabolism) refers to the chemical alteration of drugs and foreign compounds in the body. Biotransformation leads to products of drug with increased polarity, which will allow the drug to be eliminated. Biotransformation occurs in many tissues or organs including liver, digestive system, lung, skin, and kidney, but for most drugs the liver is the major site of it.

There are two broad types of biotransformation, called phase I and phase II (Figure 2-1).

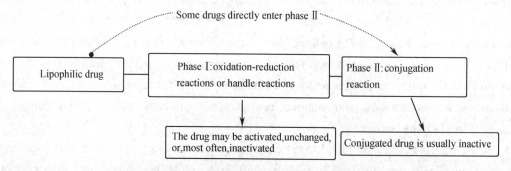

Figure 2-1   The biotransformation of drugs

Phase I reactions   Phase I reactions are also called oxidation-reduction (氧化还原) reactions or handle reactions. These reactions convert lipophilic molecules into more polar molecules by introducing or unmasking a polar function group, such as OH, or NH_2, which increase, decrease, or leave unaltered the drug's pharmacologic activity. They facilitate excretion or further biotransformation of the drug through phase II reactions.

Phase II reactions   Phase II reactions are also called conjugation (结合) reaction with an endogenous substrate, such as glucuronic acid, sulfuric acid, acetic acid or an amino acid results in polar, usually more water-soluble compounds that are most often therapeutically inactive. Drugs already possessing an OH, NH_2 or-COOH group may enter Phase II directly and become conjugated without prior phase I metabolism.

In many cases, metabolism of a drug results in its conversion to compounds that have little or no pharmacologic activity. In other cases, biotransformation of an active compound may lead to the formation of metabolites that also have pharmacologic actions. A few compounds (prodrugs) have no activity until they undergo metabolic activation.

$$Drug \longrightarrow Inactive\ metabolite\ (s)$$
$$Drug \longrightarrow Active\ metabolite\ (s)$$
$$Prodrug \longrightarrow Drug$$

Within the cells of the liver is a group of enzymes that specifically function to metabolize foreign (drug) substances. These enzymes are referred to as the drug microsomal metabolizing system (DMMS). The DMMS utilizes cytochrome (细胞色素) P450 enzymes (CYP) that are major enzyme systems involved in phase I reactions. The main function of this system is to take lipid-soluble drugs and chemically alter them so that they become water-soluble compounds. Water-soluble compounds can be excreted by the kidneys. Lipid-soluble compounds are repeatedly reabsorbed into the blood.

Interaction at CYP is an important pharmacokinetic mechanism that can affect clinical use of drugs. Knowledge of CYP isoforms involved in metabolism of drugs and the type of interaction can guide clinical selection of drugs and explain adverse drug interactions. Interactions may take the form of competition, inhibition, or induction.

Some drugs can enhance the quantities and activity of CYP, (e.g., phenobarbital and alcohol) when they are taken repeatedly. By stimulating this system, the drugs actually increase the number of CYP in the system; this process is referred to as enzyme induction. With an increase in the number of enzymes, there is a faster rate of drug metabolism. Consequently, the duration of drug action is decreased for all drugs metabolized by the microsomal enzymes.

Other drugs can inhibit the quantities and activity of CYP [e.g., chloromycetin (氯霉素) and isoniazid (异烟肼)] to cause enzyme inhibition. This action slows the metabolism of all other drugs metabolized by these enzymes. This will increase the duration and intensity of the drugs inhibited. Enzyme induction and enzyme inhibition are common causes of adverse drug interactions.

2.4   Drug excretion

Drug excretion refers to the removal of drug from the body. Generally, only hydrophilic molecules are excreted effectively. Lipophilic drugs must be metabolized to hydrophilic drug metabolites to be excreted. Drug may be excreted via a number of routes, such as renal (urine), bile (feces), and respiratory (exhaled gases), the kidneys are the most important organs for drug excretion. Changes in excretion rates will affect the plasma concentration of drugs and their metabolites and thus play an important role in the design of drug regimens.

2.4.1   Renal excretion

Renal excretion is quantitatively the most important route of excretion for most drugs and drug metabolites. The kidney permits elimination because the vascular wall structure in the region of the glomerular capillaries allows unimpeded passage into urine of blood solutes having molecular weights (MW) < 5000.

Renal excretion involves three processes: glomerular (肾小球) filtration, tubular (肾小管) secretion, and(or) tubular reabsorption.

(1) Glomerular filtration   Drugs enter the kidney through renal arteries, which divide to form a glomerular capillary plexus. Free drug (游离型药物) flows through the capillary slits into the Bowman space as part of the glomerular filtrate. Lipid solubility and pH do not influence the passage of drugs into the glomerular filtrate. However, variations in the glomerular filtration rate (GFR, 肾小球滤过率) and protein binding of drugs do affect this process.

(2) Tubular secretion   Secretion primarily occurs in the proximal tubules by two energy-requiring active transport systems: one for anions and one for cations. Each of these transport systems shows low specificity and can transport many compounds. Thus, competition between drugs for these carriers can occur within each transport system.

(3) Tubular reabsorption   As a drug moves toward the distal convoluted tubule, its concentration increases and exceeds that of the perivascular space. The drug what is uncharged may diffuse out of the nephric lumen, back into the systemic circulation.

The sum of these processes determines the extent of net renal drug excretion. In order to make the drug excreted, the drug or drug metabolite must be water soluble and preferably in an ionized form. As mentioned, acid drugs are mostly ionized in alkaline urine and basic drugs are mostly ionized in an acid urine. In the case of barbiturate or aspirin overdose (acid drugs), alkalization of the urine with sodium bicarbonate will hasten elimination of either drug in the urine.

2.4.2   Biliary excretion(胆汁排泄)

Biliary excretion involves active secretion of drug molecules or their metabolites from hepatocytes into the bile. The bile then transports the drugs to the gut, where the drugs are excreted. The efficiency of biliary excretion is quite variable. There is another pathway involving the intestinal tract, enterohepatic circulation (肝肠循环).

Enterohepatic circulation refers to the circulation of drugs from the liver to the bile, followed by entry into the small intestine, absorption by the enterocyte (肠上皮细胞) and transport back to the liver. Drugs that undergo extensive enterohepatic circulation generally have long durations of action because of this repeated cycling of the drug (liver → bile → intestines → blood → liver). Enterohepatic circulation is an especially important concept in the field of toxicology as many lipophilic xenobiotics undergo this process causing repeated liver damage [e.g., digitoxin (地高辛)].

3. Basic concepts of pharmacokinetics

In the body, drugs are absorbed, distributed, metabolized and excreted continuously with the change of time, and they are always in a dynamic change. The blood links up the four links of the process in the body and connects with the effective parts. In the study of pharmacokinetics, the dynamic changes of blood concentration are often measured, and the rate equation is selected for analysis, and the parameters of pharmacokinetics are calculated.

3.1   Blood concentration-time curve

Blood samples were collected at different times after administration to measure the concentration of blood drugs. Take time as abscissa and blood concentration as ordinate to draw blood concentration-time curve (Figure 2-2).

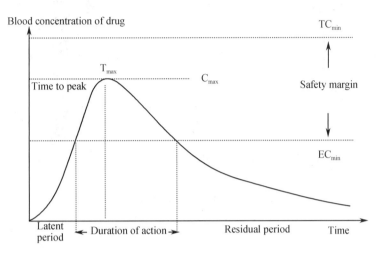

Figure 2-2　Blood concentration-time curve

C_{max} = maximal drug level obtained with the dose;T_{max} = time at which C_{max} occurs;EC_{min}= maximal effective concentration;TC_{min}= maximal toxic concentration;Time to peak = time from administration to C_{max}

3.2　Compartment model

In the pharmacokinetics, in order to facilitate the dynamic analysis, it is usually assumed that the human body is a system, which is divided into several compartments (i.e., compartment model), and the rate of drugs entering and leaving each compartment is equal. This is an empirical (经验性的) model that does not explain actual mechanisms by which drug is absorbed, distributed, and eliminated from body. Groups of tissues that have similar blood flow and drug affinity (亲和力) are represented by a single compartment. Thus, a compartment is not a real anatomic region within body.

Since drug can enter and leave body, the model is characterized as an open model. The commonly used models are open one compartment model and open two compartment model.

(1) Open one compartment model (一室模型)　The body is regarded as a uniform whole, and the drugs are distributed to the body fluids and tissues and organs immediately after entering the blood circulation, and the dynamic balance is achieved rapidly. This system is called open one compartment mode. The single-phase decrease of blood concentration resulted in the elimination of the reaction. open one compartment mode is most commonly used in pharmacokinetic studies.

(2) Open two compartment model (二室模型)　Divide the body into central (including) and peripheral chambers. At first, the drug enters the central chamber and reaches equilibrium at the moment of the central chamber, and then transfers to the peripheral chamber. At this time, the concentration of the drug in the blood drops rapidly. After the transfer reaches equilibrium, the concentration of the drug in the blood drops slowly, and the rate of decline is determined by the elimination. The rapid decline phase of blood drug concentration is called partial phase (α phase), and the slow decline phase is called elimination phase (β phase). The transport between the central and peripheral chambers is reversible, but the drug can only be eliminated from the central chamber. The kinetic process of most drugs *in vivo* accords with the open two compartment model (Figure 2-3).

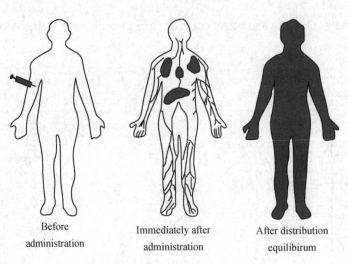

Before administration

Immediately after administration

After distribution equilibirum

Figure 2-3   Two compartment model

3.3   Elimination kinetics（消除动力学）

Drug elimination is the summation of the processes described earlier. Drug elimination proceeds in two types of time dependent patterns: first-order kinetics and zero-order kinetics.

(1) First-order kinetics（一级动力学）   When drug elimination proceeds by first-order kinetics, a constant proportion or fraction of drug is eliminated per unit time. As a result, plasma drug concentrations decline exponentially. This occurs because the elimination mechanisms adjust their activity to the prevailing drug concentration. When drug concentrations increase, elimination mechanisms can accept more drug. Important: as long as elimination proceeds by first-order kinetics the fraction of drug eliminated per unit time remains constant regardless of the starting concentration. As a result, for drugs that are eliminated by first-order kinetics: the time to eliminate the drug is independent of dose and increasing dose or frequency of administration produces predictable rises in plasma concentrations (Figure 2-4).

(2) Zero-order kinetics（零级动力学）   Zero-order kinetics is also called saturation（饱和）kinetics. The enzyme is saturated by a high free-drug concentration, and the rate of metabolism remains constant over time. A constant amount of drug is metabolized per unit of time, and the rate of elimination is constant and does not depend on the drug concentration. Plasma concentrations decline in linear fashion. As a result, a progressively smaller proportion of drug is eliminated as plasma concentrations increase (Figure 2-5). In other words, the proportion of drug eliminated depends on the starting concentration. Zero-order kinetics makes prediction of drug concentrations over time problematic.

(3) Elimination rate constant (K_{el}, K_e)   The elimination rate constant describes the fraction of drug eliminated per unit of time or the rate at which plasma concentrations will decline during the elimination phase. The slope of the plasma concentration time curve is the elimination rate constant (K_{el}).

$$K_{el} = slope = concentraion/time$$

The elimination rate constant (proportion per unit time) can be used to calculate the time necessary to eliminate a certain proportion of drug (inverse of rate constant).

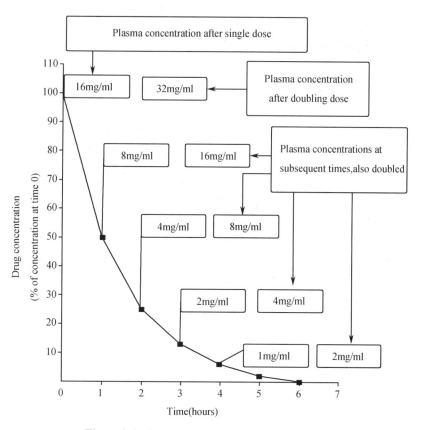

Figure 2-4　Drug elimination: first-order kinetics

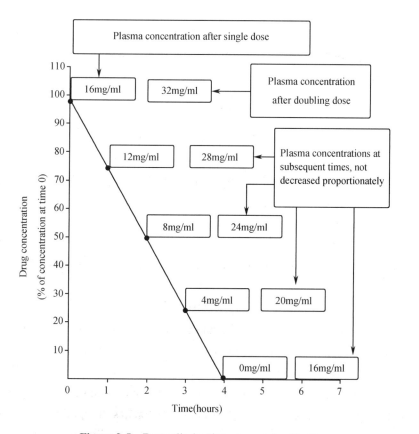

Figure 2-5　Drug elimination: zero-order kinetics

3.4 Kinetic parameters

3.4.1 Bioavailability(*F*)

Bioavailability (生物利用度) is the measure of the fraction of a dose that reaches the systemic circulation. Intravascular administration (e.g., IV) does not involve absorption, and there is no loss of drug. *F*=100%. With extravascular administration [e.g., per os (PO; oral), intramuscular (IM), subcutaneous (SC), inhalation], less than 100% of a dose may reach the systemic circulation because of variations in bioavailability. Determining bioavailability is important for calculating drug dosages for non-intravenous routes of administration. The route by which a drug is administered, as well as the chemical and physical properties of the agent, affects its bioavailability.

$$F=\frac{A(the\ dose\ that\ reaches\ the\ systemic\ circulation)}{D\ (dose)}\times100\%$$

Absolute bioavailability:

$$F=\frac{AUC_{PO}}{AUC_{IV}}\times100\%$$

Relative bioavailability:

$$F=\frac{AUC\ (test\ drug)}{AUC\ (standard)}\times100\%$$

AUC = area under the curve; PO = oral; IV = intravenous bolus; AUC_{IV} = horizontally striped area; AUC_{PO} = vertically striped area.

3.4.2 Apparent volume of distribution(V_d)

Apparent volume of distribution represents the theoretical volume in liters into which a drug is dissolved to produce the plasma concentration observed at steady state. It is calculated as the quotient of the amount of drug administered and the steady state plasma concentration.

$$V_d=\frac{Amount\ of\ drug\ in\ the\ body}{C_0}$$

V_d = volume of distribution; C_0 = the plasma concentration at time zero.

V_d is low when a high percentage of a drug is bound to plasma proteins. V_d is high when a high percentage of a drug is being sequestered in tissues. This raises the possibility of displacement by other agents. Changes in V_d influence drug plasma concentrations and may necessitate changes in dosage or result in toxicity.

3.4.3 Elimination half-life($t_{1/2}$)

Half-life is the time for plasma concentrations to decline to one half their starting value. Half-life is calculated as:

$$t_{1/2}=0.693/K_{el}$$

where 0.693 is a constant derived from the natural log (ln) (because the decay is exponential for first-order kinetics) of the ratio of drug concentration at the beginning and end of one half-life, which by definition is 2 (100%/50%) (ln 2 = 0.693).

Thus, the half-life is inversely related to the elimination rate constant because $t_{1/2}$ estimates the time needed to eliminate a specific proportion (50%) of drug. This makes the $t_{1/2}$ a very useful parameter that can be used to estimate the followings. ①Time for the drug to be completely eliminated from the body.

Four to five half-lives are necessary to reduce drug concentration by 95% to 97%. ②Duration of action of the drug. The longer the half-life of the drug, the longer the plasma concentration of the drug will remain above the minimally effective concentration. ③Time to achieve steady state. On continuous or repeated administration, approximately 4 to 5 half-lives are required to reach steady state. ④Appropriate dosage interval to achieve steady state concentrations.

3.4.4   Clearance(*CL*)

Clearance estimates the amount of drug cleared from the body per unit of time. Total *CL* is a composite estimate reflecting all mechanisms of drug elimination and is calculated as:

$$CL = \frac{V_d}{K_{el}} = 0.693 \times \frac{V_d}{t_{1/2}}$$

Clearance is inversely related to half-life. The higher the clearance, the shorter the half-life and vice versa. Clearance can be used to calculate the rate at which drug must be added to the circulation to maintain the dosage rate.

3.5   Multiple dose concentration-time curve

In the clinical treatment, most drugs reach the effective treatment concentration through repeated administration and maintain at a certain level. At this time, the blood concentration is called the steady state plasma concentration (Figure 2-6).

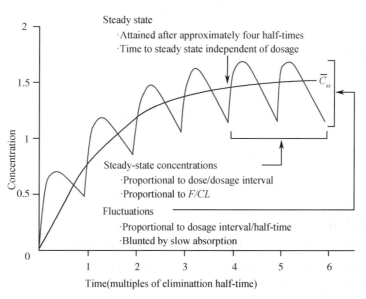

Figure 2-6   Fundamental pharmacokinetic relationships for repeated administration of drugs

(1) Steady state plasma concentration   The fluctuation of blood concentration was increased, and the curve of concentration time was zigzag. After 4-5 $t_{1/2}$, the sawtooth curve fluctuated in a certain level range, that is to say, the steady-state plasma concentration. Importance are as follows. ①The plateau value (坪值) concentration is directly proportional to the dose. ②The fluctuation range of the upper and lower limit of the steady state plasma concentration is directly proportional to the total amount of each medication under the condition that the total amount of daily medication is constant; for the drugs with the effective concentration close to the middle toxic concentration, it is more appropriate to take more times. ③The time to reach a stable average concentration will be determined by clearance and half-life.

(2) Loading dose　In clinical practice, it is desirable to raise plasma concentrations above therapeutic levels rapidly, we can use a large dose at the beginning, that is the loading dose (负荷剂量). By the loading dose, the blood concentration can quickly reach the steady state plasma concentration, and then use the maintenance amount to supplement the elimination of drugs from the body. If 2 times of the maintenance amount (double the first amount) can be given at the first application, the steady state plasma concentration will be reached at the first half-life.

重 点 小 结

重点内容	主要掌握
药物跨膜转运	被动转运 主动转运
药物体内过程	吸收：与给药途径相关 分布：血浆蛋白结合、器官血流量、体液 pH、体内屏障 代谢：肝药酶 P450 系统 排泄：肾排泄、胆汁排泄、呼吸道排泄
药物代谢动力学基本概念	血药浓度 – 时间曲线、房室模型、药物消除类型 药物代谢动力学参数：生物利用度、表观分布容积、药物清除率、半衰期 多次给药血药浓度 – 时间曲线：稳态血药浓度、负荷量

目 标 检 测

一、选择题

（一）单项选择题

1. 在碱性尿液中弱碱性药物（　　　）

　　A. 解离少，再吸收少，排泄快　　　B. 解离多，再吸收少，排泄慢

　　C. 解离少，再吸收多，排泄慢　　　D. 排泄速度不变

　　E. 解离多，再吸收多，排泄慢

2. 药物的吸收与下列哪个因素无关（　　　）

　　A. 给药途径　　　　　　　　　B. 溶解性　　　　　　　　　C. 药物剂量

　　D. 肝肾功能　　　　　　　　　E. 局部血液循环

3. 某药的血浆蛋白结合部位被另一药物置换后，其作用（　　　）

　　A. 不变　　　　B. 减弱　　　　C. 增强　　　　D. 消失　　　　E. 不变或消失

医药大学堂
WWW.YIYAODXT.COM

4. 有关药物从肾脏排泄的正确叙述是（　　）

   A. 改变尿液 pH 可改变药物的排泄速度

   B. 与血浆蛋白结合的药物易从肾小球滤过

   C. 解离的药物易从肾小管重吸收

   D. 药物的排泄与尿液 pH 无关

   E. 药物的血浆浓度与尿液中的浓度相等

5. 按一级动力学消除的药物，其 $t_{1/2}$（　　）

   A. 随给药剂量而变　　　　　　B. 固定不变

   C. 随给药次数而变　　　　　　D. 口服比静脉注射长

   E. 静脉注射比口服长

6. 某药 $t_{1/2}$ 为 24 小时，若按一定剂量每天服药 1 次，约第（　　）天可达稳态血药浓度

   A. 2　　　　　　B. 3　　　　　　C. 0.5　　　　　　D. 1　　　　　　E. 5

（二）多项选择题

7. 药物血浆半衰期（　　）

   A. 与制定药物给药方案有关　　　B. 与调整药物给药方案有关

   C. 与消除速率常数有一定的关系　D. 与了解药物自体内消除的量及时间有关

   E. 与口服给药的峰浓度有关

8. 了解血浆半衰期对临床用药的参考意义是（　　）

   A. 了解一次给药后，药物在体内达到的血药浓度峰值

   B. 了解连续给药后血药浓度达到稳态的时间

   C. 了解给药的适当时间间隔

   D. 了解药物的最低有效浓度

   E. 了解药物在一定时间内消除的相对量

9. 药物表观分布容积的意义是（　　）

   A. 提示药物在血液及组织中分布的相对量

   B. 可了解肾脏的功能

   C. 用以估计体内总药量

   D. 用以估计欲达到有效血药浓度时应给剂量

   E. 反映机体对药物吸收和排泄的速度

二、思考题

尝试理解药物代谢动力学参数在指导临床用药中的意义。

（殷玉婷）

Chapter 3　Pharmacodynamics

 学习目标

1. **掌握** 药物基本作用及双重性；药物量－效关系及量－效曲线；药物作用机制（受体作用）。
2. **熟悉** 药物作用的选择性；治疗指数与安全范围。
3. **了解** 药物受体学说；受体类型及细胞内信号转导系统；受体的调节。

Pharmacodynamics (药物效应动力学) can be defined as the study of the biochemical and physiological effects of drugs and their mechanisms of action. The objectives of the analysis of drug action are to delineate the chemical or physical interactions between drug and target cell and to characterize the full sequence and scope of the actions of each drug. Such a complete analysis provides the basis for both the rational therapeutic use of a drug and the design of new and superior therapeutic agents. Basic research in pharmacodynamics also provides fundamental insights into biochemical and physiological regulation.

1. Basic action of drug

1.1　Drug action and pharmacological effects (药物作用与药理效应)

Drug action refers the action of a drug on the body, this is a primary action. It takes place on the level of molecule. So it expresses the specificity, for example, interaction between drugs and receptors. Pharmacological effect (药理效应) refers the response of the body to the drug. Drugs are categorized by the type of action causing on the body. There are four types of responses. ①Stimulation (兴奋) or depression (抑制). These are drugs that either increase or depress cellular activity. ②Replacement (替代). These are drugs that replace an essential body compound such as insulin or estrogen. ③Antibacterial effects. These drugs interfere with bacterial cell and limit bacterial growth or eliminate the bacteria, such as penicillin.

As the different construction and function of the living organism, the drug action also expresses the different selectivity and characteristic.

Selectivity of drug (药物作用的选择性): selectivity refers to the specific or extensive extent of the effects of drugs on the body. The drugs with high selectivity, with a specific target and narrow range of effects, can specifically affect the function of the body's local or few organ tissues. For example, cardioside (强心苷) mainly excites myocardium (心肌), while phenobarbital (苯巴比妥) inhibits the central nervous system. The low-selectivity drugs have many action sites and wide range of effects, which can affect the function of whole body or multiple organs. Atropine (阿托品) shows low selectivity as it can obviously affect the function of heart, blood vessels, smooth muscle, glands and central nervous system, etc.

1.2   The dual characteristics of drug action (药物作用的双重性)

The effects of drugs on the body show duality. On one hand, the effect of drugs on the body is called therapeutic effect, which accords with the purpose of drug use and is beneficial to improve the physiological, biochemical or pathological process of the patient. On the other hand, it can produce adverse effects on the body and is not in accordance with the purpose of drug use.

1.2.1   Therapeutic effect(治疗作用)

Therapeutic effect of drug differs its pharmacological effect, it only includes the part of the pharmacological effect that are beneficial to the treatment of disease. The therapeutic effect can be divided into three types.

(1) Etiological treatment (对因治疗)   The treatment aims to eradicate the pathological factor. It is a completely therapeutic method, such as the antibiotics is used to treat bacterial infection.

(2) Symptomatic treatment (对症治疗)   The treatment aims to reduce or improve the symptoms, such as the rescue of shock, higher fever, pang, and convulsion so on.

(3) Supplement therapy (replacement therapy) [补充治疗(替代治疗)]   The treatment aims to supplement the deficiency of nutritional fraction (营养组分) or endogenous active material (内源活性物质), such as hormones.

1.2.2   Adverse reaction(不良反应)

Any drug, no matter how trivial its therapeutic actions, has the potential to produce harmful effects, Adverse reactions are a cost of modern medical therapy. "Mechanism-based" adverse reactions are relatively easily predicted by preclinical and clinical pharmacology studies. But not all of the adverse reaction could be avoided. A few adverse reactions are irreversible，which is called drug induced-disease, such as the neurogenic deafness (神经源性耳聋) induced by gentamicin (庆大霉素).

(1) Side reaction (副作用)   A reaction unrelated to the therapeutic aim occurs at the therapeutic dose. For example, atropine can cause dry mouth, palpitations, constipation and other side effects when used to relieve gastrointestinal cramp.

(2) Toxic reaction (毒性反应)   It occurs while the drug is overdosed and result in accumulation of the drug in the body. It is a serious reaction and should be avoided. The acute toxic reaction frequently damages the circulation, nervous and respiratory system. The chronic toxic reaction commonly damages liver, kidney, bone marrow and endocrine system. Chronic toxicity can also be shown as carcinogenic (致癌), teratogenic (致畸) and mutagenic (致突变) effects, because the drug affects the DNA of cells, thus genetic abnormalities occur in the process of division, inducing teratogenesis and canceration.

(3) Residual effect (后遗效应)   The reaction occurs under the threshold concentration after withdrawal of the drug. It refers the residual reaction of the given drug. For example, after taking the phenobarbital (苯巴比妥), the patient can manifest tired, drowse on the next morning.

(4) Withdrawal reaction (停药反应) It also can be called rebound reaction (反跳反应) and results from a sudden withdrawal of the drug or uncontrol of the disease. For example, sudden withdrawal of clonidine can result in the sharp raise of the blood pressure.

(5) Allergic reactions (变态反应) If the patient was previously sensitized to the drug, a drug might trigger the patient's immunologic mechanism (免疫机制) that results in allergic symptoms. Antibodies in patients are produced as the drug being administered to create the sensitivity. The next time the drug is given to the patient, the drug reacts with the antibodies and results in the production of histamine. Histamine causes allergic symptoms to occur. There are four types of allergic reactions. ①Anaphylactic (过敏). This is an immediate allergic reaction that can be fatal. ②Cytotoxic reaction (细胞毒反应). This is an autoimmune response that results in hemolytic anemia (溶血性贫血), thrombocytopenia (血小板减少症), or lupus erythematosus (红斑狼疮). In some cases, it takes months for the reaction to dissipate. ③Immune complex reaction (免疫复合反应). This is referred to as serum sickness and results in angioedema (血管性水肿), arthralgia (关节痛), fever, swollen lymph nodes (淋巴结肿大), and splenomegaly (脾肿大). The immune complex reaction can sustain up to three weeks after the drug is administered. ④Cell mediated. This is an inflammatory skin reaction (炎症性皮肤反应) that is also known as delayed hypersensitivity.

(6) Idiosyncrasy (特异质反应) This is an abnormal response that is unpredictable and unexplainable, which could result from the patient overresponding or underresponding to the drug or the drug having an effect that is different from what is expected. This is related to the congenital hereditary factor, for example, the patient with the congenital lack of G-6PD easily develops to hemolysis (溶血).

(7) Drug dependence (药物依赖性) This can be either a physical or psychological dependency. With a physical dependency, the patient experiences an intense physical disturbance when the drug is withdrawn. With psychological dependency, the patient develops an emotional reliance on the drug. The most common addictive drugs include two categories: one is anesthetized analgesics (麻醉镇痛药), such as morphine (吗啡), pethidine (哌替啶) and so on, the other category is sedative hypnotics such as phenobarbitalxe (苯巴比妥).

2. Relation between drug dose and clinical response

About the dose response relationship (量–效关系), we can deal with receptors as molecules and show how receptors can quantitatively account for the relation between dose or concentration of a drug and pharmacological responses. According to the occupation theory, as the increase of the drug concentration or dose, the receptors are gradually occupied. The response reaches the maximum when all the pharmacological receptors are occupied. As Figure 3-1 shows when drug concentration is changed into the logarithm (对数), the dose-response curve become the symmetrical curve (对数曲线).

2.1 Graded dose-response relations (量反应量–效关系)

This response expresses a continuously augment or decreases in the quantity, like the blood pressure, blood cells count and so on. In the dose response relationship curve, there are two important terms:

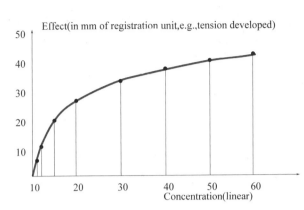
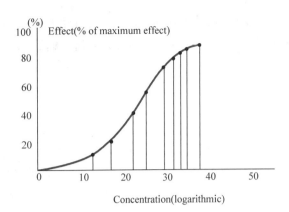

Figure 3-1   Concentration-effect relationship

pharmacological potency and maximal efficacy (Figure 3-2).

2.1.1   Potency

Potency(效价强度) refers to the concentration (EC_{50}) or (ED_{50}) of a drug required to produce 50% of the drug's maximal effect. Potency of a drug depends in part on the affinity (K_D) of receptors for binding the drug and in part on the efficiency with drug receptor interaction is coupled to response. In this group drugs (Figure 3-3), drug B is the most potent one because the ED_{50} or EC_{50} is less than drug A, C and D.

2.1.2   Efficacy(maximal efficacy)[效能(最大效应)]

Efficacy is the maximal responses induced by drugs. Efficacy of a drug depends on drug's intrinsic activity.

For clinical use, it is helpful to distinguish between a drug's potency and its efficacy. The clinical effectiveness of a drug depends not on its potency (EC_{50} or ED_{50}), but on its maximal efficacy.

The efficacy of a drug is obviously crucial for making clinical decisions when a large response is needed. Drug A, C and D (Figure 3-3) have equal maximal efficacy, while the maximal efficacy of drug B is the minimum among drug A, B, C, D.

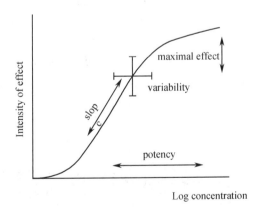

Figure 3-2   Potency, efficacy and slope

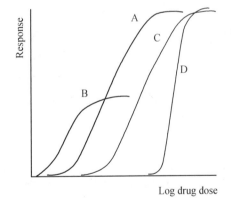

Figure 3-3   Graded dose-response curves for four drugs, illustrating different pharmacologic potencies and different maximal efficacies

2.1.3   Slope

The slope (斜率) of the concentration-effect curve reflects the pharmacodynamics of a drug, including the shape of the curve that describes drug binding to its receptor. The steepness of the curve dictates the range of doses that are useful for achieving a clinical effect. Aside from this fact, the slope of the concentration-effect curve has more theoretical than practical usefulness.

2.2 Quantal dose-effect curves (质反应量–效曲线)

The concentration of a drug that produces a specified effect in a single patient is termed the individual effects, and the defined effect is either present or absent, which is named quantal response (质反应). For example, for prevention of convulsion (抗惊厥)-effective and invalid, individual effective concentrations usually are lognormally distributed, which means that a normal variation curve is the result of plotting the logarithms of the concentration against the frequency of patients achieving the defined effect. To take accumulative frequency distribution of individuals achieving the defined effect as a function of drug concentration-percent curve or the quantal concentration-effect curve (Figure 3-4.).

The dose of a drug required to produce a specified effect in 50% of the population is the median effective dose (ED_{50}) (半数有效量). In preclinical studies of drugs, the median lethal dose, as determined in experimental animals, is abbreviated as LD_{50}. The ratio of the LD_{50} to ED_{50} is an indication of the therapeutic index (治疗指数), which is a statement of how selectivity

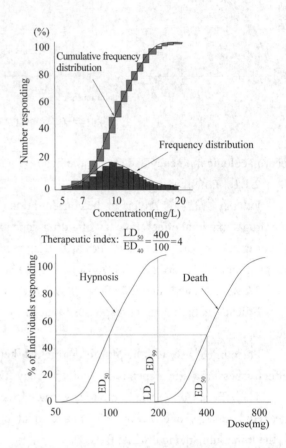

Therapeutic index: $\dfrac{LD_{50}}{ED_{40}} = \dfrac{400}{100} = 4$

Figure 3-4　Frequency distribution curves and quantal concentration-effect and dose-effect curves

the drug is in producing, it is desired versus its adverse effects. In clinical studies, the dose, or preferable the concentration, of a drug required to produce toxic effects can be compared with the concentration required for the therapeutic effect in the population to evaluate the clinical therapeutic index.

3. Mechanism of drug action

The effects of most drugs result from their interaction with organism, tissue, cell and macromolecules (大分子). These interactions alter the function of the pertinent component and thereby initiate the biochemical and physiological changes that are characteristic of the response to the drug.

(1) Physicochemical reaction (理化反应)　Mannitol increases the delivery of Na^+ and water by increasing the osmotic pressure of the proximal tubule and the loop of Henle. Antacids is used to neutralize the gastric acid (中和胃酸) and to treat digestive ulcer.

(2) Interfere cellular metabolism (干扰细胞代谢)   To supply the vital metabolite material to correct the deficiency. For example, insulin is used to treat diabetes mellitus. Flurouracil (氟尿嘧啶) as a false metabolite incorporates into DNA and RNA of the cancer cell to exert its antitumor action.

(3) Interfere the transportation of physiological metabolite (干扰生理物质转运)   Some drugs exert their action by interfering the transportation of inorganic ions, for example, diuretics realizes its diuretic action by inhibition of the exchange of Na^+-K^+, K^+-H^+ in the renal tubule.

(4) Interfere the enzymatic activity (影响酶的活性)   Neostigmine competitively inhibits cholinesterase; omeprazole irreversibly inhibits the proton pump.

(5) Act on the ion channel (作用于离子通道)   Antiarrhythmic quinidine (抗心律失常的奎尼丁) blocks the Na^+ channel on the membrane of myocardial muscle. Vasodilator drugs of the dihydropyridine type (二氢吡啶型血管扩张药物) inhibits the opening of L-type calcium channels.

(6) Interfere the metabolism of nucleic acid (影响核酸代谢)   Just like most of anticancer drugs.

(7) Receptor (受体)   To see next section "Drug and receptor".

4. Drug and receptors

4.1   Concept and characteristics

4.1.1   The concept of receptors

The receptor refers the component of a cell or organism that interacts with a drug and initiates the chain of biochemical events leading to the drug's observed effects.

4.1.2   The characteristics of the receptors

(1) Receptors are simple entities, principally characterized by their affinity for binding drug and endogenous ligands (first messenger) such as neurotransmitters, steroid and hormones.

(2) Receptors also are complex molecules whose structures and biochemical functions determine the concentration-effect relation as well as selectivity of ligands or drugs.

(3) Receptors exhibit high affinity for their ligands or ligand drug (most of ligands exert their pharmacological effects at 1 pmol-1 nmol levels).

(4) The exertion of the regulatory function of the receptor depends on the second messenger by that the chemical signals are enlarged, differentiated and integrated.

(5) The receptors are saturable. When the binding of the receptor-ligands reached the maximal volume, the binding is no longer augmented.

(6) The binding of ligand-receptor expresses a reversibility that means this binding may be disassociated and replaced by other colleague ligands.

4.1.3   Types of receptors

(1) Ligand-gated channels receptor (离子通道受体)   Receptors for several neurotransmitters form agonist-regulated, ion-selective channels in the plasma membrane, termed ligand-gated ion channels, which convey their signals by altering the cell's membrane potential or ionic composition. This group includes the nicotinic cholinergic receptor; the GABA receptor for gamma-aminobutyric acid; and receptors for glutamate, aspartate, and glycine. They are all multisubunit proteins, with each subunit predicted to span the plasma membrane several times. Symmetrical association of the subunits allows them to form a segment of the channel wall and to cooperatively control channel opening and closing (Figure 3-5A).

(2) G-Protein coupled receptor (G蛋白偶联受体, GPCR)   A large superfamily of receptors that accounts for many known drug targets interacts with distinct heterotrimeric GTP-binding regulatory proteins known as G proteins. G proteins are signal transducers that convey information (i.e.,agonist binding) from the receptor to one or more effector proteins. GPCRs include a number of biogenic amines, eicosanoids and other lipid-signaling molecules, peptide hormones, opioids, amino acids such as GABA, and many other peptide and protein ligands. G protein-regulated effectors include enzymes such as adenylyl cyclase, phospholipase C, phosphodiesterases, and plasma membrane ion channels selective for Ca^{2+} and K^+. Because of the huge quantities and physiological importance, GPCRs are widely used targets for drugs (Figure 3-5B).

(3) Receptors as enzymes (酶活性受体)   The largest group of receptors with intrinsic enzymatic activity are cell surface protein kinases, which exert their regulatory effects by phosphorylating (磷酸化)diverse effector proteins at the inner face of the plasma membrane. Phosphorylation can alter the biochemical activities of an effector or its interactions with other proteins. Most receptor protein kinases target tyrosine residues in their substrates; these include receptors of insulin, many cytokines and diverse peptides, and proteins that direct growth or differentiation. A few receptor protein kinases also phosphorylate serine or threonine residues (Figure 3-5 C).

Another family of receptors that are functionally protein kinases contains a modification of the structure described above. Protein kinase-associated receptors lack the intracellular enzymatic domains but, in response to agonists, bind and(or) activate distinct protein kinases on the cytoplasmic face of the plasma membrane. Receptors of this group include several receptors for neurotrophic peptides and the multisubunit antigen receptors on T and B lymphocytes.

(4) Cytosolic receptor (细胞核受体)   Some receptors, such as those of corticosteroids, thyroid hormone, retinoic acid, and vitamin D, could link to and interact with DNA. The receptors are located intracellularly and so agonists must pass through the cell membrane in order to get to their receptor, the complex can bind to specific DNA sequences and so alter the expression of specific genes. As a result, secondary transduction involves an increase or decrease in the synthesis of various proteins (Figure 3-5 D).

4.2   Intracellular signal transduction (细胞内信号转导)

Physiological signals also are integrated within the cell as a result of interactions between second-messenger pathways. Compared with the number of receptors and cytosolic signaling proteins, there are relatively few recognized cytoplasmic second messengers. Well-studied second messengers include cyclic AMP and cyclic GMP, Ca^{2+}, inositol phosphates, diacylglycerol, and nitric oxide. Second messengers influence each other directly, by altering the other's metabolism, and indirectly, by sharing intracellular targets.

4.2.1   Cyclic AMP(cAMP,环磷酸腺苷)

Cyclic AMP, the prototypical second messenger, is synthesized by adenylyl cyclase under the control

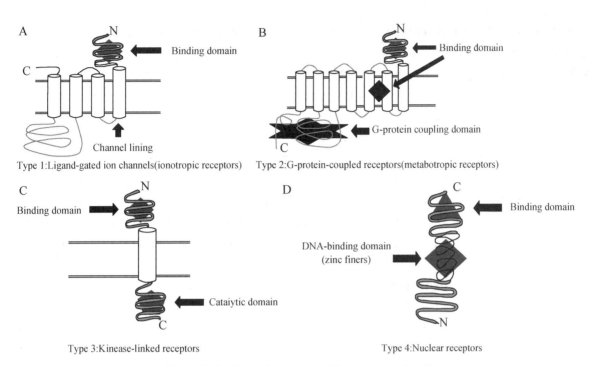

Figure 3-5   General structure of four receptor families

of many G protein-coupled receptors; stimulation is mediated by G_s and inhibition by G_i. There are at least ten tissue-specific adenylyl cyclase isozymes, and each has unique pattern of regulatory responses. Several adenylyl cyclase isozymes are either stimulated or inhibited by G protein $\beta\gamma$ subunits, which allows G proteins other than G_s to modulate cyclase activity. Some isozymes are stimulated by Ca^{2+} or Ca^{2+}-calmodulin complexes. Cyclic AMP is eliminated by a combination of hydrolysis, catalyzed by cyclic nucleotide phosphodiesterases, and extrusion by several plasma membrane transport proteins. Phosphodiesterases (磷酸二酯酶) form yet another family of important signaling proteins whose activities are regulated by controlled transcription as well as by second messengers (cyclic nucleotides and Ca^{2+}) and interactions with yet other signaling proteins. In most cases, cyclic AMP functions by activating cyclic AMP-dependent protein kinases, a relatively small group of closely related proteins. In addition to activating a protein kinase, cyclic AMP also directly regulates the activity of plasma membrane cation channels, which are particularly important in olfactory neurons. Cyclic AMP signals are thus propagated throughout the biochemical behavior of the target cell.

4.2.2   Calcium

Intracellular Ca^{2+}, another second messenger, offers several interesting comparisons with cyclic AMP. The release of Ca^{2+} into the cytoplasm is mediated by diverse channels: plasma membrane channels regulated by G proteins, membrane potential, K^+ or Ca^{2+} itself, and channels in specialized regions of endoplasmic reticulum (内质网) that respond to the second messenger inositol trisphosphate (IP_3), or, in muscle, to cell depolarization (去极化). Ca^{2+} is removed both by extrusion and by reuptake into the endoplasmic reticulum. Ca^{2+} propagates its signals through a much wider range of proteins than does cyclic AMP, including metabolic enzymes, protein kinases, and Ca^{2+}-binding regulatory proteins that regulate still other ultimate and intermediary effectors.

4.2.3   Guanylyl cyclase system(鸟苷酸环化酶系统)

Guanylyl cyclase catalyses the conversion of GTP to cGMP. This cGMP goes on to cause activation of protein kinase G ,then in turn phosphorylates contractile protein and ion channels. Transmembrane guanylyl cyclase is exhibited by the atrial natriuretic peptide receptor upon the binding of atrial natriuretic peptide.Cytoplasmic guanylyl cyclase activity is exhibited when bradykinin activates receptors on the membrane of endothelial cells (内皮细胞) to generate nitric oxide (一氧化氮), which then acts as a second messenger to activate guanylyl cyclase within the cell.

4.2.4 Inostitol phosphate system(磷酸肌醇系统)

It is also called phospholipase/inositaol phosphate system or calcium/ phosphoinositides (磷酸肌醇). Activation of M_1，M_3，5-HT$_2$，peptide and α_1-adrenoceptors, via Gq, causes activation of phospholipase C (PLC),a membrane-bound enzyme, which increases the rate of degradation of phosphatidylinosital (4,5) bisphosphate into diacylglycerol (DAG) and inositol (1,4,5) triphosphate (IP$_3$). Well-studied second messenger system involves hormonal stimulation of phosphoinositide hydrolysis (磷酸肌醇水解).

4.3 Drug-receptor interactions

$$[D]+[R] \xrightarrow{k_1} [DR] \xrightarrow{k_2} E$$

$[D]$ and $[R]$ mean drugs and receptors respectively; $[DR]$ means the complex of $[D]$ and $[R]$; E means the response produced by binding of drug to receptor.

The rate at which the forward reaction occurs is dependent upon the interaction $[D]$ and the receptor concentration $[R]$:

$$\text{Forward rate} = k_1[D][R]$$

The rate at which the backward reaction occurs is mainly dependent upon the interaction between the drug and the receptor $[DR]$:

$$\text{Backward rate} = k_2[DR]$$

When the reaction reached equilibration:

$$[DR] \text{ production} = [DR] \text{ dissociation}$$

Productive rate of $[DR]$ equals the rate dissociation of $[DR]$:

$$k_1[D] \times [R] = k_2[DR]$$

Because $[R]=[R_\tau]-[DR]$, $[R]$ is free receptor, $[R_\tau]$ is total receptor and $[DR]$ is binding receptor.

$$k_1([R_\tau]-[DR]) \times [D] = k_2[DR]$$

$$([R_\tau]-[DR]) \times [D] = \frac{k_2}{k_1}$$

Suppose $\dfrac{k_2}{k_1}=k_D$, k_D is defined as the dissociation constant, it expresses the affinity of the drug for receptor. The lower the k_D is, the higher the affinity is.

$$([R_\tau]-[DR]) \times [D] = k_D[DR]$$

$$[R]=[R_\tau]-[DR]$$

So

$$k_D = \frac{[R][D]}{[DR]}$$

This is to say, when the reaction reaches equilibration(平衡), the dissociation constant equals the product of drug and free receptor is divided by total receptors.

$$\text{From } ([R_\tau]-[DR]) \times [D] = k_D[DR]$$

$$[R_\tau] \times [D] - [DR] \times [D] = k_D[DR]$$

$$[R_\tau] \times [D] = (k_D + [D]) \times [DR]$$

$$\frac{[DR]}{[R_\tau]} = \frac{[D]}{k_D + [D]}$$

Take E as the effect of the concentration of drug, the E produced when the total receptors are occupied as E_{max}. According to the occupation theory:

$$\frac{E}{E_{max}} = \frac{[DR]}{[R_\tau]} = \frac{[D]}{k_D + [D]}$$

When $[D] = 0$, $E=0$, $[D]>k_D$, $[DR] \to [R_\tau]$, $E= E_{max}$.

When $[D]=k_D$, $\frac{[DR]}{[R_\tau]} = 50\%$, $E = \frac{E_{max}}{2}$

Conclude: k_D is the drug concentration (mol) by which 50% of the total receptor may be occupied. Suppose pD_2 (Affinity index) $=-\log k_D$, the larger pD_2 is, the higher the affinity is.

The final drug response depends on not only the affinity but also the intrinsic activity (α). The α is termed the ability of drug which binds and activates the receptor as well as produces a subsequent response.

$$\frac{E}{E_{max}} = \alpha \frac{[DR]}{[R_\tau]}$$

So we must consider α when we evaluate the response of drugs.

4.4　Classification of drugs acting on the receptor

4.4.1　Agonist

Agonists (激动药) refer to the drugs that have not only affinity but also intrinsic activity, so they can activate receptors and produce a subsequent response (Figure 3-6).

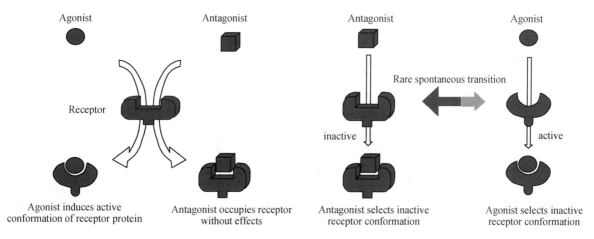

Figure 3-6　Molecular mechanisms of drug-receptor interaction

(1) Full agonists (完全激动药)　Full agonists have high efficacy and are able to produce a maximal response while occupying only a small percentage of the receptors available. In other word, these drugs have a high affinity and $\alpha= 1$.

(2) Partial agonist (部分激动药)　Partial agonist have low efficacy and unable to elicit the maximum response even if they are to occupy all the available receptor. Therefore, these drugs have lower affinity and α<1.

4.4.2 Antagonist

Antagonists (拮抗药) bind to receptors but do not activate them, they do not induce a conformational change and thus have no efficacy. However, because antagonists occupy the receptor, they prevent agonists from binding and therefore block their action.

(1) Competitive antagonists (竞争性拮抗药)　These drugs bind to receptors reversibly and effectively produce a dilution of the receptors. A parallel shift is produced to the right of the agonist dose-response curve. The competitive antagonist can be quantified in terms of the dose ratio. The dose ratio is the ratio of the concentration of agonist producing a given response in the presence and absence of a certain concentration of antagonist. The antagonist parameter (pA_2) is termed the negative logarithm of the concentration of the antagonist that is required when the given effect of the agonist in the absence of the antagonist is realized by a doubled concentration of the agonist. Making the assumption that the competitive antagonist is acting in a totally reversible manner then the pA_2 is equal to the negative logarithm of the K_D for the antagonist (Figure 3-7A).

(2) Non-competitive antagonists (非竞争性拮抗药)　These are also known as irreversible antagonists, their presence also produce a shift to the right of the agonist dose-response curve, but depress the maximum response. This means that the antagonist's effects cannot be overcome by the addition of greater doses of agonist (Figure 3-7B).

4.4.3 Spare receptor

There are some drugs that possess higher activity, its maximum response can be obtained when the partial receptors are occupied. This excess of receptors is called spare receptor (储备性受体) and is served

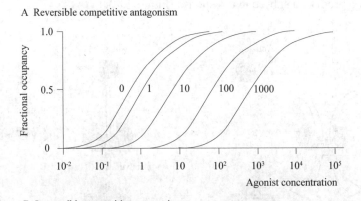

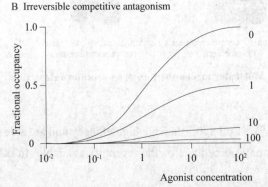

Figure 3-7　Hypothetical agonist concentration-occupancy curves in the presence of reversible and irreversible competitive antagonists

to sharpen the sensitivity of the cell to small changes in agonist concentration .

4.5　Receptor regulation

Receptor-mediated (受体调节) responses to drugs and hormonal agonists often "desensitize" with time. After reaching an initial high level, the response gradually diminishes over seconds or minutes, even in the continued presence of the agonists. This desensitization (脱敏) is usually reversible. Thus, 15 minutes after removal of the agonist, a second exposure to agonist results in a response similar to the initial response. For instance, agonist-induced desensitization of the nicotinic acetylcholine receptor (烟碱乙酰胆碱受体).

The ready reversibility of desensitization differs from the slower onset and more prolonged effect of receptor down-regulation (受体下调), an agonist-induced decrease in receptor number (which is often seen with receptor tyrosine kinase). Down-regulation, which is produced by agonist-induced decrease in receptor biosynthesis and increases in receptor internalization and degradation (内化和降解), usually occurs over hours to days, internalization may play several different roles in receptor regulation.

重 点 小 结

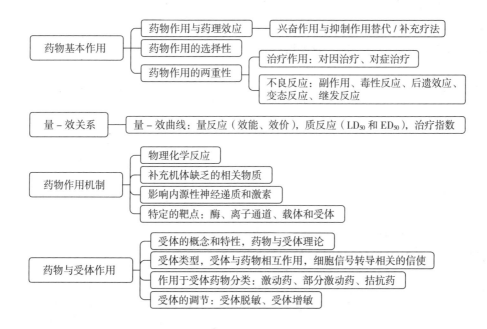

目 标 检 测

一、单项选择题

1. 变态反应是在下列哪种剂量下产生的（　　　）
   A. 治疗量　　　　　　　　　　B. 大剂量
   C. 与剂量无关　　　　　　　　D. 停药后的残存剂量
   E. 无效量

题库

2. 用药后可造成机体病理性损害，并可预知的不良反应是（　　　）
   A. 继发反应　　 B. 特异质反应　　 C. 毒性反应　　　 D. 变态反应　　　 E. 副作用

3. 后遗效应是指（　　　）
   A. 血药浓度有较大波动时产生的生物效应
   B. 药物剂量过大引起的效应
   C. 血药浓度低于有效血药浓度时的效应
   D. 血药浓度高于有效血药浓度时的效应
   E. 仅可能出现于极少数人的反应

4. 决定药物副作用多少的主要因素是（　　　）
   A. 药物的理化性质　　　　　　 B. 药物的选择作用
   C. 药物的安全范围　　　　　　 D. 患者的年龄和性别
   E. 给药途径

5. 关于受体激动剂的特点叙述正确的是（　　　）
   A. 能与受体结合　　　　　　 B. 必须占领全部受体
   C. 有很强的内在活性　　　　 D. 使药物的构象发生改变
   E. 与受体有亲和力且有内在活性

6. 受体拮抗剂与受体（　　　）
   A. 有亲和力，无内在活性　　　 B. 既有亲和力又有内在活性
   C. 无亲和力，有内在活性　　　 D. 既无亲和力又无内在活性
   E. 具有较强的亲和力，仅有较弱的内在活性

二、名词解释

1. 效价
2. 效能

三、思考题

1. 作用于受体的药物分类及其异同点有哪些？
2. 从药物与受体相互作用的角度论述拮抗剂的特点。

（周玖瑶）

Chapter 4 Introduction to the autonomic nervous system

 学习目标

1. **掌握** 作用于传出神经系统药物作用的方式。
2. **了解** 传出神经系统解剖分类、化学递质、传出神经受体及其生理效应。

1. The autonomic nervous system

The autonomic nervous system (ANS) is also called the visceral nerves. They are the branches of the cranial and spinal motor nerves that innervate cardiac and smooth muscle (involuntary) of the internal organs and glands which are not under conscious control, are regulated by the hypothalamus and the medulla oblongata. They are so named because it is autonomous; it functions independently of the conscious or somatic nervous system. The ANS regulates the activities of the internal organs and glands that are under involuntary or unconscious control. Before discussing the pharmacology of the autonomic nervous system, it is helpful to briefly review the general organization of the nervous system and the major anatomic and physiologic features of the autonomic nervous system.

The ANS is divided into two major subcategories: the sympathetic autonomic nervous system (SANS) and the parasympathetic autonomic nervous system (PANS). Both the PANS and SANS have ganglia (神经节), between the CNS and the end organ, but the somatic system does not. An important anatomic difference between the SANS and PANS is that the ganglia of the former lie in two paraventral chains (腹侧链) adjacent to the vertebral column (脊柱), whereas most of the ganglia of the PANS system are located in the organs innervated.

Most of the time, the SNS and the PNS systems are opposing to each other (Table 4-1). The neurotransmitters (神经递质) bind to and stimulate various autonomic receptor sites that are located on the cell membranes of the internal organs and glands. This produces the characteristic effects that are associated with each division of the ANS.

Table 4-1 Effects of sympathetic and parasympathetic stimulation

Organ	Sympathetic effect	Parasympathetic effect
Adrenal medulla	Release of epinephrine	—
Arteries	Vasoconstriction (exceptions are the coronary arteries and arteries to skeletal muscle, which are dilated)	Most arteries are not supplied by parasympathetic nerves
Heart	Increases heart rate and AV conduction. Increases contractility	Decreases heart rate and AV conduction. Slight decrease in contractility
Intestines, GI motility, and secretions	Decreased	Increased
Postganglionic neurotransmitter	Norepinephrine released	Acetylcholine released
Pupil of the eye	Dilation (mydriasis)	Constriction (miosis)
Respiratory passages, lower	Bronchodilation	Bronchoconstriction
Urinary bladder	Relaxation	Contraction
Urinary sphincter	Contraction	Relaxation

2. Neurotransmitters

Communication between nerve cells, and between nerve cells and effector organs, occurs through the release of specific chemical signals (neurotransmitters) from the nerve terminals. This release is triggered by the arrival of the action potential at the nerve ending, leading to depolarization (去极化). An increase in intracellular Ca^{2+} initiates fusion of the synaptic (突触) vesicles (囊泡) with the presynaptic membrane and release of their contents. The neurotransmitters rapidly diffuse across the synaptic cleft, or synapse, between neurons and combine with specific receptors on the target cell.

2.1 Acetylcholine

Acetylcholine (ACh) is the neurotransmitter at both nicotinic (烟碱) and muscarinic (毒蕈碱) receptors in tissues that are innervated. Note that all direct transmission from the CNS (preganglionic and motor) uses ACh, but postganglionic transmission in the SANS system may use one of the organ-specific transmitters described below.

ACh is formed from choline (胆碱) and activated acetate (acetyl coenzyme A, 乙酰辅酶A), a reaction catalyzed by the choline acetylase (胆碱乙酰化酶). The highly polar choline is taken up into the axoplasm by the specific choline-transporter (CHT) localized to membranes of cholinergic axons terminals and a subset of storage vesicles. During persistent or intensive stimulation, the CHT ensures that ACh synthesis and release are sustained. The newly formed ACh is loaded into storage vesicles by the vesicular ACh transporter (VAChT).

During activation of the nerve membrane, the permeability of synapse to Ca^{2+} increases, and Ca^{2+}

flows in a large amount, which makes the vesicle and presynaptic membrane fuse to form a model hole, and then the vesicle contents are discharged into the synaptic space through the hole, which combines with the cholinergic receptor on the post synaptic membrane, and makes the effector produce physiological effect.

Released ACh is rapidly inactivated and hydrolyzed to choline and acetic acid (乙酸) by a specific acetylcholinesterase (AChE, 乙酰胆碱酯酶), localized to pre-junctional and post-junctional membranes.

2.2　Norepinephrine and epinephrine

When norepinephrine and epinephrine are the neurotransmitters, the fiber is termed adrenergic. In the sympathetic system, norepinephrine mediates the transmission of nerve impulses from autonomic postganglionic nerves to effector organs(note: A few sympathetic fibers, such as those involved in sweating, are cholinergic, and, for simplicity).

Tyrosine (Tyr) is actively transported into nerve endings and is converted to dihydroxyphenylalanine (DOPA, 多巴) via tyrosine hydroxylase. This step is rate limiting in the synthesis of NE. DOPA is converted to dopamine (DA, 多巴胺) via L-aromatic amino acid decarboxylase (DOPA decarboxylase，多巴脱羧酶). DA is taken up into storage vesicles where it is metabolized to NE via dopamine β-hydroxylase (DβH，多巴胺β-羟化酶).

Presynaptic membrane depolarization opens voltage-dependent Ca^{2+} channels. Influx of this ion causes fusion of the synaptic granular membranes, with the presynaptic membrane leading to NE exocytosis into the neuroeffector junction. NE then activates post-junctional receptors, leading to tissue-specific responses depending on the adrenoceptor subtype activated.

Termination of NE actions is mainly due to removal from the neuroeffector junction back into the sympathetic nerve ending via an NE reuptake transporter system（uptake 1, 再摄取1）. At some sympathetic nerve endings, the NE released may activate pre-junctional alpha adrenoceptors involved in feedback regulation, which results in decreased release of the neurotransmitter. Metabolism of NE is by catechol-O-methyltransferase (COMT) in the synapse or MAO-A in the pre-junctional nerve terminal （uptake 2, 再摄取2）.

3. Autonomic receptors

3.1　Muscarinic and nicotinic receptors

ACh binds to muscarinic and nicotinic receptors, abbreviated M and N. The major receptor types are muscarinic (M_{1-3}), ganglionic nicotinic (N_N) and endplate nicotinic (N_M). M receptors are on organs that receive parasympathetic innervations. N receptors are in ANS ganglia and function as nerve to nerve neurotransmitters. N receptors are also important in nerve to muscle communication (the neuromuscular junction).

ACh is the neurotransmitter at all N receptors, at the M receptors innervated by postganglionic fibers of the PANS, and the thermoregulatory sweat glands innervated by the SANS.

3.2 α receptors and β receptors

NE (and epinephrine) binds to alpha and beta receptors (α and β). Another name for epinephrine is adrenaline, so these receptors are also commonly referred to as adrenergic receptors. The most important with regard to drug actions are four major subtypes (α_1, α_2, β_1, β_2, β_3).

The action of α_1 receptor stimulation is the contraction of smooth muscle; β_1 receptors are located mainly on the heart and mediate cardiac stimulation, an increase in heart rate and force of contraction. β_2 receptors are located on smooth muscle and produce relaxation of smooth muscle.

4. Manipulating the autonomic nervous system

We can strengthen or weaken the SNS or the PNS to change the balance between the two systems. The main pharmacological difference between the sympathetic nerves and the parasympathetic nerves is the neurotransmitter released from the postganglionic nerve ending of each division.

For strengthening parasympathetic, we can increase stimulation of the M receptors by giving an agonist or inhibiting the breakdown or removal of endogenous (the body's own) ACh.

For weakening parasympathetic, we can decrease M receptor stimulation by giving an antagonist.

For strengthening sympathetic we can increase stimulation of the α and β receptors via administration of an agonist (sympathomimetic) that stimulates these receptors, inhibition of the breakdown or removal of endogenous NE or epinephrine or inhibition of synaptic NE reuptake by the presynaptic cell, leading to increased NE in the synaptic cleft.

For weakening sympathetic we can decrease stimulation of the α and β receptors via administration an antagonist that blocks these receptors or a drug that turns down the ganglion.

Depending on the clinical situation being treated, it is possible to selectively increase or decrease the function of a particular organ or system. The following chapters will discuss the individual drug classes and major pharmacologic features.

重 点 小 结

重点内容	主要掌握
自主神经系统概况	自主神经系统解剖分类
	交感神经和副交感神经生物效应
神经递质	乙酰胆碱
	去甲肾上腺素、肾上腺素
受体	胆碱受体
	肾上腺素受体
作用于自主神经系统的方式	直接作用
	间接作用

目 标 检 测

题库

一、选择题

（一）单项选择题

1. β_1 受体阻滞产生的效应是（　　　）
   A. 骨骼肌松弛
   B. 血管扩张
   C. 内脏平滑肌松弛
   D. 支气管平滑肌松弛
   E. 心肌收缩力减弱

2. N_2 受体阻滞产生的效应是（　　　）
   A. 骨骼肌松弛
   B. 血管扩张
   C. 内脏平滑肌松弛
   D. 支气管平滑肌松弛
   E. 心肌收缩力减弱

3. 支气管哮喘是下列哪个受体效应引起的（　　　）
   A. M 受体兴奋
   B. β_2 受体兴奋
   C. N_2 受体兴奋
   D. β_2 受体阻滞
   E. α_1 受体阻滞

（二）多项选择题

4. 关于自主神经系统，叙述正确的有（　　　）
   A. 交感神经系统主司休息状态；副交感神经主要拮抗交感神经的作用，主司应激状态
   B. 交感神经系统的神经纤维发自 T_1~L_2 脊髓侧角
   C. 第二级神经元的胞体位于神经节内，称为神经节前（突触前）神经元
   D. 副交感神经系统由 Ⅲ，Ⅶ，Ⅸ，Ⅹ 脑神经和骶髓的 S_2~S_4 构成
   E. 第一级神经元的胞体在脑内的灰质或脊髓

二、思考题

自主神经系统药物作用方式有哪几种？

（殷玉婷）

Chapter 5　Cholinergic agonists

学习目标

1. **掌握** 毛果芸香碱的药理作用、临床应用及注意事项。
2. **熟悉** 乙酰胆碱的药理作用。
3. **了解** 胆碱受体激动药的分类及代表药。

Cholinergic agonists are the name given to a group of medicines that mimic the actions of acetylcholine by binding directly to cholinoceptors [muscarinic (毒蕈碱) or nicotinic(烟碱)]. These agents can be divided on the basis of chemical structure into esters of choline (胆碱酯类) and alkaloids (生物碱). They also can be classified pharmacologically by their spectrum of action depending on the type of receptor muscarinic or nicotinic that is activated. A few of them are highly selective for the muscarinic or for the nicotinic receptor. Many have effects on both receptors, acetylcholine is typical.

1. Muscarinic and nicotinic receptor agonists

Acetylcholine (乙酰胆碱)

Acetylcholine is secreted by cholinergic neurons in the CNS, autonomic ganglia (自主神经节), adrenal medulla (肾上腺髓质), and the neuromuscular junction. As an endogenous neurotransmitter, it has very important physiological functions, and it's important to be familiar with the pharmacological effects and mechanisms of the transmitter although its broad-ranging actions render it of very limited therapeutic value.

【Pharmacodynamics】

(1) Cardiac effects Administration of ACh mimics the cardiac effects of the parasympathetic nervous system with reduced contractility, sinus rate (窦性心率), and AV nodal conduction (房室结传导). The result is reduced cardiac output and heart rate.

(2) Vascular effects and blood pressure Intravenous injection of ACh results in vasodilation (血管舒张) apparently by eliciting release of nitric oxide and thus activating the nitric oxide mechanism of local blood flow regulation. This reduces systemic vascular resistance and in the context of reduced cardiac output, described above, combines to produce a drop in systemic arterial pressure, yielding hypotension (低血压). This effect of ACh appears to be mediated by cholinergic receptors on the vascular wall itself.

(3) GI and GU effects　Theoretically one would expect activation of muscarinic receptors in the GI and GU tract (胃肠道) to enhance GI secretions, GI Motility (胃肠动力), as well as boost contraction of the bladder's detrusor muscle, thus promoting micturition (排尿).

(4) Ocular effects　When administered by eye drops, ACh induces miosis (缩瞳) by enhancing contraction of the pupillary sphincter muscle (瞳孔括约肌).

【Clinical indications】There are almost no contemporary therapeutic uses for acetylcholine due to its rapid inactivation by cholinesterases and its diverse non-specific effects as described above.

Carbachol (卡巴胆碱)

Carbachol is a choline carbamate and a positively charged quaternary ammonium (季铵) compound that can bind and activate acetylcholine receptors. It is not well absorbed in the gastro-intestinal tract and does not cross the blood-brain barrier. It is primarily used topically in the eye to induce miosis of the pupil. This is done prior to certain ophthalmological surgeries and in the medical treatment of glaucoma(青光眼). When used topically in this form there are few systemic adverse effects.

2. Muscarinic receptor agonists

Pilocarpine (毛果芸香碱)

Pilocarpine is a naturally occurring alkaloid which is extracted from the South American shrub named "Pilocarpus jaborandi". It is a selectively muscarinic receptor agonist that binds to muscarinic-M_3 receptors and results in contraction of smooth muscles and stimulation of various exocrine glands.

【Pharmacokinetics】The drug is available in the form of eye drops, tablets, suspensions and gel. It has a slow onset of action which is about 10 to 15 minutes but has a longer duration of action about 6 to 8 hours, and therefore can be given thrice a day. It is inactivated at neuronal synapses and in plasma and is excreted in urine.

【Pharmacodynamics】

(1) Eyes (Figure 5-1)

1) Miosis　Pilocarpine produces miosis through contraction of the iris sphincter muscle (虹膜括约肌).

2) Decrease intraocular pressure (IOP，眼内压)　Pilocarpine contracts the ciliary muscle, causing increased tension on the scleral spur and opening of the trabecular meshwork spaces to facilitate outflow of aqueous humor (房水). Outflow resistance is reduced, lowering IOP. Miosis relieves appositional angle narrowing and closure, which lowers IOP in certain types of angle-closure glaucoma.

3) Spasms of accommodation (调节痉挛)　Pilocarpine stimulate the muscarinic receptors on the ciliary muscle to trigger contraction, which leads to relaxation of the lens, thus allowing for focusing on near objects.

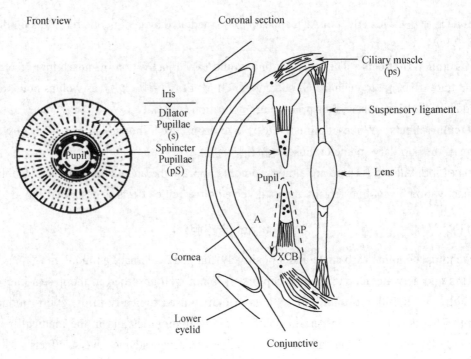

Figure 5-1　Effects of Pilocarpine on eyes

(2) Glandular secretion Pilocarpine, in appropriate dosage, can increase secretion by the exocrine glands. The sweat, salivary, lacrimal, gastric, pancreatic, and intestinal glands and the mucous cells of the respiratory tract may be stimulated.

【Clinical indications】

(1) Treatment of glaucoma [open-angle and acute angle-closure(开角型及闭角型青光眼)] Pilocarpine drops cause contraction of the ciliary muscle which opens the trabecular meshwork spaces to increase the outflow of aqueous humor through the canal of Schlemm (巩膜静脉窦), thereby lowering intra-ocular pressure. It also cause miosis by causing contraction of the iris sphincter muscle. This can be beneficial as well in lowering intraocular pressure in certain types of angle-closure glaucoma. The drug also can reduce the elevated intraocular pressure in patients with primary open-angle glaucoma.

(2) Treatment of dry mouth Pilocarpine is effective for the treatment of radiation-induced dry mouth by stimulating salivary gland function.

【Adverse reactions】Excessive sweating (diaphoresis) is a frequent side effect of pilocarpine. Other side effects include: nausea, vomiting, diarrhea (腹泻), salivation (流涎), flushing, increased urinary frequency.

3. Nicotinic receptor agonists

Agonists of the nAChR include nicotine (尼古丁), epibatidine (地棘蛙素), and choline. Nicotinic agonists have no important role in therapeutics. The stereotypical nicotinic agonist—nicotine itself—is used as a recreational stimulant by many people via various routes of administration. After administration of doses commonly used for this purpose there is little or no effect on peripheral nicotinic synapses. The general stimulatory effect of small doses of nicotine is the result of nicotine promoting the release of a large number of CNS neurotransmitters. This stimulating effect of low-dose nicotine is reversed when nicotine is administered at higher doses. Peripheral effects include tachycardia, increased arterial pressure and reduction of gastrointestinal motility. The light-headed feeling experienced by naive smokers is due to stimulation of nicotinic receptors located on sensory nerve fibers, principally chemoreceptors in the carotid body. Nicotine is quite toxic (0.5-1.0mg/kg in mammals) and higher doses can cause serious adverse reactions and even death.

重 点 小 结

药物	受体类型	药理作用	临床应用	不良反应
乙酰胆碱	M 受体、N 受体	抑制心脏、舒张血管、刺激腺体、收缩平滑肌	药理学研究工具药，无临床实用价值	—
卡巴胆碱	M 受体、N 受体	似乙酰胆碱、作用久	青光眼	调节痉挛、头痛、结膜充血
毛果芸香碱	M 受体	眼 (缩瞳、降眼压、调节痉挛)，促腺体分泌	青光眼口腔黏膜干燥症	瞳孔缩小、调节痉挛；全身毒性反应，如出汗、流涎、呕吐等

目 标 检 测

题库

一、单项选择题

1. 毛果芸香碱对眼的作用是（　　　　）
   A. 瞳孔缩小，升高眼内压，调节痉挛　　　　B. 瞳孔缩小，降低眼内压，调节痉挛
   C. 瞳孔扩大，升高眼内压，调节麻痹　　　　D. 瞳孔扩大，降低眼内压，调节麻痹
   E. 瞳孔缩小，降低眼内压，调节麻痹

2. 毛果芸香碱的缩瞳机制是（　　　　）
   A. 阻断虹膜 α 受体，开大肌松弛　　　　B. 阻断虹膜 M 胆碱受体，括约肌松弛
   C. 激动虹膜 α 受体，开大肌收缩　　　　D. 激动虹膜 M 胆碱受体，括约肌收缩
   E. 抑制胆碱酯酶，使乙酰胆碱增多

3. M-R 受体激动药无下列哪种作用（　　　　）
   A. 缩瞳、降低眼内压　　　　B. 腺体分泌增加
   C. 胃肠、膀胱平滑肌兴奋　　　　D. 骨骼肌收缩
   E. 心脏抑制、血管扩张、血压下降

4. 与毒扁豆碱相比，毛果芸香碱不具备下列哪种特点（　　）
　　A. 遇光不稳定　　B. 维持时间短　　C. 刺激性小　　　　D. 作用较弱　　　　E. 水溶液稳定
5. 毛果芸香碱降低眼内压的机制是（　　）
　　A. 减少房水生成　　　　　　　B. 收缩局部血管
　　C. 促进房水回流　　　　　　　D. 扩张局部血管
　　E. 降低血管通透性
6. 与毛果芸香碱相比，毒扁豆碱用于治疗青光眼的优点是（　　）
　　A. 作用强而久　　　　　　　　B. 水溶液稳定
　　C. 毒副作用小　　　　　　　　D. 不引起调节痉挛
　　E. 不会吸收中毒

二、多项选择题

7. 毛果芸香碱的药理作用有（　　）
　　A. 缩瞳　　　　　　　　　　B. 降低眼内压　　　　　　C. 调节痉挛
　　D. 汗腺、唾液腺分泌增加　　E. 汗腺、唾液腺分泌减少
8. 毛果芸香碱可用于治疗（　　）
　　A. 尿潴留　　　　　　　　　B. 重症肌无力　　　　　　C. 角膜炎
　　D. 青光眼　　　　　　　　　E. 阿托品中毒

（周　园）

Chapter 6 Anticholinesterase agents and cholinesterase reactivators

PPT

 学习目标

　　1.掌握　可逆性抗胆碱酯酶药的药理作用及临床用途；难逆性抗胆碱酯酶药有机磷酸酯类农药的中毒机制、中毒途径、解救原则及措施。
　　2.熟悉　胆碱酯酶作用及胆碱酯酶复活药碘解磷定（PAM）的作用和用途。
　　3.了解　氯解磷定（PAM-Cl）的作用特点。

An anticholinergic agent is a substance that blocks the action of the neurotransmitter acetylcholine at synapses in the central and the peripheral nervous system. The function of acetylcholinesterase (AChE) (胆碱酯酶) in terminating the action of acetylcholine (ACh) at the junctions of the various cholinergic nerve endings with their effector organs or postsynaptic sites is considered. These agents inhibit parasympathetic nerve impulses by selectively blocking the binding of the neurotransmitter acetylcholine to its receptor in nerve cells. Drugs that inhibit AChE are called anticholinesterase agents. They cause ACh to accumulate in the vicinity of cholinergic nerve terminals and thus are potentially capable of producing effects equivalent to excessive stimulation of cholinergic receptors throughout the central and peripheral nervous systems.

1. The hydrolysis reaction of cholinesterase

In biochemistry, a cholinesterase is a family of esterase (脂酶) that lyses choline-base esters, several of which serve as neurotransmitter. Thus, it is either of two enzymes that catalyze the hydrolysis of these cholinergic neurotransmitters, such as breaking acetylcholine into choline (胆碱) and acetic acid. These reactions are necessary to allow a cholinergic neuron to return to its resting state after activation (Figure 6-1). In muscle contraction, acetylcholine must be broken down by a choline esterase. Once the ACh is bound, the hydrolytic reaction occurs at a second region of the active site called the esteratic subsite. Here, the ester bond of ACh is broken, releasing acetate and choline. In addition to two subsites of active center, AChE contains one or more "peripheral" anionic sites (阴离子场) distinct from the choline-binding pocket of the active site. It serves for binding ACh and other quartenary ligands acting

医药大学堂
WWW.YIYAODXT.COM

45

as uncompetitive inhibitors that bind at a site clearly distinct from that occupied by the monoquarternary competitive inhibitors. This site is involved in the substrate inhibition characteristics of AChE.

Choline is then either temporarily trapped within the junctional folds of the muscular endplate or immediately taken up again by the high affinity choline uptake (HACU) system on the presynaptic membrane. Acetate, however, becomes covalently bonded to serine residues

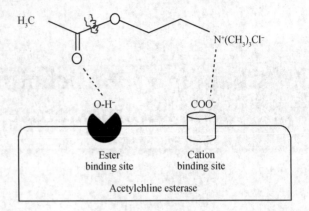

Figure 6-1　Schematic representation of AChE binding sites

within the esteratic subsite, forming a temporary acetylated form of AChE. A molecule of water then reacts with this intermediate, liberating the acetate group, which diffuses into the surrounding medium. What remains is an active form of the enzyme, ready to react with a newly released molecule of ACh. AChE is a serine hydrolase (丝氨酸水解酶) mainly found at neuromuscular junctions and cholinergic brain synapses. Its principal biological role is termination of impulse transmission at cholinergic synapses by rapid hydrolysis of the neurotransmitter ACh to acetate and choline (Figure 6-2).

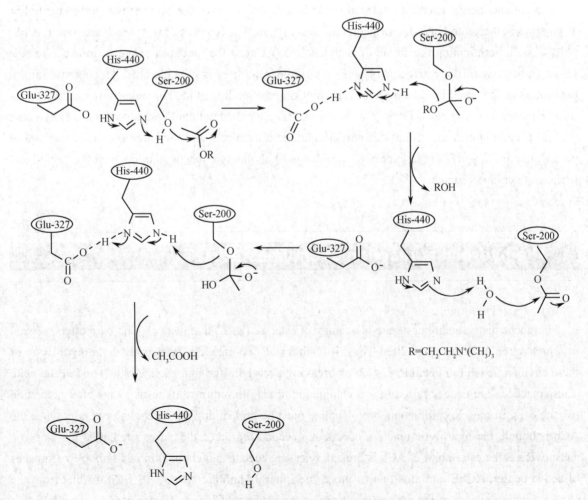

Figure 6-2　Mechanism of ACh hydrolysis catalyzed by AChE

2. Cholinesterase inhibitor

A cholinesterase inhibitor suppresses the action of the enzyme. Among the most common acetylcholinesterase inhibitors are phosphorus-based compounds, which are designed to bind to the active site of the enzyme.

2.1 Reversible inhibitor

Neostigmine (新斯的明)

Neostigmine is a medication used to treat myasthenia gravis (重症肌无力), Ogilvie syndrome, and urinary retention without the presence of a blockage.

【Pharmacokinetics】Neostigmine does not cross the blood-brain barrier and enter the CNS, but it does cross the placenta. The oral bioavailability of these hydrophilic ionised compounds is low. In spite of the short elimination half-life of pyridostigmine, intraindividual variations in plasma concentration during a dose interval are small in myasthenic patients receiving oral maintenance therapy, probably as a result of slow absorption from the gastrointestinal tract.

【Pharmacodynamics】Neostigmine bind to the anionic and ester site of cholinesterase. The drug blocks the active site of acetylcholinesterase so the enzyme can no longer break down the acetylcholine molecules before they reach the postsynaptic membrane receptors. This allows the threshold to be reached so a new impulse can be triggered in the next neuron.

【Clinical indications】

(1) **Reversible acetylcholinesterase inhibitors in alzheimer's disease treatment**   AD is associated with loss of cholinergic neurons (胆碱能神经) in the brain and the decreased level of ACh. The major therapeutic target in the AD treatment strategies is the inhibition of brain AChE. The different physiological processes are related to AD damage or destroy cells that produce and use ACh, thereby reducing the amount available to deliver messages to other cells. Cholinesterase inhibitor drugs can boost cholinergic neurotransmission in forebrain regions and compensate for the loss of functioning brain cells.

(2)**Others**   It is used to improve muscle tone in people with myasthenia gravis. Another indication for use is the conservative management of acute colonic pseudo-obstruction, or Ogilvie's syndrome, in which patients get massive colonic dilatation in the absence of a true mechanical obstruction.

【Adverse reactions】Long-term use may increase the risk of both cognitive and physical decline. Possible effects of anticholinergics include: poor coordination, dementia decreased mucus (黏液) production in the nose and throat; consequent dry, sore throat, dry-mouth and so on. Elderly patients are at a higher risk of experiencing CNS side effects.

Donepezil (多奈哌齐)

Donepezil is a selective, reversible AChE inhibitor.

【Pharmacokinetics】It is available as disintegrating tablet and oral solution, being 100% oral bioavailability with ease crossing the blood-brain barrier and slow excretion. As it has a half-life of about 70 hours, it can be taken once a day.

【Pharmacodynamics】Donepezil binds and reversibly inactivates the cholinesterase, thus inhibiting hydrolysis of acetylcholine. This increases acetylcholine concentrations at cholinergic synapse. In addition to its actions as an acetylcholinesterase inhibitor, donepezil has been found to act as a potent agonist of the σ_1 receptor, and has been shown to produce specific antiamnestic effects in animals mainly via this action (Figure 6-3).

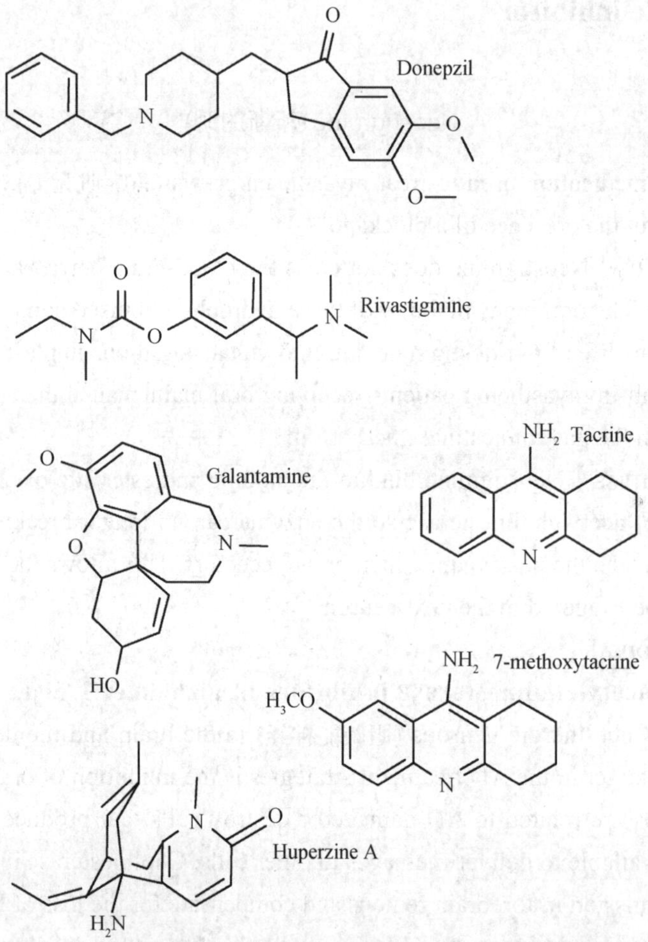

Figure 6-3 Selected reversible AChE inhibitors in pharmacotherapy of AD

【Clinical indications】Donepezil binds to the peripheral anionic site exerting not only symptomatic effects in the AD treatment, but also causative ones delaying the deposition of amyloid plaque.

【Adverse reactions】In clinical trials the most common adverse events leading to discontinuation were nausea (恶心), diarrhea (腹泻), and vomiting (呕吐). Other side effects included difficulty sleeping, muscle cramps and loss of appetite. Donepezil should be used with caution in people with heart disease, cardiac conduction disturbances, chronic obstructive pulmonary disease, asthma, severe cardiac arrhythmias and sick sinus syndrome.

Carbamates (氨基甲酸酯)

Carbamates are organic compounds derived from carbamic acid (NH_2COOH). These reversible AChE inhibitors have been applied as pesticides, then as parasiticides in veterinary medicine, and in prophylaxis of organophosphorus compounds (OPs) poisoning as well. As a potent AChE inhibitor, this therapeutic agent reduces ACh hydrolysis rate, and thereby increases its level in damaged neurosynaptic clefts improving nerve impulse transmission. Besides, pyridostigmine is capable to prevent the irreversible binding of OP to AChE. Consequently, it is applied as a prophylactic against nerve agent intoxication. Furthermore, rivastigmine is a carbamate with probably the most meaningful pharmacological application, being validated in the symptomatic treatment of AD.

2.2 Irreversible inhibitor

Organophosphorus compounds (有机磷化合物)

OPs are esters or thiols derived from phosphoric, phosphonic, phosphinic or phosphoramidic acid. In medicine and agriculture, the word "organophosphates" refers to a group of insecticides and nerve agents that inhibit AChE. The OPs exert their main toxicological effects through non-reversible phosphorylation of esterase in the central nervous system. The typical symptoms of acute poisoning (急性毒性) are agitation, muscle weakness, muscle fasciculations, miosis, hypersalivation, sweating.

【Pharmacodynamics】Mechanism of AChE inhibition induced by OPs, reactivation, spontaneous hydrolysis, and aging of the phosphorylated enzyme.

【Clinical indications】OPs, except their use as toxic compounds, have been applied in ophthalmology as therapeutic agents in the treatment of chronic glaucoma, an eye disease in which the optic nerve is damaged in a characteristic pattern. The disease is associated with increased fluid pressure in the eye and can permanently damage vision in the affected eye and lead to blindness if left untreated.

【Adverse reactions】The primary target of OP action is AChE, and the main mechanism of toxicity in acute OP exposure involves the specific irreversible inhibition of this enzyme activity in the nervous system and blood, manifesting as a cholinergic crisis with excessive glandular secretions and weakness, miosis (瞳孔缩小) and fasciculation of muscle, which may lead to death. OPs may affect liver, kidney, muscles, immune, and hematological system, causing many human body disorders.

2.3 Cholinesterase reactivator (胆碱酯酶活化剂)

Detoxification of organophosphorus and carbamate insecticides are based on enzymatic hydrolysis. Carbamates and OPs are polar compounds accumulating in fatty tissues and can be eliminated by their conversion to water soluble compounds. Carbamates are most effectively decomposed by carboxylesterases (CESs), the esterases are capable to hydrolyze carboxyl esters. The mechanism of the CESs catalyzed hydrolysis of carboxyl esters consists in the reversible acylation of a serine residue in the active center of the protein, releasing the covalently acylated enzyme and the alcohol moiety of the carboxyl ester. However, much more efficient route of OPs detoxification is hydrolysis by PTEs, esterases of an unknown physiological role. The mechanism of PTEs action is based on the bond cleavage between the phosphorous atom and the leaving group (-X) of OPs（Figure 6-4）.

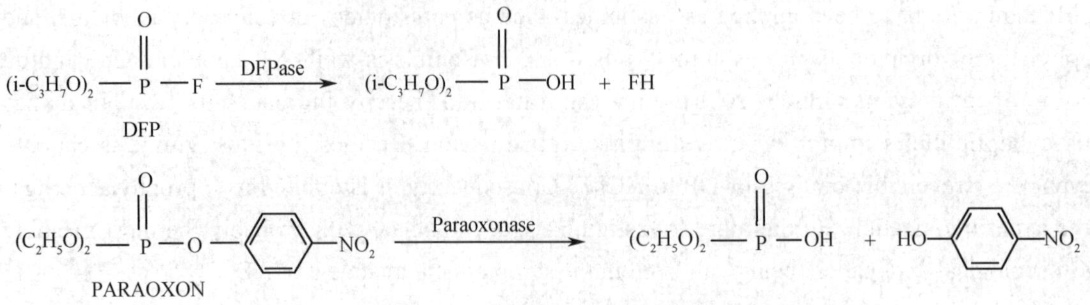

Figure 6-4   OPs hydrolysis catalyzed by known DFPase and paraoxonase

Pralidoxime (解磷定)

Pralidoxime, usually as the chloride or iodide salts, belongs to a family of compounds called oximes that bind to organophosphate-inactivated acetylcholinesterase. It is used to treat organophosphate poisoning in conjunction with atropine and diazepam. Pralidoxime is typically used in cases of organophosphate poisoning. Pralidoxime binds to the other half of the active site and then displaces the phosphate from the serine residue. The conjoined antidote (解毒剂) then unbinds from the site, and thus regenerates the fully functional enzyme. Some phosphate-acetylcholinesterase (磷酸化乙酰胆碱酯酶) conjugates continue to react after the phosphate docks to the esteric site, evolving into a more recalcitrant state. Pralidoxime is often used with atropine to help reduce the parasympathetic effects of organophosphate poisoning.

重 点 小 结

类别	药物	药理作用	临床应用	不良反应
胆碱酯酶抑制药	可逆性抗胆碱酯酶药：新斯的明	逆转肌肉松弛、结膜充血，增加胃酸分泌	重症肌无力，腹胀气，尿潴留，阿尔茨海默病	肌纤维震颤，肌张力下降
	难逆性抗胆碱酯酶药：有机磷酸酯类	治疗急性中毒、慢性中毒	—	—
胆碱酯酶复活药	碘解磷定	恢复 AChE 活性	减轻 N 样症状	局部轻微疼痛，头痛，恶心及心动过速

目 标 检 测

一、单项选择题

1. 新斯的明的禁忌证是（　　　）
   A. 重症肌无力 　　　　　　　　　　B. 术后腹胀气和尿潴留
   C. 阵发性室上性心动过速 　　　　　D. 青光眼
   E. 机械性肠梗阻

2. 毒扁豆碱主要用于治疗（　　　）
   A. 重症肌无力 　　　　　　B. 青光眼 　　　　　　C. 腹胀气
   D. 尿潴留 　　　　　　　　E. 阵发性室上性心动过速

3. 氯解磷定对有机磷农药中毒的哪一种症状缓解最快（　　　）
   A. 大小便失禁 　　　　　　B. 血压下降 　　　　　　C. 骨骼肌震颤
   D. 中枢神经兴奋 　　　　　E. 瞳孔缩小

4. 当发生有机磷酸酯类急性中毒时，常用的解毒药物为（　　　）
   A. 碘解磷定＋氯解磷定 　　B. 氯解磷定＋阿托品 　　C. 阿托品
   D. 碘解磷定 　　　　　　　E. 氯解磷定

二、多项选择题

5. 阿托品用于有机磷酸酯类中毒的解救，以下叙述正确的是（　　　）
   A. 能直接中和体内积聚的 ACh 　　B. 能迅速解除 M 样症状
   C. 能迅速控制肌束颤动 　　　　　D. 能缓解部分中枢神经系统的中毒症状
   E. 应使用大剂量，达到阿托品化

6. 新斯的明对骨骼肌兴奋作用强是由于（　　　）
   A. 直接兴奋 N_1 受体 　　　　　B. 直接兴奋 N_2 受体 　　　C. 抑制胆碱酯酶
   D. 促进运动神经末梢释放 ACh 　　E. 促进骨骼肌细胞钙内流

（王宏婷）

Chapter 7　Cholinergic antagonists

学习目标

1．掌握　阿托品的药理作用、临床应用和不良反应。

2．熟悉　山莨菪碱和东莨菪碱的作用特点；骨骼肌松弛药的分类、作用特点及用途。

3．了解　神经节阻滞药的作用及用途。

Anticholinergic drug is a kind of drugs, which can combine with cholinoceptors but cannot produce or just produce little cholinergic action, and then inhibit cholinergic neurotransmitters (胆碱能神经递质) or cholinomimetics connection with the acceptor in order to produce the effect of anticholinergic. It is also called the cholinoceptor blocker (胆碱受体阻滞药). According to the different of clinical application and the selectivity about M acceptors and N acceptors, anticholinergic drugs include three kinds such as M cholinoceptor blocker, N_1 cholinoceptor blocker and N_2 cholinoceptor blocker.

1.　M cholinoceptor blocker

1.1　Atropine alkaloid

Atropine alkaloids，such as atropine, scopolamine and anisodamine, can be extracted from plants, and they have similar chemical structures (Figure 7-1). Oxygen bridge (氧桥) has a central sedative effect, and hydroxyl can weaken the central sedative effect of oxygen bridge. Both of scopolamine and anisodine (樟柳碱) contain oxygen bridges, but anisodine has an extra hydroxyl group at the site of the tropin acid, so scopolamine is the strongest of the drugs for central sedation, and anisodine has a weaker central sedation than scopolamine. Neither atropine nor

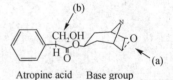

Atropine acid　　Base group

Figure 7-1　Basic chemical structure of atropine and its anlogues

Atropine: (a) no oxygen; Scopolamine: (a) oxygen; Homatropine: (a)no oxygen, (b)hydroxmethy is replaced by hydroxyl

anisodamine has an oxygen bridge, and anisodamine has one extra hydroxyl group on the tropin ring, therefore its central sedation is weakest.

Atropine (阿托品)

Atropine is the main alkaloid extracted from *Atropa belladonna* L.(颠茄), *Datura stramonium* Linn. (曼陀罗) and scopolamine of Solanaceae (茄科). The unstable scopolamine is naturally present in plants, and it can be the stable racemic scopolamine, which is produced from extract, atropine.

【Pharmacokinetics】Atropine is absorbed quickly by the ways of mouth, the blood concentration will reach a peak within an hour after taking the drug, and its effects can last up to three hours. After the patient taking it, atropine can be widely distributed throughout the body and can pass through the placenta (胎盘) into the fetal circulation (胎盘循环). About half of atropine that enters the body is excreted in its original form through the urine, while the rest of the metabolites are excreted in the urine.

【Pharmacodynamics】Atropine can competitively antagonize the activation of M-cholinergic receptors by acetylcholine or cholinergic agonists (胆碱能激动剂). Atropine has a fairly high selectivity for the M receptor, but the N_1 receptor in the ganglia (神经节) can also be blocked in a large dose or toxic dose. However, Atropine has a low selectivity to various subtypes of M receptors, for example, it can block M_1, M_2 and M_3 receptors. Atropine has a wide range of effects, and its sensitivity is varied from organ to organ. With the dose increases, the following effects occur in sequence.

(1) Suppresses gland (腺体) secretion   A small dose of atropine can significantly inhibit salivary gland and sweat gland secretion, and at the same time, respiratory tract and lacrimal gland secretion can be greatly reduced, and then resulting mouth dry and skin dry. However, high doses of Atropine can inhibit gastric secretion (胃液分泌), and the gastric acid secretion is mainly regulated by gastrin (胃泌素), therefore, atropine on gastric acid secretion has less impact while it has the most significant effect on sweat glands and salivary glands.

(2) The eyes

1) Dilating pupil (瞳孔扩大)   The atropine can block M receptors on the muscle sphincter pupillae (瞳孔括约肌), relax the circular muscle，and make it withdraw to the periphery (边缘), and then dilate pupils.

2) Raising intraocular (眼内) pressure   After the pupil has been dilated, the iris(虹膜) retreats to the periphery, and causes the root of iris becoming thicken. Then, the interspace of anterior chamber angle (前房角) become narrow, causing the backflow of aqueous humor (房水) blocked, and then the aqueous humor accumulates with each other and the eye pressure elevate.

3) Paralysis of accommodation (调节麻痹)   Atropine causes the ciliary muscle to relax and retreat to the outer edge, so that tensing the suspensory ligament and flattening the lens crystalline (晶状体), making its refraction reduce and only suitable for looking at a distant object, but cannot clearly image near objects on the retina. Therefore, people cannot see the near objects clearly.

(3) Relaxing smooth muscle   This kind of drug that called atropine, can not only relax many visceral smooth muscles but also has a special effect on those symptoms such as the relax of visceral smooth muscle that is hyperactive or spastic (痉挛性). Atropine can relieves intestinal colic (绞痛), because it has the ability to suppress the intense spasm of the gastrointestinal smooth muscle (胃肠道平滑肌), and the rage reduction of amplitude has some relationship with frequency. The atropine also has some effect on the detrusor of bladder (膀胱逼尿肌).

(4) Exciting the heart and expanding small vessels

1) Exciting the heart   The atropine, which has the ability to stimulate the heart is primarily through the following ways. At first, the therapeutic dose of atropine (0.4-0.6mg), which can slow the heart rates slightly and briefly of some patients, generally four to eight times per minute. This kind of situation may be reduced by the blocking presynaptic membrane M_1 receptors effect of atropine, and then making the number of ACh raise. However, Higher doses of atropine (1-2mg) make the M_2 receptors of the pacemaker of sinoatrial node (窦房结) blocked, then relieving the vagal nerve inhibit effect on the heart and speeding up the heart rate. The degree of heart rate acceleration depends on vagal nerve (迷走神经) tension, and the effect of heart rate acceleration is significant in young adults who with the high vagal nerve tension.

2) Expanding small vessels   Regular doses of atropine have no effect on blood vessels while the large doses of Atropine can expand blood vessels and improve the body's microcirculation, improving the situation of histanoxia (组织缺氧症).

(5) Exciting central nervous system   Atropine can make the medulla oblongata (中央延髓) and the high brain center exciting, and the intensity of action is dependent on the dose. The effect of the rapeutic dose of atropine is not obvious to excite central. Higher doses can mildly excite the brain and Medulla Oblongata, and higher dose of Atropine makes central excitation significantly enhanced, and the symptom of dysphoric (烦躁不安) will occur. Toxic dosage can cause obviously central toxic symptom, such as that patients may produce hallucination (幻觉), disorientation (定向障碍) and even convulsion (惊厥). Sustained high-dose is easy to switch from excitement to depression, resulting coma (昏迷), bulbar paralysis (延髓麻痹)and death.

【Clinical indications】

(1) Relieve the smooth muscle spasm (痉挛)   Atropine can relieve the spasm of smooth muscle and is suitable for various kinds of internal organs angina (内脏绞痛). Such as gastrointestinal colic and irritation sign of bladder such as frequency of urination and urgency of urination, the atropine has a better effect on those kinds of symphony. But the atropine was less effective in treating biliary colic (胆绞痛) and renal colic, both of which are often treated with atropine in combination with morphine (吗啡). Atropine can also be used to treat enuresis (遗尿症) by relaxing the bladder detrusor.

(2) Suppresses gland secretion   Atropine can be used before general anesthesia (麻醉) in order to reduce the secretion blocks respiratory passages and inhibit the aspiration pneumonia (吸入性肺炎) occur. It can also be used to cure severe night sweats (盗汗) and salivation (流涎).

(3) Ophthalmology (眼科)

1) Iridocyclitis (虹膜睫状体炎)   Atropine (0.5%-1%)can be used to cure iridocyclitis and relax the iris sphincter and ciliary muscle to make them having a rest, and this way is beneficial to the reduction of inflammation. At the same time, atropine can also have the effect on preventing the iris and the lens to stick together.

2) Examination of ocular fundus (眼底)   Atropine can be used when you make an eye check and need to expand your pupillary. However, the atropine, which expanding pupillary effect can be able to maintain 1or 2 weeks and the effect of adjusting paralytic (调节麻痹) also to be able to maintain 2 or 3 days, making eyesight restores slower. Therefore, atropine has been replaced by homatropine (后马托品) which has a less effect on eyes in daily life.

3) Optometry (验光)   To adjust the ciliary muscle paralysis and make the lens fixed in order to

correctly test the lenticular diopter (晶状体屈光度). But the effect of atropine action is too long, now it is just used to children optometry. Children has a very strong ciliary muscle regulation function. Therefore, the atropine plays an important role in regulating paralysis.

(4) Bradyarrhythmia (缓慢型心律失常)   Atropine is commonly used in the treatment of bradyarrhythmia, such as sinus atrial block (窦房阻滞) and atrioventricular block (房室传导阻滞) caused by excessive excitation of the vagal nerve, it can also be used to treat ventricular ectopic rhythm caused by sinus node dysfunction (窦房结功能障碍).

(5) Shock   Atropine can be used to cure the infectious shock caused by epidemic cerebrospinal meningitis (流行性脑脊髓膜炎), toxic bacillary dysentery (中毒性细菌性痢疾) and toxic pneumonia (中毒性肺炎), it may relieve the vasospasm (血管痉挛), peripheral vasodilation and improve microcirculation. The shock with tachycardia (心率过速) or high fever, should not use the atropine to treat.

(6) Organophosphate poisoning (有机磷中毒)   Atropine has detoxification function for organophosphate poisoning and some toadstools poisoning.

【Adverse reactions】Atropine has a wide range of pharmacological effects and a number of side effects. The most common symptom is including constipation (便秘), sweating decreased, dry mouth, nose and throat, blurred vision, erubescence (皮肤潮红) and difficulty of urination. Especially the elderly patients have a high risk to have acute retention of urine (急性尿潴留), gastrointestinal motility (胃肠动力) and gastroesophageal (胃食管) reflux. However, the symptom such as an allergic rash, herpes and elevated intraocular pressure are rare. The most important is that Atropine is banned in patients who have glaucoma and benign prostatic hyperplasia. Because atropine have the ability to constricts the sphincter muscle of membranous urethra (尿道括约肌) and make urination become more difficult.

Scopolamine (东莨菪碱)

【Pharmacodynamics】Scopolamine has similar pharmacological effects to atropine, and it has effects on the central and peripheral (中枢和外周) areas. Scopolamine also has a stronger salivary suppression effect than atropine, especially when it was used in a small dose, it usually has the effect to slow the heart rate rather than speeding it up. But unlike the atropine, scopolamine can inhibit the cerebral cortex, resulting in lethargy and forgetfulness. The scopolamine, as a peripheral anticholinergic drug, has a stronger inhibitory effect on the secretion of ocular smooth muscle (眼平滑肌) and glands than atropine. It has not antispasmodic effect on smooth muscle, but also with the ability to block ganglion (神经节) and neuromuscular junction (神经-肌肉接头), and a weaker effect on central nervous system.

【Clinical indications】Scopolamine also has a stronger salivary suppression effect than atropine, especially when it was used in a small dose, it usually has the effect to slow the heart rate rather than speeding it up, and sedation was the main effect. Scopolamine is clinically used as a preanesthetic agent (麻醉前药物), preventing motion sickness, carsickness and Parkinson's disease. The effect may be related to inhibition of vestibular nerve (前庭神经) function or cerebral cortex (大脑皮质), and inhibition of gastrointestinal peristalsis.

【Adverse reactions】The adverse effect of Scopolamine is similar to Atropine, and there are some serious adverse effects, such as withdrawal symptoms. Long-term use of scopolamine eye preparations can cause localized stimulus, leading to conjunctivitis, vascular congestion, edema and eczema dermatitis (湿疹性皮炎). High doses of scopolamine can cause dizziness, restlessness, tremors, fatigue and difficulty moving. Children are more likely to have the symphony such as disorientation, irritability, confusion, hallucinations, and tremors than adults.

Anisodamine (山莨菪碱)

【Pharmacodynamics】Anisodamine is a kind of alkaloid isolated from the plant anisodamus. It has been synthesized by artificial and can relieve the spasm of smooth muscle. Although the effect of anisodamine is weaker than atropine, it has a highly selective and few side effects. So it is now used instead of atropine to cure the gastrointestinal colic (胃肠绞痛).

【Clinical indications】Anisodamine can also inhibit platelet aggregation (血小板聚集), and has a strong role in improving microcirculation (微循环).Therefore, it is used to cure various kinds of infections by toxic shock. Anisodamine is also can be used to treat some other illness such as penicillin anaphylaxis (青霉素过敏性休克), diabetes, psoriasis, heroin dependence, neuropathic micturition.

【Adverse reactions】It is contraindicated in the patient who has the symptoms such as intracranial hypertension (颅内高压), malignant tumor (恶性肿瘤), acute cerebral hemorrhage (急性脑出血) and glaucoma (青光眼). After taking anisodamine, people often suffer from dry mouth, red complexion and blurred vision. Sometimes there will be a rapid heartbeat and even have a dysuria (排尿困难) symptoms.

1.2 Semisynthetic derivative

Atropine has a long-time effect on ophthalmology when used to cure eyes illness, and it is also used in internal medicine but with many side effects. In view of these shortcomings, we change its chemical structure, and then a lot of substitutes have been synthesized. There are mainly two kinds, namely dilating pupil medicine and antispasmodic (解痉药). In recent years, a new type of M_1 receptor blocker, which can selectively inhibits gastric acid secretion and is used in peptic ulcer disease (消化性溃疡), has been one kind of new drug.

1.2.1 Synthesis mydriatic(合成散瞳药)

The pupillary dilatation and regulative paralytic effect of homatropine were shorter than that of atropine, and the regulative paralytic effect will disappear in 24-36 hours after using it, which is suitable for general ophthalmologic examination (眼科检查). The peak of the regulative paralytic effect of homatropine appears faster than atropine, especially for children. The tropicamide (托吡卡胺) is characterized by its quick onset and short duration.Table 7-1 is a comparative of the effects of various drugs.

Table 7-1 Comparison of the effects of atropine and synthetic mydriatic for pupil dilation and paralysis accommodation

Drug	Concentration(%)	Pupil dilation		Paralysis accommodation	
		Peak (min)	Recovery (day)	Peak (min)	Recovery(day)
Atropine	1.00	30.00-40.00	7.00-10.00	1.00-3.00	7.00-12.00
Homatropine	1.00	40.00-60.00	1.00-3.00	0.25	1.00-3.00
Tropicamide	1.00	20.00-40.00	0.25	0.25	<0.25
Cyclopentolate (环喷托酯)	1.50	30.00-50.00	1.00	1.00	0.25-1.00

1.2.2　Synthesis spasmolytic(合成解痉药)

【Clinical indications】

(1) Quaternary ammonium antispasmodic (季铵盐解痉剂)　The most commonly used drug is propineterine (丙胺太林), which has the following characteristics: Oral administration has poor absorption, having difficult to penetrate the blood-brain barrier and rarely has central effect. However, injection administration has a strong spasmolytic effect on gastrointestinal smooth muscle and has the different degree ganglia block function. The toxic dose of propylamine can cause nerve muscle to transmit block and aspiration paralytic (呼吸麻痹).Propineterine can be used for stomach peptic ulcer (十二指肠溃疡), gastrointestinal spasm and vomiting during pregnancy. Commonly used drugs include propantheline bromide [溴丙胺太林 (普鲁本辛)], oxyphenonium bromide (溴化羟苯乙胺), valethamate bromide (溴化戊乙胺酯), glycopyrrolate (格隆溴铵) and diponium bromide (地泊溴铵). All of these drugs can be used as an adjunct to ease the spasm of the visceral smooth muscle and cure peptic ulcer.

(2) Tertiary amine antispasmodic (叔胺解痉药)　This kind of drugs include dicycloverine, oxyphencyclimine, etc. Benactyzinehydrochloride (盐酸贝那替秦) is the representational drug of tertiary amine gene, which has a high liposolubility, is easy to be absorbed by oral administration and has obvious effect on spasmolysis and inhibition to gastric juice secretion. In addition, it is also has the antipsychotic effect and suitable for the patients who have ulcer disease, hyperacidity of stomach, hyperperistalsis of intestine or bladder irritation symptoms (膀胱刺激症状) of anxiety disorder.

1.3　Selectivity M-cholinoceptor blocker

This kind of drug can block the M_1 receptor selectivity, such as pirenzepine and telenzepine. The pirenzepine selectively blocks M_1 receptors on gastric parietal cells and inhibits the secretion of gastric acid and pepsin (胃蛋白酶). It is mainly used in the treatment of stomach and peptic ulcer. Taking it by the ways of oral will have a poor absorption, it has a very low bioavailability and if you take it with food, the bioavailability will improve, so, it should be taken before meals. It cannot penetrate through the blood-brain barrier easily. Therefore, it does not have the central excitatory effect like atropine.

2. N_1 cholinoceptor blocker

N_1 cholinoceptor blocker, which is known as mecamylamine (美卡拉明), having the ability that selectively bind to N_1 choline receptors in ganglion cells and competitively block ACh bind with receptor, making ACh cannot depolarize the ganglion cells. Thus blocking the transmission of nerve impulses through the ganglion cells, it's also called a ganglionic blocker (神经节阻滞药).

【Pharmacodynamics】

(1) The cardiovascular system　The sympathetic nervous system takes an advantage on dominating blood vessels. Therefore, after the medication causes the arterioles to dilate, the peripheral resistance (外周阻力) to reduce as well as the superior vein to dilate. Then, the return heart blood volume (回心血量) and the cardiac output reduce, as a result the blood pressure drop significantly.

(2) The eyes Parasympathetic nervous system (副交感神经) is dominant in the ciliary muscles (睫状肌) and iris, and has the effect of mydriasis (散瞳) and paralysis after taking this kind of drug.

(3) Smooth muscle and glands The gastrointestinal tract, eye, bladder and other smooth muscle and glands are dominated by parasympathetic nervous system (副交感神经系统), therefore, the symptoms such as bladder smooth muscle relaxation and urinary retention will occur after taking drug. It can also inhibit sweat glands (汗腺) and salivary glands secretion, causing dry mouth and other symptoms.

【Clinical indications】Ganglionic blockers have been used to treat hypertension in the past, but because of their extensive effects, many side effects and their fast and strong antihypertensive effect (抗高血压作用). Nowadays they are less commonly used to treat the hypertension. The drug is mainly used as an anesthetic auxiliary medicine (辅助麻醉药) to play the role of controlled hypotension. Because its hypotensive effect is strong and fast, when dosage is improper, it may cause heart, brain, kidney and other organs blood supply insufficiency, or make reflex blood pressure regulation failure and lead to postural hypotension. Therefore, it is contraindicated (禁忌) in patients who have coronary artery insufficiency (冠状动脉功能不全), cerebral sclerosis (脑硬化症), and renal dysfunction (肾功能不全).

3. N₂ cholinoceptor blocker

N₂ choline receptor blockers, which is also called muscle relaxants (肌松药). It can bind to N₂ receptors on the membrane of the motor endplate (运动终板膜) of the neuromuscular junction, blocking the normal transmission of nerve impulses at the neuromuscular junction and leading to muscle relaxation. Therefore it can be used as an anesthetic adjuvant in general anesthesia. Muscle relaxants can be used under general anesthesia (全身麻醉) to obtain muscle relaxation required for surgery and reducing the use of general anesthetics. According to the different Pharmacodynamics, muscle relaxants can be divided into depolarizing (non-competitive) muscle relaxants and non-polarizing (competitive) muscle relaxants.

The characteristics of this kind of drugs include following symphony: to begin with, short-term fasciculation (肌束震颤) occurs initially, which is related to the inconsistent depolarization (去极化) time of skeletal muscle in different parts of the body. Then, the symptom such as rapid tolerance can occur with continuous use of drugs. Finally, anti-AChE drug cannot antagonize the relaxant effect of this drug on muscle, however, anti-AChE drug even strengthens the relaxant effect of this drug on muscle.

3.1 Depolarizing muscular relaxants (去极化型肌松药)

This kind of drugs is represented by succinylcholine, which binds to the N₂ choline receptor on the membrane of the motor endplate to produce a similar but longer lasting depolarization of acetylcholine, inhibiting the endplate unresponsive effect to acetylcholine. As a result, the skeletal muscles are flabby (松弛).

Succinylcholine(琥珀胆碱)

It was quickly hydrolyzed to succinylcholine by butyrylcholinesterase (丁酰胆碱酯酶) in plasma and liver, so the effect of muscle relaxation was significantly weakened. Then, after further hydrolyzed to succinic acid and choline, the effect of muscle relaxants is completely gone.

【Pharmacodynamics】The pharmacological action of succinylcholine appears quickly and its duration is short. Due to the difference of depolarization time in different parts of skeletal muscle, uncoordinated fasciculation often occurs and then rapidly turns to relaxation. This occurs mainly in the neck, limbs and abdominal muscles, but the role of respiratory muscle relaxation is the least obvious.

【Clinical indications】Intravenous injection of succinylcholine in our body makes the drug act quickly and briefly, having a strong paralysis effect to the laryngeal muscle. Therefore, this method is suitable for endotracheal intubation (气管内插管术), tracheoscopy (气管镜), esophagoscope (食管镜) and other short-term operation. The intravenous drip is suitable for the operation which needs a long time.

【Adverse reactions】

(1) **A strong sense of suffocation**   Because the succinylcholine can cause a strong sense of suffocation (窒息感), it is contraindicated in conscious patients. It's usually given after an IV thiopental (静脉输入硫喷妥钠). Since succinylcholine varies greatly among individuals (个体差异), the rate of drip must be controlled according to the response to achieve a satisfactory degree of muscle relaxation.

(2) **Raising intraocular pressure**   Succinylcholine causes the extra skeletal muscles to contract briefly, raising intraocular pressure, which is contraindicated in patients undergoing Glaucoma and cataract extraction.

(3) **To be poisoned**   Specific patients with hereditary decrease of plasma cholinesterase activity and patients with organophosphate poisoning are highly sensitive to succinylcholine and easy to be poisoned.

3.2   Except for depolarizing muscle relaxants (非去极化型肌松药)

Except for depolarizing muscle relaxants, also known as competitive muscle relaxants, bind to N_2 choline receptors on the membrane of the motor nerve endplates and competitively block the depolarization of ACh and relax skeletal muscles. It can make a short-term drop in blood pressure, heart rate, bronchospasm (支气管痉挛) and excessive saliva secretion. However, due to the limited source of this drug and there are more side effects in it, it is now used rarely.

【Pharmacodynamics】

(1) **Muscle relaxation**   Tubocurarine binds to the N_2 receptors on the membrane of skeletal muscle cells, competitively blocking the action of ACh and causing muscle relaxation. Tubocurarine relaxes the muscles from the eyes, resulting in drooping eyelids (睑下垂), strabismus(斜视), aphasia (失语症), and difficulty in chewing and swallowing, followed by relaxation of the muscles of the neck, trunk, limbs and intercostal (肋间) muscles even causing paralysis of the inhalation muscles (吸入肌) which can lead to death.

(2) **Histamine release**   Tubocurarine can cause some symptoms such as bronchospasm (支气管痉挛), low blood pressure, histamine-like rash (组胺样疹块), and salivation.

(3) **Ganglion block**   Common dosage of tubocurarine can partially block the ganglia and adrenal

medulla(肾上腺髓质), causing a drop in blood pressure, and leading heart rate increased.

【Clinical indications】In recent years, the relatively safe drugs such as pipecuronium (泮库溴铵), vecuronium (维库溴铵) and atracurium (阿曲库铵) can be used as general anesthesia adjuvant, and also can be used in thoracic (胸腔) and abdominal surgery and tracheal intubation (气管插管).

【Adverse reactions】

(1) Regular dosage of tubocurarine can cause heart rate to rise, blood pressure to drop, excessive bronchospasm and saliva (唾液) production.

(2) Overdose tubocurarine can cause respiratory paralysis, it can rescue with neostigmine. It is contraindicated in patients who with symptoms of myasthenia gravis (重症肌无力), severe shock, and respiratory insufficiency (呼吸肌功能不全).

重 点 小 结

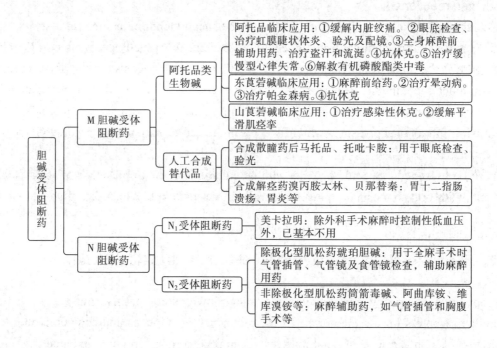

目 标 检 测

一、选择题

（一）单项选择题

1. 在治疗量就有明显中枢镇静作用的药物是（　　）

   A. 阿托品   B. 毛果芸香碱   C. 山莨菪碱

   D. 东莨菪碱   E. 卡巴胆碱

2. 阿托品可产生下列哪种药效（　　）

   A. 使骨骼肌松弛   B. 引起内脏平滑肌松弛   C. 治疗青光眼

   D. 治疗室上性心动过速   E. 增加汗腺分泌

3. 阿托品禁用于（　　　）
A. 虹膜睫状体炎　　　　　　　B. 有机磷中毒　　　　　　　C. 酸中毒
D. 青光眼　　　　　　　　　　E. 休克
4. 与阿托品相比，东莨菪碱的特点是（　　　）
A. 中枢作用强　　　　　　　　B. 常用于有机磷中毒　　　　C. 对眼的作用强
D. 对胃肠道平滑肌作用强　　　E. 对心脏作用强
5. 以下哪种药物可竞争性阻断 N_2 受体（　　　）
A. 筒箭毒碱　　　　　　　　　B. 毛果芸香碱　　　　　　　C. 琥珀胆碱
D. 东莨菪碱　　　　　　　　　E. 美卡拉明
6. 东莨菪碱治疗帕金森病主要是由于（　　　）
A. 外周性抗胆碱作用　　　　　B. 中枢性抗胆碱作用
C. 直接松弛骨骼肌作用　　　　D. 血管扩张作用
E. 运动神经终板持久的去极化作用

（二）多项选择题
7. 下列哪些疾病是阿托品的禁忌证（　　　）
A. 青光眼　　B. 心动过缓　　C. 虹膜炎　　D. 盗汗　　E. 前列腺肥大

二、思考题

琥珀胆碱过量为什么不能用新斯的明解救？

（白　莉）

Chapter 8　Adrenoceptor agonists

 学习目标

1.**掌握**　去甲肾上腺素、肾上腺素、异丙肾上腺素的作用机制、药理作用、临床应用及主要不良反应。

2.**熟悉**　肾上腺素受体激动药按作用方式及对受体选择性的分类。

3.**了解**　麻黄碱、多巴胺的作用机制、药理作用及临床应用；各种拟肾上腺素药的体内过程。

The adrenoceptor agonists are a large group of drugs with chemical structure and pharmacological action similar to adrenaline and noradrenaline. They can bind to adrenaline receptor and activate the receptor to produce adrenaline-like effect, so they are also known as adrenomimetic drug. Most of them are structurally catecholamine, and mimic the effect of sympathetic nervous system stimulation, so sometimes called sympathomimetic drugs or sympathomimetic amines. According to their selectivity to different subtypes of adrenoceptors, they can be divided into three categories: α-adrenoceptor agonists; α, β-adrenoceptor agonists; β-adrenoceptor agonists.

1. α-adrenoceptor agonists

Noradrenaline (去甲肾上腺素)

Noradrenaline (NA; norepinephrine, NE) is the primary neurotransmitter released from noradrenergic nerve terminal, and is one of the catecholamine-type hormone secreted in a small amount from adrenal medulla (肾上腺髓质). Officinal noradrenaline is a synthetic product which is unstable in light and air, especially in neutral and alkaline solution where it is oxidized and discolored rapidly in the presence of oxygen and divalent metal ions such as calcium. It is relatively stable in acid solution and commonly used as heavy tartrate.

【Pharmacokinetics】Due to the strong vasoconstriction at the site of injection, noradrenaline is poorly absorbed after administrated subcutaneously or intramuscularly, and is destroyed by alkaline intestinal fluid in the gut if given orally. The preferred route is intravenous infusion with a rapid onset of action and shorter duration. Exogenous noradrenaline is not easy to pass through the blood-brain barrier and rarely reaches the brain tissue. Most of them are inactivated by catechol-O-methyltransferase (COMT，儿茶酚-O-甲基转移酶) and monoamine oxidase (MAO，单胺氧化酶) metabolism and the metabolite can be excreted by urine.

【Pharmacodynamics】 Norepinephrine can activate α receptor strongly but shows no selectivity to α_1 and α_2 receptors. It has a weak effect on β_1 receptor, while almost no effect on β_2 receptor.

【Pharmacological action】

(1) Blood vessel　Noradrenaline constricts both arteries and veins by activating α_1 receptor located on vascular smooth muscle. However, the vasoconstrictor effect is more pronounced in the arterial resistance vessels. The most obvious vasoconstriction is found in skin and mucosa, followed by renal vessels. Contraction also occurs in the brain, liver, mesentery (肠系膜)and even skeletal muscle vessels.

Norepinephrine dilates coronary vessel, because: ①Norepinephrine excites heart and increases myocardial metabolites such as adenosine (腺苷), and so on, which causes coronary vasodilation. ②The increase of coronary flow due to the increase of blood pressure and coronary perfusion pressure. ③Norepinephrine activates the α_2 receptor of the presynaptic membrane of the noradrenergic nerve endings (神经末梢突触前膜) in the vascular wall, therefore inhibits the release of noradrenaline.

(2) Heart　In isolated cardiac tissue, norepinephrine stimulates the heart to increase heart rate and contractility of myocardium by activating the β_1 receptor, causing increased cardiac output. *In vivo*, however, due to enhanced vagal reflexes (迷走神经反射) mediated by raised blood pressure overcome the direct positive chronotropic effects of norepinephrine on the heart, the heart rate may be slowed down and the cardiac output may be decreased. But, at very high doses, norepinephrine increases the cardiac rhythm, which may cause arrhythmia.

(3) Blood pressure　At a small dose, norepinephrine excites heart to increase the systolic pressure (收缩压). While the diastolic pressure (舒张压) is not significantly increased due to the weak vasoconstriction effect of norepinephrine, so the pulse pressure difference (脉压) is increased. However, at a large dose, the norepinephrine causes a significant rise in peripheral resistance due to intense vasoconstriction of most vascular beds, including the kidney. Consequently, both systolic and diastolic pressures are increased, and the pulse pressure difference is decreased (Figure 8-1).

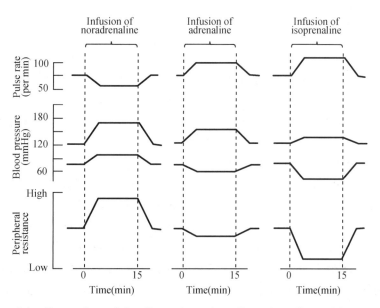

Figure 8-1　Comparison of the effects of noradrenaline, adrenaline and isoprenaline

(4) Other effects　Norepinephrine has a weak effect on the metabolism of the body, and only when the dose is high, the blood glucose will be elevated.

【Clinical indications】

(1) Shock and hypotension　Noradrenaline is only limited to the early stage of neurogenic shock and hypotension (神经源性休克和低血压) after pheochromocytoma resection (嗜铬细胞瘤切除术) or drug poisoning.

(2) Hemostasis of upper gastrointestinal hemorrhage (上消化道出血的止血)　After diluted, noradrenaline can be taken orally to make the blood vessels of esophagus and gastric mucosa contracted and make local hemostasis.

【Adverse reactions】

(1) Local tissue ischemic necrosis (局部组织坏死)　Local tissue ischemic necrosis can be caused by too long intravenous infusion time, too high concentration or drug leakage from the blood vessels. If the leakage or injection site is found with pale skin, the injection site should be stopped or replaced, hot compress should be carried out, and phentolamine, a α receptor blocker, should be used for local infiltration injection to dilate the blood vessels.

(2) Acute renal failure (急性肾衰竭)　If the infusion time is too long or the dosage is too large, the renal blood vessels will contract violently, which will result in oliguria (少尿), anuria (无尿) and even renal parenchyma (肾实质) injury. Therefore, the urine volume should be kept above 25ml per hour during the administration.

【Contraindications】Patients and pregnant women with hypertension, arteriosclerosis (动脉硬化), organic heart disease (器质性心脏病), oliguria, anuria and severe microcirculation disorders are prohibited.

2. α and β-adrenoceptor agonists

Adrenaline (肾上腺素)

Adrenaline(Adr), also known as epinephrine, is the main hormone of adrenal medulla. Officinal adrenaline usually is extracted from adrenals of cattle, sheep and other domestic animals or is synthesized. Similar to noradrenaline, epinephrine is oxidized and discolored rapidly on exposure to air or light and decomposed in neutral, especially in alkaline solution.

【Pharmacokinetics】Dosage delivery routes for epinephrine include intravenous, inhalation, nebulization, intramuscular injection, and subcutaneous injection. Adrenaline will be inactivated in the alkaline intestinal fluid, intestinal mucosa and liver, which makes it hardly reach the effective blood concentration if oral administration. Similar to that of noradrenaline, epinephrine is extensively metabolized with only a small amount excreted unchanged through the kidney.

【Pharmacodynamics】Epinephrine is a potent agonist at all α and β adrenoceptors. At low dose, β receptor is more sensitive to the epinephrine. Whereas at high dose, effects produced by α receptor activation are more prominent.

【 Pharmacological action 】

(1) Heart   Epinephrine strengthens the contractility of the myocardium (positive inotropic，正性肌力), increases heart rate (positive chronotropic, 正性频率) and accelerates the conduction through activating the β_1 and β_2 receptors of the myocardium, conduction system and sinoatrial node (窦房结). Therefore, cardiac output, myocardial metabolism and myocardial oxygen consumption are increased. If overdose or the intravenous injection is too fast, epinephrine may cause cardiac arrhythmia (心律失常), premature contraction (期前收缩) and even ventricular fibrillation (室颤). Especially for those patients with myocardial ischemia, hypoxia and heart failure (心衰), epinephrine may aggravate the disease or cause rapid cardiac arrhythmia.

(2) Blood vessel   The action of epinephrine on blood vessels depends on the distributed density of α_1 and β_2 receptors and the dosage of the drug. Due to high density of α_1 adrenoceptors, the vasoconstriction of smaller arteries and the anterior sphincter of the precapillary (毛细血管前括约肌) caused by epinephrine is most obvious, although veins and large arteries also respond to the drug. Among all of vessels, the density of α_1 receptors in the vascular smooth muscle of the skin, mucosa, kidney, gastrointestinal tract is dominant, so the vasoconstriction of the skin and mucosa is the strongest, and the visceral blood vessels, especially the renal blood vessels also contract significantly. Whereas, the vasoconstriction of the brain and lung is very weak, sometimes they are passively dilated due to the rise of blood pressure. Differently, adrenaline often relaxes the vessels of skeletal muscle and liver when used at small dose by activating β_2 receptor, a dominantly distributed receptor in the vessels of skeletal muscle and liver. However, at a large dose, adrenaline causes vasoconstriction of skeletal muscle due to vasodilation of skeletal muscle mediated by β_2 receptor is overcome by the vasoconstriction action of α_1 receptor that are also present in the vascular bed. Adrenaline also relaxes coronary arteries, which may be associated with the following factors. ①Adrenaline dilates coronary artery by acting on β_2 receptor of coronary artery. ②Adrenaline causes the increase of myocardial contractility and myocardial metabolites such as adenosine, which causes coronary vasodilation.

(3) Blood pressure   When adrenaline is given by slow intravenous infusion or by subcutaneous injection, the systolic pressure is increased moderately due to increased cardiac contractile force and a rise in cardiac output. Peripheral resistance decreases owing to the dominant vasodilator action of adrenaline on β_2 receptors of the skeletal muscle, which counteracts or exceeds the effect of the contraction of the blood vessels of the skin and mucous membrane mediated by α receptors. Consequently, the diastolic blood pressure is not changed or decreased and the pulse pressure difference increases. As such, the blood of all parts of the body will be redistributed, which is conducive to meet the need for energy supply of the body in the emergency state. At higher rates of infusion, both the systolic and diastolic pressure increase due to the excitation of the heart and the contraction of the blood vessels of the skin and mucous membrane and other tissues. Therefore, the typical change of blood pressure mediated by adrenaline is biphasic response, which is obvious pressor effect appears rapidly after administration followed by a longer and weaker depressor effect. If α receptors antagonist is given before epinephrine administration, the pressor effect of epinephrine can be reversed to a significant depressor response by the excitatory effect of epinephrine on β_2 receptor in blood vessels.

(4) Smooth muscle   The effect of epinephrine on smooth muscle in different organ and tissue mainly depends on the type of adrenergic receptor in muscle. By activating β_2 receptor of bronchial smooth muscle, epinephrine relaxes bronchus and inhibits mast cells from releasing histamine and other allergic substances. Through activating α receptors, epinephrine contracts the bronchial mucosal blood vessels and reduces the permeability of the capillaries, which eliminates the edema of the bronchial mucosa. The effect of epinephrine on uterine smooth muscle is related to sexual cycle, filling state and dosage. In general, it can inhibit uterine tension and contraction at the end of pregnancy, relax the bladder detrusor and shrink the deltoid and sphincter, which may result in dysuria and urinary retention.

(5) Metabolism　Adrenaline has a number of important influences on metabolic processes. Under the therapeutic dose, adrenaline increases the oxygen consumption and blood glucose levels through activation of α receptor and β_2 receptor or decreasing glucose uptake in peripheral tissues by inhibition of insulin release. Adrenaline activates triglyceride enzyme to accelerate fat decomposition and increase free fatty acids in blood, which may be related to the activation of β_1 and β_3 receptor.

(6) Central never system　At the therapeutic dose, adrenaline is not easy to pass through the blood-brain barrier, so no obvious central excitation is observed. However, when the dose is large, adrenaline may cause central excitation symptoms, such as excitement, vomiting, myotonia (肌强直), and even convulsion (惊厥).

【Clinical indications】

(1) Cardiac arrest (心脏骤停)　When intracardiac administration, adrenaline may be used to restore cardiac rhythm in patients with cardiac arrest caused by accidents, drug poisoning, infectious diseases and heart conduction block in the process of drowning, anesthesia and operation. For the sudden cardiac shock caused by electric shock, adrenaline should be used with defibrillator or lidocaine together.

(2) Allergic diseases

1) Anaphylactic shock (过敏性休克)　Adrenaline is the drug of choice for the treatment of type1 hypersensitivity reaction in response to allergens. The pharmacodynamics includes the followings. ①Through activating α receptor, adrenaline contracts precapillary and reduces capillary permeability. ②Adrenaline improves heart performance and relieves bronchospasm through its agonist activities on β_1 and β_2 receptor. ③Adrenaline reduces release of anaphylactic mediators and dilates coronary artery, which may quickly relieve clinical symptoms of anaphylactic shock and save patients' lives. The prefer route is intramuscular injection or subcutaneous injection. In severe cases, it should be diluted 10 times with normal saline and injected intravenously and slowly to avoid adverse reactions such as a sudden rise of blood pressure and arrhythmia.

2) Bronchial asthma (哮喘)　Adrenaline is a powerful bronchodilator. However, due to serious adverse reactions, it is only used for an acute asthma attack.

3) Angioneurotic edema and serum diseases (血管神经性水肿和血清病)　Adrenaline can rapidly relieve the symptoms of allergic diseases such as angioneurotic edema, serum diseases, urticaria and hay fever (荨麻疹和花粉症).

(3) Local application　Adrenaline is usually added to local anesthetics in a proportion of 1∶250 000 (the dosage does not exceed 0.3mg once) to delay the absorption of local anesthetics and prolong the duration of local anesthetics. Very weak solutions of adrenaline (1∶100 000) can also be used topically on the surface of nasal mucosa and gingiva for local hemostasis.

(4) Glaucoma (青光眼)　Adrenaline may be useful in the treatment of glaucoma, which can reduce intraocular pressure by promoting aqueous outflow and desensitizing β receptor mediated intraocular response.

【Adverse reactions】

(1) Common adverse reactions　The main adverse reactions for systemically administered epinephrine include anxiety, apprehensiveness, restlessness, tremor, weakness, dizziness, sweating, palpitations, pallor, nausea and vomiting, headache, and respiratory difficulties. These symptoms occur in some persons receiving therapeutic doses of epinephrine, but are more likely to occur in patients with heart disease, hypertension, or hyperthyroidism (甲状腺功能亢进症).

(2) Cardiovascular   Epinephrine can trigger cardiac arrhythmias, even ventricular fibrillation, angina, hypertension, ventricular ectopy and stress cardiomyopathy (室性异位与应激性心肌病).

(3) Hemorrhage (出血)   Rapid rises in blood pressure associated with epinephrine use is easy to cause cerebral hemorrhage, particularly for elderly patients with cardiovascular disease.

【Contraindications】Epinephrine is forbidden in patients with hypertension, cerebral arteriosclerosis (脑动脉硬化), organic heart disease, diabetes (糖尿病) and hyperthyroidism.

Dopamine (多巴胺)

Dopamine (DA) is the immediate metabolic precursor of norepinephrine biosynthesis. Officinal dopamine is the synthetic product.

【Pharmacological action】Dopamine can activate α, β and peripheral dopamine receptors (D receptor). In addition, it promotes the release of norepinephrine from nerve endings.

(1) Cardiovascular   The effect of dopamine on cardiovascular system is related to the concentration of drug. At low concentration, it mainly binds to dopamine receptor located in renal, mesenteric and coronary beds and activates adenylate cyclase to increase the level of cAMP in cells, which leads to vasodilation. Larger dose of dopamine can act on the β_1 receptor of the heart and increase the cardiac contractility and cardiac output.

(2) Blood pressure   Larger dose of dopamine exerts a stimulatory effect on the β_1 receptor and D receptor, which can increase cardiac output and decrease the resistance of renal and mesenteric vascular. As a consequence, the systolic blood pressure is increased, but the diastolic blood pressure has no obvious change or is increased slightly, thereby, the pulse pressure difference increases. With dosage increasing continuously, dopamine can cause vasoconstriction and pressor effect by activating α receptor of blood vessels to increase total peripheral resistance, which can be antagonized by α receptor blocker.

(3) Renal   Low concentration of dopamine promotes sodium excretion and diuresis by dilating renal blood vessels, increasing renal blood flow and glomerular filtration rate. At high dose, α receptor of renal vessels can be excited, which can make renal vessels contract obviously.

【Clinical indications】Dopamine, when given by continuous infusion, is the drug of choice for various kinds of shock, such as septic shock (感染性休克), cardiogenic shock (心源性休克). Before dopamine is administered to patients in shock, hypovolemia (低血容量) and the acidosis (酸中毒) should be corrected and the changes of cardiac function should be monitored during the administration. In addition, dopamine combined with diuretics is also used to treat acute renal failure and severe congestive heart failure, primarily in patients with low or normal peripheral vascular resistance and in oliguria patients.

Ephedrine (麻黄碱)

Ephedrine is an alkaloid extracted from Ephedra and now has been synthesized. It can activate adrenergic receptor directly by activating α_1, α_2, β_1 and β_2 receptors in different tissues, and indirectly by promoting the release of noradrenaline from adrenergic nerve endings. Compared with epinephrine, ephedrine has the following characteristics: ①Ephedrine is stable in chemical properties and is effective when oral administration. ②Longer-acting and less potent than epinephrine. ③Ephedrine can penetrate into CNS and causes mild stimulation of CNS. ④Ephedrine is easy to produce rapid tolerance.

【Clinical indications】

(1) As a bronchodilator, ephedrine is used to prevent asthma attack and treat mild asthma but is less effective for an acute asthma attack.

(2) Solutions of ephedrine (0.5%-1.0%) can be used topically to eliminate the nasal obstruction (鼻塞) caused by the congestion of the nasal mucous membrane, which can obviously improve the swelling of the mucous membrane.

(3) Ephedrine is used primarily to treat mild hypotension and bradycardia (心率减慢) associated with epidural and subarachnoid anesthesia (硬膜外和蛛网膜下腔麻醉).

(4) To relieve the skin and mucosa symptoms of urticaria and angioneuroedema.

3. β-adrenoceptor agonists

Isoprenaline (异丙肾上腺素)

Isoprenaline, also known as isoproterenol, is a synthetic product and often used as its hydrochloride or sulfate.

【Pharmacological action】 Isoprenaline is a potent, nonselective β receptor agonist with very low affinity for α receptor. Therefore, isoproterenol has powerful effects on all β receptors, but almost no action at α receptor.

(1) **Cardiovascular** Isoprenaline exerts a strong stimulation on the β_1 receptor of the heart, causing positive inotropic and positive chronotropic effects, which shortens systolic and diastolic phase. Compared with epinephrine, the effects of isoproterenol on accelerating heart rate and conduction are stronger, which increases significantly myocardial oxygen consumption and may cause arrhythmia, but less causes ventricular fibrillation.

(2) **Blood vessels and blood pressure** Through acting on β_2 receptor, isoproterenol dilates the blood vessels in skeletal muscle, renal, mesenteries, and even coronary arteries. Among of them, the dilation of skeletal muscle blood vessels is the most significant, followed by coronary artery, and the dilation of mesentery and kidney blood vessels is weak. Because of its cardiac stimulatory action, the systolic blood pressure is increased, but the diastolic blood pressure is decreased slightly due to reduced peripheral resistance. Consequently, the coronary blood flow increased. But if intravenous administration, isoproterenol can cause a significant decrease in diastolic blood pressure, which reduces the perfusion pressure of coronary artery, therefore the effective coronary blood flow may not be increased.

(3) **Smooth muscle of bronchus** Through activating β_2 receptor, isoproterenol relaxes the smooth muscle of bronchus, which is stronger than adrenaline. The release of histamine (组胺) and other allergic substances are also inhibited by isoproterenol. Differently, it has no contractile effect on the blood vessels of bronchial mucosa, so the effect of eliminating mucosal edema is not as good as adrenaline.

Isoproterenol also produces tolerance after long-term use.

(4) Others　The effect of isoproterenol on promoting lipolysis is similar to that of adrenaline, but its effect on increasing blood glucose is weaker than that of adrenaline.

【Pharmacokinetics】Isoproterenol is readily absorbed when given sublingually or inhaled as an aerosol. While, oral administration is easy to lose efficacy due to the binding with sulfuric acid group (硫酸基) in intestinal mucosa. Isoproterenol is mainly metabolized by COMT in liver and other tissues, but less metabolized by MAO and also less taken up by noradrenergic nerve, so its effect lasts longer than adrenaline.

【Clinical indications】

(1) Cardiac arrest　Combined with noradrenaline or metaraminol, isoproterenol injected intracardiacally is suitable for the treatment of cardiac arrest caused by a slow ventricular rhythm, high atrioventricular block or sinoatrial node failure.

(2) Atrioventricular block (房室传导阻滞)　Sublingual administration or intravenous infusion of isoproterenol is used to treat grade Ⅱ and Ⅲ atrioventricular block.

(3) Bronchial asthma　Sublingual or spray administration of isoproterenol is effective to control acute attack of bronchial asthma.

(4) Shock　Isoprenaline was used to treat septic shock with high central venous pressure and low cardiac output, but it largely has been replaced by other sympathomimetic drugs.

【Adverse reactions and contradictions】Palpitations, tachycardia, headache, and dizziness are common during isoprenaline administration. Cardiac ischemia, tachycardia and even dangerous ventricular fibrillation may occur, particularly in patients with asthma and with underlying coronary artery disease. It is forbidden to be used for patients with coronary heart disease, myocarditis (心肌炎) and hyperthyroidism.

重 点 小 结

分类	药物	对不同肾上腺素受体作用比较			作用方式	
		α受体	β₁受体	β₂受体	直接作用于受体	释放递质
α受体激动药	去甲肾上腺素	+++	++	+/-	+	
	间羟胺	++	+	+	+	+
	去氧肾上腺素	++	+/-	+/-	+	+/-
	甲氧明	++	-	-	+	-
α及β受体激动药	肾上腺素	++++	+++	+++	+	
	多巴胺	+	++	+/-	+	+
	麻黄碱	++	++	++	+	+
β受体激动药	异丙肾上腺素	-	+++	+++	+	
	多巴酚丁胺	+	++	+	+	+/-

目 标 检 测

一、选择题

（一）单项选择题

1. 上消化道出血患者可给予（　　）
   A. 去甲肾上腺素口服　　　B. 去甲肾上腺素静脉注射　　　C. 去甲肾上腺素肌内注射
   D. 肾上腺素皮下注射　　　E. 肾上腺素口服
2. 能通过血脑屏障兴奋中枢引起失眠的拟肾上腺素是（　　）
   A. 麻黄碱　　　B. 肾上腺素　　　C. 去甲肾上腺素
   D. 多巴胺　　　E. 异丙肾上腺素
3. 临床可用于治疗支气管哮喘、房室传导阻滞以及休克的拟肾上腺素药是（　　）
   A. 肾上腺素　　　B. 去甲肾上腺素　　　C. 多巴酚丁胺
   D. 异丙肾上腺素　　　E. 麻黄碱
4. 能增加肾血流量、防治肾衰竭的拟肾上腺素药是（　　）
   A. 麻黄碱　　　B. 去甲肾上腺素　　　C. 多巴胺
   D. 肾上腺素　　　E. 去氧肾上腺素

（二）多项选择题

5. 去甲肾上腺素能使神经兴奋，引起（　　）
   A. 心肌收缩力增强　　　B. 支气管舒张　　　C. 皮肤黏膜血管收缩
   D. 脂肪、糖原分解　　　E. 瞳孔扩大肌收缩 (扩瞳)
6. 可作用于 α 和 β 受体的拟肾上腺素药有（　　）
   A. 去甲肾上腺素　　　B. 异丙肾上腺素　　　C. 肾上腺素
   D. 麻黄碱　　　E. 多巴胺

二、思考题

试从作用机制比较去甲肾上腺素、肾上腺素及异丙肾上腺素对血压的影响。

（张海宁）

Chapter 9 Adrenoceptor antagonist drugs

 学习目标

1. **掌握** 酚妥拉明、酚苄明的临床应用、不良反应及禁忌证。
2. **熟悉** β受体阻断药的药理作用及临床应用。
3. **了解** 普萘洛尔、拉贝洛尔的作用特点。

Adrenoceptor antagonists are also named antiadrenergic drugs or adrenoceptor blocking drugs, which antagonize their receptors and then show important effects. Some adrenoceptor antagonists are of great clinical value. The drugs possessing effects vary dramatically could be categorized into α receptor antagonists and β receptor antagonists according to the different selectivity of drugs to α and β receptor. The major effects of the pharmacologic antagonist drugs are produced by occupying α_1, α_2, or β receptors outside the central nervous system and preventing their activation by catecholamines (儿茶酚胺类) and related agonists.

For pharmacologic research, α_1 and α_2 adrenoceptor antagonist drugs have been very useful in the experimental studying of autonomic nervous system function. In clinical therapeutics, nonselective α adrenoceptor antagonists have been used in the treatment of pheochromocytoma (嗜铬细胞瘤) (tumors that secrete catecholamines), and α_1 selective antagonists are used in primary hypertension (原发性高血压) and benign prostatic hyperplasia (良性前列腺增生症). β receptor antagonist drugs have been found useful in a much wider variety of clinical diseases and are firmly used in the treatment of hypertension, ischemic heart disease (缺血性心脏病), arrhythmia (心律失常), endocrinologic and neurologic disorders (内分泌及神经系统疾病), and other conditions.

1. α-receptor antagonist drugs

α receptor antagonists may be reversible or irreversible in their interaction with these receptors. Reversible antagonists can either bind to or dissociate from receptors, and the antagonism can be surmounted with sufficiently high concentrations of agonist; irreversible drugs do not disaggregate from receptors and cannot be overcame. Phentolamine and prazosin are examples of reversible antagonists, and phenoxybenzamine results in irreversible blockade by forming a reactive intermediate that covalently binds to α receptors.

The duration of effects of a reversible antagonist is largely dependent on the drug half-life (半衰期) *in vivo* and the rate at which it dissociates from its receptor. The shorter the half-life of the drug in the body, the less time it takes for the effects of the drug to dissipate. However, the effects of an irreversible antagonist may last long after the elimination of the drugs from the plasma. In the case of phenoxybenzamine, the restoration of tissue responsiveness after extensive α receptor blockade is mainly dependent on synthesis of new receptors, which may take several days. The rate of return of α_1 adrenoceptor drug effect may be particularly important in patients who have a sudden cardiovascular event or who become candidates for urgent surgery.

Because arteriolar and venous tone (动静脉张力) is determined by the effects on the receptors in vascular smooth muscle considerably, α receptor antagonist drugs cause a lowering of peripheral vascular resistance and blood pressure. These drugs can inhibit the pressor effects of common doses of α receptor agonists; actually, in the case of agonists with both α and β_2 effects (e.g., epinephrine), selective α_1 receptor antagonism may convert a pressor to a depressor response. This change of effects is named "epinephrine reversal (肾上腺素作用的翻转)", which illustrates how the activation of both α and β receptors in the same tissue may lead to opposite responses.

α receptor antagonists may cause postural hypotension (体位性低血压) and reflex tachycardia (反射性心动过速). Postural hypotension is due to the opposability of sympathetic nervous system stimulation of α_1 receptors in vascular smooth muscle, and the contraction of veins is an important component of the capacity to maintain blood pressure in the upright position since it reduces peripheral venous hydrops (外周小静脉积水). Constriction of arterioles (小动脉) in the legs may also contribute to the postural response (姿势反应). Tachycardia may be more marked with agents that block α_2 presynaptic (突触前) receptors in the heart, since the augmented release of norepinephrine will further stimulate β receptors in the heart.

Phentolamine (酚妥拉明)

Phentolamine decreases peripheral resistance in vascular smooth muscle through blockade of α_1 receptors and possibly α_2 receptors. Phentolamine activate the sympathetic nerve innervating heart in response to baroreflex (压力感受器反射) mechanisms. Phentolamine agonize muscarinic receptors, H_1 and H_2 histamine receptors. Since phentolamine potently blocks α_1 and α_2 receptors nonselectively, antagonism of presynaptic α_2 receptors may lead to enhanced release of norepinephrine from sympathetic end. Enhanced norepinephrine release may contribute to marked cardiac stimulation via unblocked β adrenoceptors.

【Clinical indications】

(1) Treatment of peripheral vasospasm (外周血管痉挛) Vasodilatation (血管舒张) induced by blocking α receptors is beneficial for Raynaud's syndrome (雷诺综合征) which is characterized by vasoconstriction due to increased sympathetic nerve activity.

(2) Treatment of Shock Vasodilation and positive cardiac effects produced by α receptor antagonist are useful for treating shock (one feature of some shocks in vasoconstriction with resultant decreased tissue perfusion).

(3) Treatment and diagnose of pheochromocytoma Phentolamine is used in the treatment of pheochromocytoma, an adrenal catecholamine-secreting tumor that may cause hypertension, tachycardia (心动过速), and arrhythmia (心律失常).

(4) Treatment of acute myocardial infarction (急性心肌梗死) and congestive heart failure (充血性心力衰竭)   The acute myocardial infarction, congestive heart failure, and an inadequacy of cardiac output can cause an increase in sympathetic tone and increase peripheral resistance. Blocking of sympathetic vasoconstriction (血管收缩) by α–adrenergic receptor antagonist can rapidly reverse these processes, i.e., decrease the cardiac work and pulmonary congestion and edema.

【 Adverse reactions 】 Adverse reactions include mainly arrhythmia and angina pain, and gastrointestinal irritation (abdominal pain, diarrhea, vomiting and aggravating ulcer).

Tolazoline (妥拉唑林)

The α–adrenergic blocking effects are similar to that of phentolamine, but somewhat less potent. Cholinomimetic effect and histamine like effects are stronger. Side effects include postural hypotension, tachycardia (reflex), arrhythmias and angina. Clinically, it is mainly used for treatment of the peripheral vasospastic disease and extravasation of norepinephrine during intravenous injection.

Phenoxybenzamine (酚苄明)

Phenoxybenzamine showed persistent and complete blockade effects through covalent bonding to the receptor, which is difficult to reverse. In the cardiovascular system, the decline of diastolic blood pressure occurs because of decreased peripheral resistance. Systolic blood pressure (收缩压) drops sharply when the patient appears an upright position (postural hypotension). Reflex tachycardia (反射性心动过速) emerges as soon as peripheral resistance decreased and following decreased venous return to the heart. Tachycardia is also caused by blockade of presynaptic α_2 receptors, which inhibit feedback control of noradrenaline release.

Prazosin (哌唑嗪)

Prazosin is an effective drug used clinically for curing hypertension as a selective α_1 adrenoceptor antagonist. There is very low affinity for α_2 receptor provides a prominent therapeutic superiority. Prazosin possesses less adverse actions that are characteristically observed with nonselective α receptor (e.g., tachycardia, positive inotropy, and renin release).

The selectivity of prazosin for α_1 adrenoceptors avoids increased reflex release of noradrenaline, and then, this may prevent the tachycardia observed with the nonselective α receptor antagonists. Tachycardia, mediated by reflex baroreceptor mechanisms, may occur occasionally.

Diastolic pressure (舒张压) falls because of decreased peripheral resistance and reduction of circulating blood volume (due to venous pooling of blood in the large veins), inducing decreased venous return. Orthostatic hypotension occurs owing to α_1 receptor blockade in the large veins. "First-dose phenomenon (首剂现象)" of specific adverse reactions of prazosin comprises dizziness or syncope(晕厥) and lead to loss of consciousness. The adverse effect may be preventable by starting with a low dose and increasing the dosage slowly.

Yohimibine (育亨宾)

Yohimbine, a α_2 selective antagonist, is an indole alkaloid. It has no significant clinical use. Theoretically, it could be useful in autonomic insufficiency by promoting neurotransmitter release through blockade of presynaptic α_2 receptors. Yohimbine may improve symptoms in some patients with painful diabetic neuropathies (糖尿病神经病变). It has been suggested that yohimbine improves male sexual function; however, evidence for this effect in humans is limited. At present, it is mainly used as a tool drug in experimental researches.

2. β-receptor antagonist drugs

The β adrenoceptors are classified as β_1 and β_2 receptors. A subclassification of β adrenoceptor antagonists into nonselective and selective was necessitated by the fact that drugs such as propranolol block both β_1 and β_2 receptors, while other drugs such as metoprolol (美托洛尔) selectively block the β_1-receptors with only minor effects on β_2 adrenoceptors.

【Classification】

(1) Nonselective β receptor antagonists ①Full blockers：propranolol, timolol (噻吗洛尔), sotalol (索他洛尔), and nadolol (纳多洛尔). ②Blockers with intrinsic sympathomimetic activity (ISA)：alprenolol (阿普洛尔), oxprenolol (氧烯洛尔), and pindolol (吲哚洛尔).

(2) Selective β_1 adrenergic blockers ①Full blockers：metoprolol and atenolol. ②Blockers with intrinsic activity：acebutolol (醋丁洛尔).

(3) Mixed β and α receptor blockers Labetalol is one of the agents.

【Pharmacodynamics】

(1) Effects on the cardiovascular β receptor antagonist drugs decrease chronically blood pressure in patients with hypertension. The mechanisms involved may include effects on the heart and blood vessels, suppression of the renin-angiotensin system (肾素-血管紧张素系统), and perhaps effects in the central nervous system or elsewhere. β receptor antagonist drugs are of major clinical importance in the treatment of hypertension. In contrast, conventional doses of these drugs do not usually cause hypotension in healthy individuals with normal blood pressure.

β receptor antagonists have prominent effects on the heart (Figure 9-1). The negative inotropic and chronotropic effects (负性肌力和负性频率作用) are predictable from the role of adrenoceptors in regulating these functions. Slowed atrioventricular conduction (房室传导) with an increased PR interval (PR间期) is a related result of adrenoceptor blockade in the atrioventricular node (房室结). These effects are beneficial to the treatment of some patients' diseases but may have adverse effects on other patients. In the vascular system, the β receptor antagonist drug opposes β_2 mediated vasodilation (血管舒张). This may acutely lead to a rise in peripheral resistance, resulted from unopposed α receptor stimulating following by the lowered blood pressure due to the fall in cardiac output induced sympathetic nervous system discharges. β receptor antagonist drugs inhibit the release of renin caused by the sympathetic nervous system. In any event, while the acute effects of these drugs may include a rise in peripheral resistance, chronic drug administration can reduce peripheral resistance in patients with hypertension.

(2) Effects on smooth muscle of respiratory tract The airway resistance increased, especially in the patients with asthma, because of the blockade of β_2 receptors in bronchial smooth muscles. The effect is less on normal people.

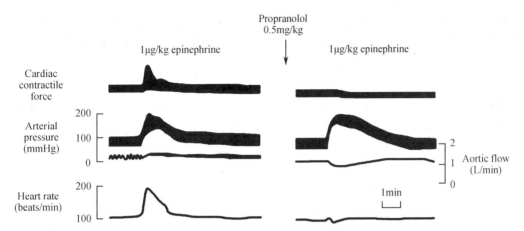

Figure 9-1   The effect in an anesthetized dog of the injection of epinephrine before and after propranolol
In the presence of a β receptor antagonist, epinephrine no longer augments the force of contraction (measured by a strain gauge attached to the ventricular wall) nor increases cardiac rate. Blood pressure is still elevated by epinephrine because vasoconstriction is not blocked[Shanks RG. The pharmacology of β sympathetic blockade[J]. Am J Cardiol 1966, 18(3): 308-316.]

(3) **Intrinsic sympathomimetic activity (ISA, 内在拟交感活性)**　Some β receptor antagonists, such as, pindolol, oxprenolol have the function of partial activating β receptor. That is to say, these β receptor antagonists possess ISA. Therefore, they can bind to β receptors and weakly activate the receptors in the absence of catecholamines. These agents inhibit the effects of β receptor agonists by competing β receptors, and are beneficial for the hypertensive patients with bradycardia (心动过缓).

(4) **Effects on metabolic**　β receptor antagonists inhibit the secretion of insulin from the pancreas and prevent the hyperglycemic response to adrenaline.

(5) **Effects on eyes**　Several β receptor antagonists reduce intraocular pressure (眼内压), especially in glaucoma (青光眼). The mechanism usually reported is decreased aqueous humor (眼房水) production.

【Clinical Indications】

(1) **Angina and myocardial infarction (心绞痛和心肌梗死)**　β receptor antagonists are used in the treatment of angina pectoris through decreasing oxygen requirement of cardiac muscle. They could be used for prophylaxis of myocardial infarction.

(2) **Arrhythmia (心律失常)**　A β adrenergic blocker is used for prophylaxis of supraventricular and ventricular arrhythmias (室上性和室性心律失常) because of its decreasing cardiac rate, conductivity, contraction, and oxygen requirement.

(3) **Hypertension (高血压)**　β receptor antagonists can reduce the blood pressure of patients with hypertension by blocking cardiac β_1 receptors, then resulting in decreased cardiac output, and by blocking the positive feedback of β receptors in the presynaptic ganglion (神经节突触前膜), resulting in decreased release of noradrenaline. β receptor antagonists have no apparent effect on blood pressure in normal man.

(4) **Glaucoma**　Glaucoma is a major cause of blindness and of great pharmacologic interest because the chronic form often responds to drug therapy. The primary manifestation is increased intraocular pressure (眼内压增高) not initially associated with symptoms. Without treatment, increased intraocular pressure results in damage to the retina (视网膜) and optic nerve (视神经), with restriction of visual fields (视野) and , eventually, blindness.

β receptor antagonists, especially timolol is used for glaucoma (β receptor antagonists could effectively diminish intraocular pressure by decreasing the secretion of aqueous humor).

(5) Hyperthyroidism (甲状腺功能亢进) β receptor antagonists are used for hyperthyroidism by depressing the wide spread sympathetic stimulation.

【Adverse reactions】Major adverse reactions include worsening of preexisting asthma, heart failure caused by depressing myocardial contractility, hypoglycemia (低血糖症), and aggravation of peripheral vascular disease.

2.1 Propranolol(普萘洛尔)

Propranolol interacts with β₁ and β₂ receptors with nearly equal affinity, is deficient in intrinsic sympathomimetic activity, and does not antagonism α receptors.

Propranolol is beneficial for the treatment of hypertension and angina, and used to relieve the supraventricular and ventricular arrhythmias or tachycardias, premature ventricular contractions (室性期前收缩), digitalis-induced tachyarrhythmias, myocardial infarction, pheochromocytoma, essential tremor, and the prophylaxis of migraine (偏头痛). It also has been used for several off-label indications including Parkinsonian tremors (sustained-release only), akathisia induced by antipsychotic drugs, variceal bleeding in portal hypertension (门静脉高血压所致静脉曲张破裂出血), and generalized anxiety disorder.

2.2 Both α-and β-receptor antagonists

Labetalol (拉贝洛尔)

Labetalol is representative of a class of drugs that competitive block α₁, β₁ and β₂ receptors. Blood pressure is lowered by reduction of systemic vascular resistance without significant alteration in heart rate in cardiac output. It could be used to treat different types of hypertension. Common adverse effects include dizziness, fatigue, nausea, etc. Asthma and congestive heart failure are prohibited to use.

重 点 小 结

药物	药理作用	临床应用	不良反应
酚妥拉明	舒张血管、兴奋心脏	外周血管痉挛性疾病、静脉滴注去甲肾上腺素外漏、急性心梗、嗜铬细胞瘤	腹痛、腹泻、呕吐和诱发加重溃疡、心律失常、心绞痛
酚苄明	扩张血管、降低血压	外周血管痉挛性疾病、良性前列腺增生引起的阻塞性排尿困难、嗜铬细胞瘤	心律失常、胃肠道刺激
哌唑嗪	选择性阻断 α₁ 受体，降压	高血压、顽固性心功能不全	首剂效应、眩晕、头痛、胃肠道反应
普萘洛尔	非选择性 β 受体阻断药	心律失常、心绞痛、高血压、甲状腺功能亢进	反跳现象、诱发或加重哮喘、升高血脂

目 标 检 测

一、选择题

（一）单项选择题

1. 普萘洛尔治疗心绞痛的主要药理作用是（　　　）
  A. 降低心肌收缩力，减慢心率 B. 扩张冠脉 C. 降低心脏前负荷
  D. 降低左室壁张力 E. 以上都不是

2. 治疗外周血管痉挛性疾病可选用（　　　）
  A. β受体阻断剂 B. α受体阻断剂 C. α受体激动剂
  D. β受体激动剂 E. 以上均不行

3. 下列何药可诱发或加重支气管哮喘（　　　）
  A. 肾上腺素 B. 普萘洛尔 C. 酚苄明
  D. 酚妥拉明 E. 甲氧明

4. 下列哪种情况禁用β受体阻断药（　　　）
  A. 心绞痛 B. 快速型心律失常 C. 高血压
  D. 房室传导阻滞 E. 甲状腺功能亢进

（二）多项选择题

5. 酚妥拉明的临床应用有（　　　）
  A. 抗休克 B. 治疗难治性心肌梗死和充血性心力衰竭
  C. 治疗外周血管痉挛性疾病 D. 治疗静脉滴注去甲肾上腺素外漏
  E. 嗜铬细胞瘤诊断

6. 普萘洛尔的临床用途有（　　　）
  A. 抗心律失常 B. 治疗慢性心功能不全 C. 抗心绞痛
  D. 抗高血压 E. 治疗偏头痛

二、思考题

论述 α 受体阻断药和 β 受体阻断药的药理作用及临床应用。

（徐志立）

Chapter 10   Anxiolytic and hypnotic drugs

 学习目标

　　1．**掌握**　苯二氮䓬类药物及其代表药地西泮的药物代谢动力学特点、药理作用、机制、主要临床应用和不良反应。

　　2．**熟悉**　其他镇静催眠药的特点及临床应用。

　　3．**了解**　新型镇静催眠药的作用特点及临床应用。

There is considerable overlap in the pharmacology of drugs that have anxiolytic (抗焦虑) and hypnotic (催眠) properties. Compounds with sedative properties (镇静作用) at low doses often have hypnotic effects at higher doses. In addition, sedative drugs may have anxiolytic properties when used at doses that are too low to produce sedation. Compounds such as buspirone have been developed that have anxiolytic properties but do not sedate.

1. Biological basis

1.1　Biological basis of anxiety disorders

Anxiety disorders (焦虑症) are among the most common psychiatric syndromes (精神分裂症) and affect 15% of the general population at some time during their life. The clinical manifestations of anxiety are both psychological and physical. Anxiety is only pathological when it is inappropriate to the degree of stress to which the individual is exposed. A variety of anxiety disorders are recognized, of which the most common are generalized anxiety disorder, panic disorder (恐慌症), phobic disorder (恐惧症) and obsessive compulsive disorder (强迫症).

The symptoms vary among the anxiety disorders, but usually include apprehension (恐惧), worry, fear and nervousness. Increased sympathetic nervous system activity (交感神经系统兴奋) frequently accompanies these feelings, causing sweating, tachycardia (心动过速) and epigastric discomfort (上消化道不适).

1.2　Biological basis of insomnia

The two main types of sleep pattern are non-rapid eye movement (non-REM) sleep and rapid eye movement (REM) sleep. These sleep patterns occur in cycles, with non-REM sleep varying between light sleep (stages 1 and 2) and slow-wave sleep (stages 3 and 4). Two-thirds of sleep is usually spent in stages 2-4, characterized by continuous or intermittent delta waves (slow waves) on the electroencephalogram. These deeper stages of sleep are the recuperative phase, while most dreaming occurs during the REM sleep periods. Increasing age is associated with more nocturnal awakening and longer periods of REM sleep.

Defining insomnia is complicated by the considerable variability in the normal pattern of sleep. Most healthy adults sleep between 7 and 9 hours per night, but much shorter or even longer periods can be normal. Insomnia is considered to be present if there is repeated inability to initiate or maintain sleep, despite adequate opportunity and time for sleep. There are three major categories of insomnia, defined by duration of symptoms. Symptoms include sleep-onset insomnia (difficulty falling asleep, more common in younger people), frequent nocturnal awakening (difficulty maintaining sleep, more common in older people), early morning awakening (with difficulty getting back to sleep) and difficulty functioning in the daytime due to perceived poor sleep. Obstructive sleep apnoea is a common cause of sleep disturbance, affecting up to 10% of people who report insomnia.

The reticular formation in the midbrain, medulla and pons is responsible for maintaining wakefulness. Activity in the reticular formation is dependent on sensory input via collateral connections from the main sensory pathways. Neurotransmitter systems involved in the regulation of sleep are complex. Cortical arousal is regulated by noradrenergic pathways from the locus coeruleus, cholinergic ascending tracts from brainstem nuclei, histaminergic neurons from the tuberomammillary nucleus and serotonergic neurons from the raphe nuclei. Hypocretins are important neuropeptide transmitters found in the lateral hypothalamus which, through connections with other hypothalamic and brainstem nuclei, promote wakefulness [see also narcolepsy (嗜睡症)]. Sleep is induced by neurotransmission by GABA, melatonin and galanin (a predominantly inhibitory neuropeptide) from the anterior hypothalamus, which inhibits the arousal neurons.

2. Drugs therapy for anxiety

Drugs used to treat anxiety are called anxiolytics.

Benzodiazepines (苯二氮䓬类)

In addition to their anxiolytic effect, benzodiazepines have several other properties that are clinically useful. This section also considers drugs that are not used primarily for treatment of anxiety.

【Pharmacokinetics】 Benzodiazepines are well absorbed from the gut and their lipid solubility ensures ready penetration into the brain. The pharmacokinetics of individual benzodiazepines determines their major clinical uses. Benzodiazepines that are useful for inducing sleep [e.g., temazepam (替马西泮)] are rapidly absorbed from the gut. This produces a fast onset of sedation, then sleep. Metabolism of short-acting benzodiazepines produces inactive derivatives. A brief duration of action is desirable for hypnotics, to avoid hangover sedation in the morning long-acting benzodiazepines, such as diazepam, are metabolized in the liver to active compounds that contribute to their duration of action through relatively slow elimination from the body. Repeated dosing with long acting compounds, such as diazepam, increases the risk of accumulation and a prolonged sedative effect. The anxiolytic properties of benzodiazepines are best exploited by using a compound with a long duration of action. Smaller doses can then be used to minimize sedation, and the rebound in anxiety symptoms that can occur between doses of a short-acting drug is avoided. Diazepam, lorazepam and midazolam can also be given by intravenous injection to provide rapid sedation pre-operatively or before procedures such as endoscopy(内镜检查).

Intravenous lorazepam and diazepam are also given for emergency treatment of generalized seizures and status epilepticus. Long-acting benzodiazepines, such as clobazam, clonazepam, diazepam and lorazepam, are used in the prophylaxis of epilepsy.

【Pharmacodynamics】Benzodiazepines act by potentiating the actions of GABA, the primary inhibitory neurotransmitter in the central nervous system (CNS). They act at a regulatory site closely linked to the $GABA_A$ receptor which mediates fast inhibitory synaptic neurotransmission. GABA increases the influx of Cl^- into the neuron, hyperpolarizes the cell membrane and decreases cell excitability. Binding of a benzodiazepine to subunits of the receptor induces a conformational change in the GABA receptor that enhances its affinity for the neurotransmitter. Benzodiazepines act only in the presence of GABA to enhance GABA-mediated opening of the ion channel; they have no direct action on the channel.

The $GABA_A$ receptor has α, β and γ subunits, arranged in a group of five (usually two α, two β and one γ, although only α and β are essential) around a central pore. There are many subtypes of each subunit, and therefore many receptor configurations that show differences in their regional distributions in the brain. Benzodiazepines bind between an α and γ subunit. The presence of an $α_1$ or $α_5$ subunit confers the sedative and amnesic properties of benzodiazepines, while both $α_2$ and $α_3$ appear to be involved in the anxiolytic and muscle relaxant effects. Anticonvulsant activity (肌肉松弛作用) is conferred by several α subunits. The minority of GABA receptors with only $α_4$ or $α_6$ subunits do not bind benzodiazepines (Figure 10-1).

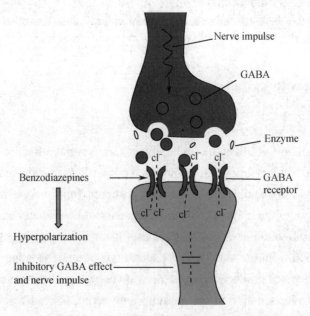

Figure 10-1   The mechanism of benzodiazepines

The increase in inhibitory neurotransmission produced by benzodiazepines has the following potentially useful effects: sedation from reduced sensory input to the reticular activating system; sleep induction at high drug concentrations; anterograde amnesia (顺行性遗忘), etc.

【Adverse reactions】At the time of peak concentration in plasma, hypnotic doses of benzodiazepines can be expected to cause varying degrees of light-headedness, lassitude, increased reaction time, motor incoordination, impairment of mental and motor functions, confusion, and anterograde amnesia. Cognition appears to be affected less than motor performance. All of these effects can greatly impair driving and other psychomotor skills, especially if combined with ethanol. The intensity and incidence of CNS toxicity generally increase with age; both pharmacokinetic and pharmacodynamic factors are involved.

When the drug is given at the intended time of sleep, the persistence of these effects during the waking hours is adverse, even though successful drug therapy can reduce the daytime sleepiness resulting from chronic insomnia. These dose-related residual effects can be insidious because most subjects underestimate the degree of their impairment.

Benzodiazepines may cause paradoxical effects. Amnesia, euphoria, restlessness, hallucinations, sleep-walking, sleep-talking, other complex behaviors, and hypomanic behavior have been reported to occur during use of various benzodiazepines. Other relatively common side effects of benzodiazepines are weakness, headache, blurred vision, vertigo, nausea and vomiting, epigastric distress, and diarrhea. Anticonvulsant benzodiazepines sometimes actually increase the frequency of seizures in patients with epilepsy.

Tolerance, decreased responsiveness to a drug following repeated exposure, is a common feature of sedative-hypnotic use. It may result in the need for an increase in the dose required to maintain symptomatic improvement or to promote sleep. Mild dependence may develop in many patients who have taken therapeutic doses of benzodiazepines on a regular basis for prolonged periods.

Buspirone (丁螺环酮)

【Pharmacokinetics】Buspirone is well absorbed from the gut and undergoes extensive first-pass metabolism in the liver. The half-life is short (2-4h).

【Mechanism of action】Buspirone is a partial agonist at presynaptic 5-HT$_{1A}$ receptors, producing negative feedback to inhibit serotonin (5–羟色胺) release. It has no effect on GABA receptors. Initial exacerbation of anxiety may occur, possibly caused by postsynaptic 5-HT$_{1A}$ receptor stimulation. The onset of the anxiolytic action of buspirone is slow, beginning after 2 weeks and reaching a maximum effect at approximately 4 weeks. The mechanism of action may involve gradual changes in neural plasticity (enhancement of neural performance or changes in neural connections). Buspirone has no sedative action and is ineffective for panic attacks.

【Adverse reactions】The frequency of adverse effects is low, with the most common effects being nausea, headaches, dizziness, nervousness, and light-headedness. Sedation and psychomotor and cognitive dysfunction are minimal, and dependence is unlikely.

3. Drugs for treating insomnia (hypnotics)

Drugs for treating insomnia are Benzodiazepines.

Zaleplon (扎来普隆), zolpidem (唑吡坦), zopiclone (唑吡酮)

These drugs are commonly referred to as Z drugs. Benzodiazepines have dose-related hypnotic effects. See above for details. Non-benzodiazepine hypnotics that modulate the $GABA_A$ chloride channel.

Mechanism of action and effects of Z compounds belong to different chemical classes but interact in a similar manner with the postsynaptic $GABA_A$ receptor on neuronal membranes. They bind to regulatory binding sites on the receptor that are close to, but distinct from, the benzodiazepine-binding site. Like the benzodiazepines, they increase GABA-mediated Cl^- influx into the cell, which inhibits neurotransmission. Zolpidem and zaleplon are selective for the α_1 subunit in the GABA receptor.

Zopiclone also acts on the α_2 subunit of the GABA receptor. Although zopiclone also possesses anxiolytic and anticonvulsant activity, its short duration of action makes it unsuitable for these indications.

【Pharmacokinetics】The Z drugs are rapidly absorbed from the gut and are metabolized in the liver. They have short half-lives (1-6h), which makes them well suited to their use as hypnotics.

【Adverse reactions】Late-night administration of zolpidem has been associated with bitter metallic taste, morning sedation, delayed reaction time, and anterograde amnesia, whereas zaleplon does not due to its rapid elimination with a half-life of approximately 1 hour. Because of the concern of physical dependence and abuse, zolpidem is approved only for the short-term treatment of insomnia.

Adverse events reported with zopiclone include anxiety, dry mouth, headache, peripheral edema, somnolence(嗜睡), and unpleasant taste.

Common adverse reactions of the Z drugs include nausea and vomiting, incoordination, drowsiness, dizziness and dependence with withdrawal symptoms.

重 点 小 结

药物	作用机制	临床应用	不良反应
地西泮以及硝西泮	能增强 GABA 能神经传递功能和突触效应，并能促进 GABA 与 $GABA_A$ 受体结合，促进 Cl^- 通道开放，Cl^- 内流增加，使神经细胞超极化，增强抑制效应	镇静、催眠、抗焦虑、抗惊厥、抗癫痫、中枢性肌肉松弛作用、癫症、神经衰弱等	嗜睡、轻微头痛、乏力、运动失调，与剂量有关，老年患者更易出现以上反应。偶见低血压、呼吸抑制、视物模糊、皮疹、尿潴留、抑郁、精神紊乱、白细胞减少。长期应用可致耐受与依赖性，突然停药有戒断症状出现
丁螺环酮	为 $5-HT_{1A}$ 受体的部分激动药，激动突触前 $5-HT_{1A}$ 受体，反馈性抑制 5-HT 释放	焦虑性激动、内心不安和紧张等急慢性焦虑状态	头晕、头痛及胃肠功能紊乱
扎来普隆	选择性激动 $GABA_A$ 受体复合物，产生中枢抑制作用	镇静催眠、抗焦虑、抗惊厥、肌肉松弛	类似苯二氮䓬类药，成瘾性较小

题库

目 标 检 测

一、单项选择题

1. 地西泮的作用机制是（　　）
　　A. 直接介导中枢神经系统细胞的钠离子内流
　　B. 抑制 Ca^{2+} 依赖的动作电位
　　C. 抑制 Ca^{2+} 依赖的递质释放
　　D. 作用于中枢神经系统细胞的苯二氮䓬受体
　　E. 抑制 GABA 神经功能

2. 中年女性，近期工作压力比较大，夜间入睡困难，常超过 2 小时。一旦入睡，睡眠质量较好，无起夜和早醒情况，用下列哪一种药物治疗比较适合（　　）
　　A. 氯氮䓬　　　　B. 劳拉西泮　　　　C. 唑吡坦　　　　D. 地西泮　　　　E. 硝西泮

3. 苯二氮䓬类药物中毒的解救药物是（　　）
　　A. 纳洛酮　　　B. 氟马西尼　　　C. 多塞平　　　　D. 佐匹克隆　　　E. 美沙酮

4. 失眠特点为易醒早醒、醒后不能入睡的患者，应该选择的药物是（　　）
　　A. 纳洛酮　　　　B. 美沙酮　　　　C. 氟马西尼　　　　D. 佐匹克隆　　　　E. 地西泮

二、多项选择题

5. 关于苯二氮䓬类药物的特点，说法正确的是（　　）
　　A. 直接开放 Cl⁻ 通道　　　　　　　　　B. 长期应用停用后具有戒断症状
　　C. 具有剂量依赖性的中枢抑制作用　　　　D. 具有镇痛作用
　　E. 具有中枢性肌肉松弛作用

（辛晓明）

Chapter 11　Drugs for psychiatric disorders

 学习目标

1. **掌握** 吩噻嗪类代表药氯丙嗪的药理作用、作用机制、临床应用及主要不良反应。
2. **熟悉** 氯氮平、丙米嗪、碳酸锂等药的药理作用、临床应用及主要不良反应。
3. **了解** 抗精神失常药的分类。

The psychiatric disorder is a mental illness diagnosed by a mental health professional that greatly disturbs your thinking, moods, and(or) behavior and seriously increases your risk of disability, pain, death, or loss of freedom, including schizophrenia, mania, depression and anxiety, and etc. The drugs for psychiatric disorders can be classified as antipsychotic drugs (抗精神病药), antidepressive drugs (抗抑郁症药), antimanic drugs (抗躁狂症药) and antianxiety drugs (抗焦虑症药) according to the clinical application.

1. Antipsychotic drugs

The term "antipsychotic drugs" conventionally refers to those used to treat schizophrenia (精神分裂症), one of the most common and debilitating forms of mental illness. Pharmacologically, most of antipsychotic drugs are dopamine receptor antagonists (多巴胺受体激动剂), although many of them also act on other targets, particularly 5-hydroxytryptamine (5-HT, 5–羟色胺) receptors, which may contribute to their clinical efficacy.

Schizophrenia is a chronic and severe mental disorder that affects how a person thinks, feels, and behaves. People with schizophrenia may experience hallucinations, delusions, and disorganized thinking and speech, and may seem like they have lost touch with reality. The symptoms of schizophrenia are divided into three categories, including positive, negative, and cognitive. The positive symptoms may include delusions, hallucinations, thought disorders, abnormal, disorganized behavior, catatonia and etc. The negative symptoms may include withdrawal from social contacts, flattening of emotional responses, anhedonia, reluctance to perform everyday tasks, difficulty beginning and sustaining activities and reduced speaking. The cognitive symptoms may include deficits in cognitive function (e.g., attention and memory). The antipsychotic drugs can be classified into several groups according to their chemical structures, including phenothiazines, thioxanthenes, butyrophenones, and etc.

1.1   First generation antipsychotics

1.1.1   Phenothizaine derivatitives(吩噻嗪类)

Chlorpromazine (氯丙嗪)

Chlorpromazine is also named Wintermine (冬眠灵), which was synthesized by a French pharmaceutical company Charpentier. Chlorpromazine is the first antipsychotic drug, that has been used to treat with schizophrenia since 1963. It is able to treat with schizophrenia, bipolar disorder, attention deficit hyperactivity disorder, nausea and vomiting, anxiety before surgery, and hiccups that do not improve following other measures.

【Pharmacokinetics】When orally administered, chlorpromazine is absorbed slowly and irregularly. When intramuscular injected (肌内注射), it is absorbed rapidly, and the plasma protein binding rate is about 90%. It can distribute in the whole body, and easily cross the blood-brain barrier. The oral bioavailability is estimated to be 30%-50% due to extensive first pass metabolism in the liver. The cytochrome P450 isoenzymes 1A2 and 2D6 are needed for metabolism of chlorpromazine. Plasma half-life is about 30 hours. It has many active metabolites, which can be detected in the urine after a long-term drug withdrawal for several weeks or even six months.

【Pharmacodynamics】

(1) Central nervous system

1) Antipsychotic effects   Chlorpromazine, as a typical antipsychotic drug, is an antagonist on different postsynaptic receptors including dopamine receptors, serotonin receptors ($5\text{-}HT_1$ and $5\text{-}HT_2$), histamine receptors (组胺受体), α_1 and α_2 adrenergic receptors (肾上腺素受体), M_1 and M_2 muscarinic acetylcholine receptors (毒蕈碱型乙酰胆碱受体). It has antipsychotic, anxiolytic, antidepressive and anti-aggressive properties and sedation effect. The symptoms of excitement and agitation can be quickly controlled after chlorpromazine treatment, and the hallucinations and delusions also gradually improved after continuous medication.

Five dopaminergic pathways are key for understanding schizophrenia and the Pharmacodynamics of antipsychotic drugs. The mesolimbic-mesocortical pathway (中脑边缘–中脑皮质通路) is the one most closely related to behavior and psychosis. The nigrostriatal pathway (黑质–纹状体通路) is involved in the coordination of voluntary movement. The tuberoinfundibular system (结节–漏斗系统) is related to the endocrine effects. The effects of medullary periventricular pathway are not defined. The incertohypothanlamic pathway (脑下丘脑通路) appears to regulate the anticipatory motivational phase of copulatory behavior in rats. Five subtypes of dopamine receptors (D_1, D_2, D_3, D_4 and D_5) have been described in the brain, consisting of two separate families, the D_1-like and D_2-like receptor groups. The D_1 and D_5 receptors are members of the D_1-like family, whereas the D_2, D_3 and D_4 receptors are members of the D_2-like family of dopamine receptors. In the brain, both D_1 and D_2 families can take effects in the nigrostriatal pathway, and D_2 family primarily affects the mesolimbic-mesocortical pathway, whereas the D_2 dopamine receptor mainly affect the tuberoinfundibular system. The dopamine hypothesis for schizophrenia indicated that the excitement of D_2 family action in the mesolimbic-mesocortical pathway paly an important role in the development of psychosis.

Currently, it proved that the typical antipsychotic agents such as phenothiazine derivatives block D_2 receptors stereo-selectively for the most part, and their binding affinity is strongly correlated with clinical antipsychotic application and extrapyramidal motor disturbances, and other side effects.

2) Antiemetic The phenothiazine derivatives have a broad spectrum effect and are effective in controlling vomiting due to a variety of causes. Chlorpromazine acts on the emetic center (催吐中枢) in the fourth cerebral ventricle of medulla oblongata (延髓), chemoreceptor trigger zone, and on peripheral receptors. It is also thought to function as a calcium channel antagonist (钙通道阻滞剂). However, chlorpromazine can not control vomiting due to vestibular stimulation.

3) Hypothermia Chlorpromazine has a strong inhibitory effect on the hypothalamic thermoregulatory center (下丘脑体温调节中枢) and interferes with its thermostatic function. It not only can reduce the body temperature of the fever, but also lower the normal body temperature. Chlorpromazine-induced hypothermia (降温) was greatly enhanced after cooling the ambient temperature. When applied simultaneously with physical cooling, it has a synergistic cooling effect.

4) Synergistic effect with central nervous depressants When applied with central nervous depressants such as general anesthetics (麻醉药), sedative hypnotics (镇静催眠药), analgesics (镇痛药), it shows a synergistic effect on the central nervous system.

(2) Autonomic nervous system Chlorpromazine can block muscarinic receptors and produce a variety of peripheral effects, including blurring of vision and increased intraocular pressure (眼内压), dry mouth and eyes, constipation and urinary retention (尿潴留). It also can block α adrenoceptors and cause orthostatic hypotension.

(3) Endocrine effects Chlorpromazine can block D_2-like family of tuberoinfundibular system, and inhibit the secretion of prolactin release inhibitor (催乳素释放抑制剂), follicle stimulating hormone release factor, luteinizing hormone release factor and ACTH. It can produce elevations of prolactin, and induce breast engorgement and lactation. It also can inhibit the production of gonadotropin (促性腺激素), glucocorticoid and pituitary growth hormone.

【Clinical indications】

(1) Schizophrenia (精神分裂症) Chlorpromazine can rapidly control hyperactive psychotic states, especially the positive symptoms (阳性症状). It can also take effect on the symptoms including excitement, restlessness, tension, hallucinations (幻觉) and delusions (妄想) induced by other mental disorders, organic psychosis and symptoms psychosis. However, negative symptoms may be worsened after treated with chlorpromazine.

(2) Epilepsy (呕吐) Chlorpromazine is used to treat nausea and vomiting induced by some diseases (e.g., cancer, radiation sickness, uremia, and so on.) and drugs (e.g., morphine and digitalis). Chlorpromazine is also used to treat intractable hiccup (顽固性呃逆). However, it can not be used to treat motion sickness caused by stimulation vestibular system or gastrointestinal tract.

(3) Artificial hibernation (人工冬眠) If used as a cocktail with pethidine (哌替啶) and promethazine (异丙嗪), it can cause "artificial hibernation". Patients with severe trauma, infection, febrile seizures, thyroid crisis, pregnancy poisoning and shock can be sedated by this cocktail.

【Adverse reactions】

(1) Common side effects The main side effects of chlorpromazine are due to its anticholinergic properties (抗胆碱能作用), which include sedation, dry mouth, constipation (便秘), urinary retention and possible lowering of seizure threshold. Appetite may be increased with resultant weight gain. Its anti sympathomimetic properties can induce low blood pressure upon standing.

(2) Extrapyramidal reactions (锥体外系反应)   These reactions occurring early during treatment with agents include Parkinson's syndrome, acute dystonia reactions (急性肌张力障碍反应), akathisia (uncontrollable restlessness, 静坐不能), and tardive dyskinesia (迟发性运动障碍). These all result directly or indirectly from D_2 receptor blockade in the nigrostriatal pathway. Extrapyramidal side effects constitute one of the main disadvantages of first generation antipsychotic drugs. Second generation drugs were thought to have less tendency to produce extrapyramidal side effects.

(3) Seizures (癫痫)   It is recognized as a complication of chlorpromazine treatment. A small number of patients have localized or generalized convulsions during medication, which can sometimes cause epileptiform discharges in EEG, and the incidence of epilepsy is increased.

(4) Metabolic and endocrine effects   Weight gain is common, and hyperglycemia (高血糖) may develop. Hyperprolactinemia (高泌乳素血症) in women results in the breast engorgement, amenorrhea galactorrhea syndrome and infertility; in men, loss of libido, impotency, and infertility may occur.

(5) Toxic or allergic reactions   These reactions commonly include rash, contact dermatitis (接触性皮炎). Agranulocytosis (粒细胞缺乏症), hemolytic anemia, and aplastic anemia occur rarely.

1.1.2   Thioxanthene derivatives(硫杂蒽类)

Chlorprothixene (氯普噻吨)

Chlorprothixene exerts strong blocking effect on postsynaptic dopamine receptors (突触后多巴胺受体) and improves mental disorders, and inhibits the ascending activation system of the brainstem reticular structure (脑干网状结构) and causes sedation, and it can also inhibit the chemosensory zone of the brain and exert antiemetic effect (antiemetic effect). The principal indications of chlorprothixene are the treatment of psychotic disorders (e.g., schizophrenia) and acute mania occurring as part of bipolar disorders. The effect of chlorprothixene on anxiety and depression is stronger than that of chlorpromazine. It shows a worse effect on control hallucinations and delusions than chlorpromazine.

1.1.3   Butyrophenone derivatitives(丁酰苯类)

Haloperidol (氟哌啶醇)

Haloperidol is a selective antagonist of D_2-like receptors and exert strong and lasting antipsychotic effect and it is classified as a highly potent neuroleptic. It has minor antihistaminic and anticholinergic properties, therefore cardiovascular and anticholinergic side-effects are seen quite infrequently, compared with less potent neuroleptics such as chlorpromazine.

1.1.4   Benzamides(苯甲酰胺类)

Sulpiride (舒必利)

Sulpiride is a selective antagonist (选择性拮抗剂) of D_2-like receptors, and exerts high affinity with D_2 receptors at mesolimbic system (中脑边缘系统). It has minor anticholinergic properties.

1.2   Second generation antipsychotics

Clozapine, Asenapine (阿塞那平), Olanzapine, Quetiapine, Paliperidone (帕潘立酮), Risperidone (利培酮), Sertindole (舍吲哚), Ziprasidone (齐拉西酮), Zotepine (佐替平) and Aripiprazole (阿立哌唑)

are atypical antipsychotics. The distinction between the typical and atypical antipsychotic drugs rests on the receptor profiles, incidence of extrapyramidal side effects, efficacy against negative symptoms, and efficacy in "treatment-resistant" group of patients.

Clozapine (氯氮平)

Clozapine can bind to serotonin receptor as well as dopamine receptor. It also is a strong antagonist of different subtypes of adrenergic, cholinergic and histaminergic receptors. Clozapine is used principally in treating treatment-resistant schizophrenia, and shows efficacy against both positive and negative symptoms. The common adverse effects for clozapine include constipation, drooling (流涎), muscle stiffness, sedation, tremors, orthostasis, hyperglycemia, and weight gain. When compared to the classical antipsychotic drugs, the causes of extrapyramidal symptoms are much less. However, the risk of agranulocytosis limits the clinic use of clozapine.

Olanzapine (奥氮平)

Olanzapine is an atypical antipsychotic drug, and it is an antagonist at different subtypes of serotonin, dopamine, α adrenergic, cholinergic and histaminergic receptors. It has high affinity for dopamine and serotonin receptors. The affinity of olanzapine for 5-HT$_2$ receptor is stronger than for dopamine receptor, and olanzapine can selectively take effect at mesolimbic pathway. The antipsychotic activity of olanzapine is mediated primarily by antagonism at dopamine receptors, specifically D$_2$. Adverse effects for olanzapine include dry mouth, dizziness, sedation, insomnia, orthostatic hypotension (体位性低血压), akathisia (静坐不能), and weight gain. It is reported to cause extrapyramidal symptoms and tardive dyskinesia, however, at a much reduced rate when compared to the classical antipsychotics.

2. Antidepressive drugs

Depression (major depressive disorder or clinical depression) is a common but serious mood disorder. It causes severe symptoms including feelings of sadness, tearfulness, hopelessness, short temper, irritation, loss of interest, memory loss, flat affect, sleep disorders, tiredness, reduced appetite and weight loss, feelings of worthlessness and etc. The deficit in function of monoamines (单胺类) is central to the biology of depression. Also, the neurotrophic and endocrine factors (the neurotrophic hypothesis) play an important role.

Currently, the antidepressant in clinical uses include selective serotonin reuptake inhibitors (5–羟色胺再摄取抑制剂), serotonin-norepinephreine reuptake inhibitors (5–羟色胺–去甲肾上腺素再摄取抑制剂, e.g., selective serotonin-norepinephrine reuptake inhibitors, tricyclic antidepressants) 5-HT$_2$ receptor modulators, tetracyclic and unicyclic antidepressants, monoamine oxidase inhibitors.

Imipramine (丙米嗪)

Imipramine is a tricyclic antidepressant (TCA, 三环类抗抑郁药), and it is a relatively strong serotonin and norepinephrine reuptake inhibitor. It also has anticholinergic, and antihistaminergic properties. It can be used to treat depression, anxiety, ADD/ADHD, enuresis and numerous other mental and physical conditions. After taking imipramine in normal people, sedation, drowsiness, decreased blood pressure, dizziness, and atropine-like effects such as dry mouth and blurred vision can be induced. After continuous medication, it can improve depression symptom produced after taking chlorpromazine. After continuous medication, the symptoms of depression can be significantly improved. Imipramine is not as commonly used today, but is sometimes used to treat major depression. It is also used to treat panic attacks, chronic pain, and Kleine-Levin syndrome. In pediatric patients it is used to treat pavor nocturnus and nocturnal enuresis.

Fluoxetine (氟西汀)

Fluoxetine is a selective serotonin reuptake inhibitor (选择性 5-HT 再摄取抑制剂 , SSRI) antidepressant. It has high affinity for monoamine receptors but lacked the affinity for histamine, muscarinic acetylcholine and α adrenoceptors. It can be used to treat depression, bipolar disorder, obsessive-compulsive disorder, bulimia nervosa, premenstrual dysphoric disorder and panic disorder. Common adverse effects include anxiety, restlessness and insomnia, as well as nausea, headache, dry mouth, sweating, blurred vision. Weight loss, trembling, weakness, skin rash, anorgasmia, itching, and a decrease in sexual drive, have also been reported. An overdose of fluoxetine or combining it with other antidepressants can lead to serotonin syndrome.

Paroxetine (帕罗西汀)

Paroxetine is a selective serotonin reuptake inhibitor antidepressant. Paroxetine shows weak effect on reuptake of NA and DA. It exhibits a weak affinity for the muscarinic acetylcholine and noradrenaline receptors, or histamine receptors. Paroxetine can be used to treat the symptoms of major depression, obsessive-compulsive disorder (OCD, 强迫症), post-traumatic stress disorder (PTSD, 创伤后应激障碍), panic disorder, generalized anxiety disorder (GAD, 广泛性焦虑症), social phobia/social anxiety disorder, and premenstrual dysphoric disorder (PMDD, 经前烦躁不安). Common adverse reactions of paroxetine include nausea, drowsiness, sweating, tremor, fatigue, insomnia, dry mouth, sexual dysfunction, dizziness, and increased or decreased appetite for constipation. Most side-effects will disappear or lessen with continued treatment. Pregnant women are advised not to take the drug due to possible fetal heart defects. Withdrawal syndromes including dizziness, sensory disturbances, sleep disturbances, irritations, tremors, nausea, sweating, and confusion occur when the drug is sudden withdrawal. It can be secreted into breast milk, and breastfeeding women must be caution.

Maprotiline (马普替林)

Maprotiline is a tetracyclic antidepressant (四环抗抑郁药). It is a strong norepinephrine reuptake inhibitor with only weak effects on serotonin and dopamine reuptake. It can be used to treat depressions of all forms and severities (endogenous, psychotic, involutional, and neurotic), the depressive phase in bipolar depression and to relieve the symptoms of anxiety, tension of insomnia. Common adverse reactions mainly include dry mouth, dizziness, fatigue, increased appetite and weight gain, hypotension, tachycardia, impaired sexual functions in men, allergic skin reactions, agitation, confusion, constipation, seizures, prolonged and painful erections, leukopenia and agranulocytosis, and etc. Liver damage and polyneuritis rarely occur.

3. Anti-manic drugs

Manic-depressive illness, also known as bipolar disorder (双相情感障碍), and anti-manic drugs (抗躁狂药) are also termed mood stabilizers. According to DSM-IV, bipolar disorders and schizophrenia are separate disease entities. Antipsychotics such as chlorpromazine, clozapine and haloperidol also show efficacy on bipolar disorder, although lithium treatment remains the "gold standard" of treatment for preventing recurrences in bipolar disorder, both types Ⅰ (with mania and major depression) and Ⅱ (with depression and hypomania).

Lithium carbonate (碳酸锂)

Lithium carbonate is shown to be useful in the treatment of the manic phase of bipolar. However, the Pharmacodynamics of lithium is not clearly understood. The main biochemical mechanisms for lithium include: ① Lithium can inhibit glycogen synthase kinase-3 (GSK-3) and deplete intracellular inositol, and provide neuroprotection, and increase neuroplasticity. ② It can inhibit Na^+-Na^+ exchange across the membrane. ③ Lithium treatment inhibits the enzyme inositol monophosphatase and leads to a depletion of free inositol and ultimately decrease of phosphatidylinositol-4,5-bisphosphate (PIP_2), the membrane precursor of inositol-1,4,5-trisphosphate (IP_3, 肌醇-1,4,5- 三磷酸) and diacylglycerol (DAG, 二酰基甘油). Lithium affects second-messenger systems involving both activation of adenylyl cyclase and phosphoinositol turnover. ④ Lithium may also increase the release of serotonin by neurons in the brain. Lithium treatment is used to treat mania in bipolar disorder, schizoaffective disorder, as well as schizophrenia. Many adverse effects associated with lithium treatment, including: ① Neurologic and psychiatric adverse effects (e.g., tremor). ② Decreased thyroid function. ③ Nephrogenic diabetes insipidus. ④ Edema. ⑤ Bradycardia-tachycardia. ⑥ Weigh gain.

重 点 小 结

类别	药物	药理作用	临床应用	不良反应
抗精神病药	典型性抗精神病药物：氯丙嗪	主要通过阻断中脑 – 边缘系统和中脑 – 皮质系统 DA 通路的 D_2 样受体而发挥抗精神病作用	精神分裂症 (主要用于Ⅰ型精神分裂症的治疗，尤其对急性患者疗效好)、呕吐、低温麻醉、人工冬眠	一般不良反应 (嗜睡、困倦、乏力、视物模糊、口干等)；锥体外系反应
	非典型性抗精神病药物：氯氮平	对脑内 5-HT_2 受体和 D_1 受体的阻滞作用较强	急性与慢性精神分裂症的各个亚型，对偏执型、青春型精神分裂症效果较好	锥体外系不良反应少且轻微

续表

类别	药物	药理作用	临床应用	不良反应
抗抑郁症药	三环类抗抑郁药：丙米嗪	主要通过抑制脑内神经元对 NA 和 5-HT 的再摄取，使突触间隙中 NA 和 5-HT 浓度增高发挥抗抑郁作用	各种抑郁症，对内源性抑郁症、围绝经期抑郁症及伴有躁狂状态的抑郁症效果较好	常见口干、便秘、排尿困难等抗胆碱作用，大剂量可致心脏传导阻滞、心律失常
抗躁狂症药	碳酸锂	①抑制糖原合酶激酶 3(GSK-3) 并消耗细胞内肌醇。②锂离子可以抑制跨膜的 Na^+-Na^+ 交换。③锂影响第二信使 IP_3 和 DAG 涉及的腺苷酸环化酶的激活和磷酸肌醇的转换。④锂可能增加大脑神经元释放 5-HT	躁狂症	不良反应较多，早期有食欲缺乏、恶心、呕吐、肌无力、肢体震颤等

目 标 检 测

题库

一、单项选择题

1. 氯丙嗪抗精神病作用的主要机制是（　　　）
　　A. 阻断黑质 – 纹状体通路 D_2 受体　　B. 阻断中脑边缘 – 中脑皮质通路的 D_2 受体
　　C. 阻断结节 – 漏斗系统 D_2 受体　　　D. 阻断肾上腺素 α 受体
　　E. 阻断 M 胆碱受体

2. 长期应用氯丙嗪治疗精神病最常见的副作用是（　　　）
　　A. 体位性低血压　　　　　B. 中枢抑制症状　　　　　C. 锥体外系反应
　　D. 糖尿病　　　　　　　　E. 过敏反应

3. 针对下列长期应用氯丙嗪出现的症状，中枢抗胆碱药不能缓解的是（　　　）
　　A. 肌肉震颤　　　　　　　B. 迟发性运动障碍　　　　C. 静坐不能
　　D. 面容呆板　　　　　　　E. 急性肌张力障碍

4. 碳酸锂的临床应用是（　　　）
　　A. 精神分裂症　　　　　　B. 抑郁症　　　　　　　　C. 焦虑症
　　D. 躁狂症　　　　　　　　E. 癫痫

5. 下列有关丙米嗪作用的叙述，错误的是（　　　）
　　A. 阻断 NA 和 5-HT 在神经末梢的再摄取　　B. 可阻断 M 胆碱受体
　　C. 对 5-HT 再摄取阻断作用强　　　　　　　D. 属于非选择性单胺摄取抑制剂
　　E. 具有抗抑郁作用

6. 下列药物中属于选择性 5-HT 再摄取抑制剂是（　　　）
　　A. 丙米嗪　　B. 氯丙嗪　　C. 帕罗西汀　　D. 氯氮平　　E. 吗氯贝胺

二、思考题

服用氯丙嗪产生锥体外系症状的原因及相关症状有哪些？

（董世芬）

Chapter 12 Drugs for neurodegenerative diseases

 学习目标

1. **掌握** 左旋多巴和卡比多巴的体内过程、药理作用、临床应用、不良反应。
2. **熟悉** 金刚烷胺、苯海索的药理作用和临床应用。
3. **了解** 治疗阿尔茨海默病药物的分类及临床应用。

Neurodegeneration is the progressive loss of structure or function of neurons. Neurodegenerative diseases mainly include Parkinson's disease (PD, 帕金森病), Alzheimer's disease (AD, 阿尔茨海默病), Huntington's disease (亨廷顿病), amyotrophic lateral sclerosis (肌萎缩侧索硬化症) and etc. The mechanism responsible for neuronal death of neurodegeneration diseases include protein aggregation (e.g., amyloidosis), excitotoxicity, oxidative stress and apoptosis.

1. Parkinson's disease

Parkinson's disease, sometimes called paralysis agitans (震颤麻痹), is a neurological disorder, which has long been characterized by the classical motor features of parkinsonism associated with Lewy bodies and loss of dopaminergic neurons in the substantia nigra (黑质). It has been recognized since the early 1800s when the physician after whom the disease is named first described it. Risk factors include age, male gender and some environmental factors. The cardinal motor symptoms of PD are tremor (震颤), rigidity (肌强直), bradykinesia/akinesia (运动迟缓/运动障碍) and postural instability, but the clinical picture includes other motor and non-motor symptoms. PD patients may also display neurobehavioral disorders (depression, anxiety), cognitive impairment (dementia), and autonomic dysfunction (e.g., orthostatic and hyperhidrosis). Non-motor symptoms may appear before motor symptoms and often predominate in the later stages of the disease. It is a chronic progressive neurodegenerative disorder that occurs mostly in older persons but that can appear in much younger patients.

The pathogenesis of PD is related to a combination of impaired degradation of proteins, intracellular protein accumulation and aggregation, oxidative stress (氧化应激), mitochondrial damage (线粒体损伤), inflammatory cascades (炎症级联反应), and apoptosis (凋亡). The pathological hallmarks of Parkinson's disease are loss of dopaminergic neurons in the substantia nigra pars compacta (SNpc, 致密部) and accumulation of misfolded α-synuclein, which is found in intra-cytoplasmic inclusions called Lewy

医药大学堂
WWW.YIYAODXT.COM

bodies. In parkinsonism, the concentration of dopamine in the basal ganglia of the brain is reduced, and pharmacologic approach is to restore dopaminergic activity or restore the normal balance of cholinergic and dopaminergic influences on the basal ganglia. Currently approved pharmacological treatments for PD, mainly including levodopa, dopaminergic receptor agonists and monoamine oxidase-B (MAO-B, 单胺氧化酶-B) inhibitors, fail to halt disease progression and provide only symptomatic relief.

Levodopa (左旋多巴)

【 Pharmacokinetics 】 After administration, levodopa is rapidly absorbed from the small intestine, and then decarboxylated to dopamine by L-aromatic amino acid decarboxylase. Plasma concentration usually peaks between 0.2 and 2 hours after an oral dose, and the plasma half-life is usually between 1 and 2 hours. The absorption of levodopa depends on the rate of gastric emptying and the pH of the gastric juice (胃液). The delayed gastric emptying and increased acidity in the stomach decrease the bioavailability of levodopa. Only about 1% of administered levodopa eventually enter the brain, where it is decarboxylated to dopamine. The rest of levodopa is metabolized extracerebrally, mainly by decarboxylation to dopamine, which can not cross the blood-brain barrier and cause adverse reactions. If used in combination with peripheral L-aromatic amino acid decarboxylase inhibitors (L-芳香族氨基酸脱羧酶抑制剂) such as carbidopa or benzrazide, the peripheral metabolism of levodopa are reduced, and more dopamine is available for entry into the brain. Levodopa is mainly metabolized in the liver and excreted by the kidneys.

【 Pharmacodynamics 】 Levodopa, the immediate metabolic precursor of dopamine, can enter the brain via an L-amino acid transporter, where it is decarboxylated (脱羧) to dopamine and does the therapeutic effect on parkinsonism. However, if given into the peripheral circulation, dopamine itself does not cross the blood-brain barrier (血脑屏障).

【 Clinical indications 】

(1) Parkinson's disease Levodopa is used alone or in combination with carbidopa to treat Parkinson's disease. The clinical efficacy is related to the severity of nigrostriatal dopaminergic neurodegeneration, which is better for mild and young patients, but worse for severe and elderly patients. It is more effective for patients with muscle rigidity and bradykinesia, but less effective for patients with muscle tremor. The onset of action is slow, and the early stage of medication is remarkable. After 2 to 3 weeks of medication, the symptoms of patients improved significantly, and the maximum effect were obtained after 1 to 6 months of medication. However, the benefits of levodopa treatment often begin to diminish after 3 to 5 years of treatment, and the reasons may be related to the progressive degeneration and loss of dopaminergic nerves in the nigro-striatum, down-regulation of receptors, and other compensational mechanisms.

Levodopa can also improve many of the clinical motor features of parkinsonism, but it is not effective for extrapyramidal reactions (锥体外系反应) caused by antipsychotics such as phenothiazines. As phenothiazines can block dopamine receptors in the brain, which inhibit the function of levodopa.

(2) Hepatic coma Levodopa can also be used for hepatic coma (肝昏迷) caused by acute liver failure.

【 Adverse reactions 】

(1) Gastrointestinal effects When levodopa is given without a peripheral decarboxylase inhibitor, anorexia (食欲缺乏), nausea and vomiting often occur in patients. The vomiting probably attributes to stimulation of D_2 receptor in the chemoreceptor trigger zone (CTZ, 催吐化学感受区) and gastrointestinal irritation effect of dopamine. When levodopa is used in combination with peripheral decarboxylase inhibitor carbidopa, adverse gastrointestinal effects are much less frequent. After continuing treatment, the adverse gastrointestinal effects tend to diminish. Peptic ulcer bleeding and perforation rarely occur.

(2) Cardiovascular effects Because of the increased catecholamine formation peripherally, adverse cardiovascular effects including tachycardia (心动过速), ventricular extrasystoles (室性期前收缩), and atrial fibrillation. Postural hypotension (体位性低血压) is common, and tends to diminish with continuing treatment.

(3) Mental disorders A wide variety of adverse mental effects may occur, including anxiety, insomnia, nightmares, hallucinations, delusions, depression, mild mania and etc. It may be necessary to reduce or withdraw the medication in severe cases.

(4) Dyskinesias and response fluctuations It has been reported dyskinesias in patients with long term use of levodopa. The common presentation is choreoathetosis (舞蹈徐动症) of the face and distal extremities. Wheezing or excessive exhalation occasionally occur. These are attributed to increase in dopamine concentration in the striatum and overexcited of DA receptors.

(5) Response fluctuations Increasing frequency of fluctuations (症状波动) occurs with continuing treatment of levodopa. In some patients, the fluctuations relate to the timing of levodopa intake (wearing-off reactions or end-of-dose akinesia). In other patients, fluctuations are unrelated to the timing of doses (on-off phenomenon). In the on-off phenomenon, off-periods of marked akinesia alternate over the course of a few hours with on-periods of improved mobility but often marked dyskinesia. The occurrence of dyskinesia may due to decrease of dopamine in the striatum. However, the exact mechanism is still unknown.

Carbidopa (卡比多巴)

Carbidopa is a peripheral aromatic-L-amino-acid decarboxylase (芳香族 L– 氨基酸脱羧酶 , AADC) inhibitor, and it is generally administered in combination with levodopa. This agent reduces peripheral metabolism to dopamine and increases the concentration of L-DOPA and dopamine in the brain. Carbidopa does not cross the blood-brain barrier, and can not be used to treat parkinsonism alone.

Selegiline (司来吉兰)

Selegiline is a monoamine oxidase inhibitor, and selectively inhibit monoamine oxidase B in the brain. Selegiline can cross the blood-brain barrier quickly after administered, andirreversibly inhibit MAO-B, and retards the breakdown of dopamine in nigra-striatum. Meanwhile, its metabolite L-methamphetamine can inhibit the reuptake of dopamine and promote the release of dopamine, which increases the dopamine concentration in the striatum and prolongs the action time. Another metabolite desmethylselegiline may have neuroprotective antiapoptotic properties.

Selegiline is also an antioxidant (抗氧化剂) that inhibits the production of superoxide anions and hydroxyl radicals during the oxidative stress of dopamine in the nigra-striatum, and protect nigro neurons and delay neuronal degeneration.

Used independently, selegiline exhibits little therapeutic benefit. However, when given in combination with levodopa, it enhances and prolongs the antiparkinsonism of levodopa and may reduce mild on-off or wearing-off phenomena, and reduce the dose of levodopa.

Tolcapone (托卡朋) and entacapone (恩他卡朋)

Tolcapone and entacapone are the second generation catechol-O-methyltransferase (COMT, 儿茶酚胺-O-甲基转移酶) inhibitors. COMT can increase plasma levels of 3-O-methyldopa (3-OMD, 3-O-甲基多巴), which may inhibit the transportation of levodopa and is associated with poor therapeutic response to levodopa. Tolcapone does not cross the blood-brain barrier and inhibit the peripheral COMT. Entacapone can cross the blood-brain barrier, that inhibit the peripheral and central COMT. When used in combination with levodopa, selective COMT inhibitors such as tolcapone and entacapone can prolong the action of levodopa by decreasing its peripheral metabolism, and decrease the clearance of the levodopa. The bioavailability of levodopa is increased. These drugs can alleviate the on-off phenomenon in patients who receiving levodopa, and prolong on-time, and reduce off-time.

Bromocriptine (溴隐亭)

Bromocriptine is an agonist of D_2 dopamine receptors and has been used as a treatment for Parkinson's disease in the past, but now is rarely used for this purpose. It has been used to treat prolactin-related reproductive system dysfunction, such as amenorrhea (闭经), galactorrhea, premenstrual syndrome, puerperal mastitis, fibrocystic breast tumor.

Ropinirole (罗匹尼罗) and pramipexole (普拉克索)

Ropinirole can directly stimulate both D_1 and D_2 receptors, and pramipexole shows high affinity for the D_3 family of receptors. These agents have been used widely for parkinsonism. They are effective as monotherapy for mild parkinsonism. When used in combination with levodopa, they are helpful in patients with advanced disease and smooth out response fluctuations.

Amantadine (金刚烷胺)

Amantadine, an antiviral agent, also shows relatively weak antiparkinsonism properties. It can improve dopaminergic function by influencing the synthesis, release, or reuptake of dopamine. Amantadine is less efficacious than levodopa, and often used in combination with levodopa. It is used for the treatment of parkinsonism, and has an improvement effect on bradykinesia, rigidity, dyskinesia, myotonia, and tremor of parkinsonism. It has a number of central nervous system side effects, include restlessness, depression, irritability, insomnia, agitation, excitement, hallucinations, and confusion.

Benzhexol (苯海索)

Benzhexol, also named artane, is well absorbed orally and easily cross the blood-brain barrier. Benzhexol is a central acetylcholine-blocking drug (中枢乙酰胆碱阻断剂). It has a remarkable therapeutic effect on tremors of parkinsonism, encephalitis, and arteriosclerosis, but it has a weak effect on muscle rigidity and slow movement. It is effective for mild parkinsonism. Benzhexol is less efficacious than levodopa, but it can be used as an adjuvant for levodopa, or those who cannot tolerate levodopa. It can be used to treat extrapyramidal adverse reactions caused by antipsychotics such as chlorpromazine. And its axial anticholinergic effect is weak, with the potency only 1/10 – 1/3 of atropine.

2. Agents used in Alzheimer's disease

Dementia is a broad category of brain diseases that cause a long-term and often gradual decrease in the ability to memory, thinking, language, judgment and behavior. The most common types of dementia include Alzheimer's disease, vascular dementia, lewy body dementia, Parkinson's disease, frontotemporal dementia and dementia induced by other nervous system diseases. AD is the most common cause of dementia, and accounts for about 70% of dementia. AD is characterized by a progressive cognitive decline. AD is associated with brain shrinkage and localized loss of neurons, mainly in the hippocampus and basal forebrain. The loss of cholinergic neurons in the hippocampus and frontal cortex is a feature of the disease, and is thought to underlie the cognitive deficit and loss of short-term memory that occur in AD. This is associated with reduced choline acetyltransferase activity and decline of central acetylcholine level. In AD, another key player is often thought to be amyloid-β (Aβ) peptide. The second form of proteinaceous deposit in the AD brain, the neurofibrillary tangle (NFT, 神经纤维缠结), is comprised of polymers of a hyperpohosphorylated form of the microtubule associated protein tau, and this may be the main downstream effector of neuronal death. The amount of NFTs in the cerebral cortex correlates strongly with cognitive decline. The "neuritic plaque", which includes both the extracellular Aβ deposition and a surrounding penumbra of degenerating neurites with pathologically-folded tau, are the most specific histopathological lesions of AD. Meanwhile, other neurotransmitter (e.g., serotonin, dopamine, norepinephrine, glutamate) abnormalities are also thought to be correlated with progress of AD.

Currently, cholinesterase inhibitors (e.g., tacrine, donepezil, rivastigmine and galantamine) and memantine are the only drugs approved for treating AD.

2.1　Central acetylcholinesterase inhibitors（中枢胆碱酯酶抑制药）

Central acetylcholinesterase inhibitors are thought to be important for treating AD because there is a reduction in activity of the cholinergic neurons. Acetylcholinesterase (AChE)-inhibitors reduce the rate at which acetylcholine (ACh) is broken down and hence increase the concentration of ACh in the brain (combatting the loss of ACh caused by the death of the cholinergic neurons).

Donepezil（多奈哌齐）

Donepezil is a second generation acetylcholinesterase inhibitor, that completely inhibits central AChE and increase the content of ACh. The efficacy has been demonstrated against patients with mild, moderate, and severe AD patients. Donepezil is rapidly absorbed orally, and the bioavailability is about 100%. It is mainly metabolized by the liver and the metabolites also show anti-AD activity, with the half-life about 70 hours. Common adverse effects include cardiovascular conditions, nausea, vomiting, peptic ulcer disease (消化性溃疡), gastrointestinal bleeding, genitourinary conditions (泌尿生殖系统疾病), neurological conditions, pulmonary conditions and etc.

Rivastigmine (卡巴拉汀)

Rivastigmine is a second generation acetylcholinesterase inhibitor. It is rapidly absorbed orally, and the plasma protein binding rate is about 40%. Rivastigmine easily crosses the blood-brain barrier. Studies have shown that it can selectively inhibit AChE activity in the cerebral cortex and hippocampus of rats, but have weak inhibition of AChE activity in the striatum and pontine, without any resistance to anti-AChE effects. Rivastigmine can improve cholinergic-mediated cognitive dysfunction in AD patients, improve cognitive abilities, such as memory, attention, and sense of direction. It can also reduce the production of Aβ precursor protein (APP, Aβ 前体蛋白). Rivastigmine tartrate capsules are indicated for the treatment of mild-to-moderate dementia of the Alzheimer's type. The main adverse reactions include nausea, vomiting, fatigue, dizziness, mental breakdown, drowsiness (嗜睡), abdominal pain and diarrhea, and etc.

Huperzine A (石杉碱–甲)

Huperzine A is a natural plant-based neuroprotectant (神经保护剂). It is an alkaloid that is extracted from Chinese club moss Huperzia serrata by Chinese researchers. Huperzine A can improve memory by improving brain levels of acetylcholine by inhibiting the production of acetylcholinesterase. The drug is rapidly absorbed orally, and bioavailability is about 96.9%. It is easy to cross the blood-brain barrier. Prototype drugs and metabolites are mainly eliminated from the kidney. Huperzine A appears to be safe and well tolerated when took in moderation. Common adverse effects include nausea, dizziness, sweating, abdominal pain, blurred vision, and etc.

2.2   Muscarinic acetylcholine receptor agonist (M乙酰胆碱受体激动剂)

Xanomeline (呫诺美林)

Xanomeline is a muscarinic acetylcholine receptor agonist with selectivity for the M_1 and M_4 subtypes. Xanomeline is well absorbed orally, crosses the blood-brain barrier, and undergoes extensive liver metabolism with at least six metabolites. It is distributed mainly in the cerebral cortex (大脑皮质) and striatum (纹状体). When orally given at a high dosage, it can remarkably improve the cognitive function and behavioral abilities of AD patients. The common adverse effects include gastrointestinal adverse effects and cardiovascular adverse reactions. As a result of hypotensive episodes and other adverse effects the oral formulation have been discontinued.

2.3   NMDA receptor antagonists (NMDA受体拮抗剂)

Memantine (美金刚)

Memantine is also approved for the treatment of AD, and it is an orally active weak antagonist at N-methyl-D-aspartate (NMDA, N- 甲基 -D- 天冬氨酸) receptors. It can work by selectively inhibiting excessive, pathological NMDA receptor activation while preserving more physiological activation. It can improve the cognitive ability in moderate or severe AD. The adverse effects of memantine include headache, dizziness, drowsiness, constipation, shortness of breath and hypertension as well as a raft of less common problems.

重 点 小 结

类别	药物	药理作用	临床应用	不良反应
抗帕金森病药	多巴胺前体药：左旋多巴	进入脑组织的左旋多巴，经脑内AADC脱羧转化为DA，补充纹状体DA的不足，产生抗帕金森病作用	帕金森病、肝昏迷	胃肠道反应、心血管反应、精神障碍、运动障碍、症状波动
	左旋多巴增效剂：卡比多巴	单独应用卡比多巴无治疗作用，其与左旋多巴合用时，可减少左旋多巴在外周被AADC脱羧转化为DA的数量，使较多的左旋多巴进入中枢而发挥作用	常与左旋多巴按剂量比1∶10组成复方多巴制剂，治疗帕金森病	—

目 标 检 测

题库

一、单项选择题

1. 与左旋多巴合用，可降低其疗效并加重其不良反应的是（　　　）
   A. 卡比多巴　　　B. 苄丝肼　　　　C. 氯丙嗪　　　　D. 东莨菪碱　　　　E. 司来吉兰
2. 左旋多巴治疗帕金森病的机制是（　　　）
   A. 增加脑内DA含量　　　　　B. 激动中枢DA受体　　　　C. 阻断中枢M受体
   D. 抑制外周脱羧酶活性　　　　E. 激动中枢M受体
3. 应用左旋多巴早期最常见的不良反应是（　　　）
   A. 胃肠道反应　　B. 精神障碍　　　C. 运动障碍　　　D. 症状波动　　　E. 肌肉震颤

二、思考题

左旋多巴治疗帕金森病的特点和机制是什么？

（董世芬）

PPT

Chapter 13   Antiepileptic drugs

 学习目标

1. **掌握** 治疗癫痫大发作、失神性发作、精神运动性发作及癫痫持续状态的首选药物。

2. **熟悉** 常用抗癫痫药苯妥英钠、乙琥胺、丙戊酸钠、地西泮的药理作用、临床应用及主要不良反应。

3. **了解** 苯妥英钠的药物代谢动力学特点及用药注意事项。

Epilepsy (癫痫) is a very common disorder, characterized by spontaneous recurring seizures, which take various forms and result from episodic neuronal discharges, the form of the seizure depending on the part of the brain affected. During the epileptic attack, the neurons in the local focus of the brain showed paroxysmal (阵发性) abnormal high-frequency discharge and spread to the surrounding areas, resulting in the transient dysfunction of the brain. Epilepsy is not a single entity, but is a family of different recurrent seizure diseases that have identically sudden, excessive and synchronous discharge of cerebral neurons. According to the clinical manifestations, epilepsy can be divided into two broad categories: partial and generalized syndromes.

1. Classification of epilepsy

1.1   Partial seizures (部分性发作)

(1) Simple partial seizures (单纯部分性发作)   Diverse manifestations determined by the region of cortex activated by seizure, which mainly show local limb movement and sensory abnormality for lasting approximate 20-60 seconds. Main characteristic is preservation of consciousness.

(2) Complex partial seizures (复杂部分性发作或精神运动性发作)   Impaired consciousness lasting 30 seconds to 2 minutes, often related to unconscious movements, such as smacking or head shaking.

1.2   Generalized seizures (全身性发作)

(1) Absence seizures (失神性发作)   A sudden loss of consciousness associated with high-voltage,

医药大学堂
WWW.YIYAODXT.COM

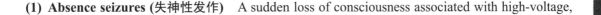

bilaterally synchronous, 3Hz-persecond spike and wave pattern in ECG, usually with some symmetrical clonic motor activity varying from eyelid blinking to jerking of the entire body.

(2) **Myoclonic seizures (肌阵挛性发作)** A transient (perhaps a second) shock-like contraction of muscles which may be restricted to part of one extremity or may be generalized.

(3) **Tonic-clonic seizures (强直–阵挛性发作)** Sudden loss of consciousness, generalized tonic-clonic convulsion, followed by a long period of comprehensive inhibition of central nervous system function, lasted for several minutes, and EEG showed high amplitude spike slow wave or spike wave.

(4) **Status epilepticus (癫痫持续状态)** Recurrent generalized tonic-clonic seizures without recovery of consciousness, dangerous to life.

2. Mechanism of epilepsy

The normal function of the central nervous system depends on a balance of excitatory and inhibitory effects. If excitation exceeds inhibition, the central nervous system tends to be hyper-excitable and the epilepsy might be produced. The most important inhibitory neurotransmitter in the brain is γ-aminobutyric acid (GABA, γ–氨基丁酸). GABA can bind to GABA receptors, which are coupled tochloride channels, and are one of the main targets of alleviating the seizure. Benzodiazepines can hyperpolarize the GABA neuron by activation of GABA receptor and result in inhibitory effects of antiepileptic and anticonvulsant.

The activation of the N-methyl-D-aspartate (NMDA, N-甲基-D-天冬氨酸) receptor is increased in several animal models of epilepsy. Some patients with epilepsy may have an inherited predisposition for faster or longer-lasting activation of NMDA channels, resulting in alteration of seizure threshold.

Sodium channel mutation, potassium channel mutation, and nicotinic acetylcholine receptor mutation are connected with a convulsion. Patients with epilepsy display elevated levels of antibody against glutamate receptor subunit. The antibody may trigger an inflammatory response that looks like encephalitis (脑炎). Some partial epilepsies in adults may be caused by focal inflammation.

At present, epilepsy treatment is still dominated by drugs, patients often need long-term medication to reduce or prevent seizures. In the extended treatment, the drug is often forced to stop or change because of its tolerance and adverse reactions.

The mechanism of antiepileptic drugs is mainly through three aspects (Figure 13-1): ①Enhance the function of GABA-ergic nerve. ②Interfering with the function of Na^+ and Ca^{2+} channels of nerve cells, so as to reduce the excitability of nerve cell membrane. ③Decreasing the conduction of excitatory glutamatergic nerve.

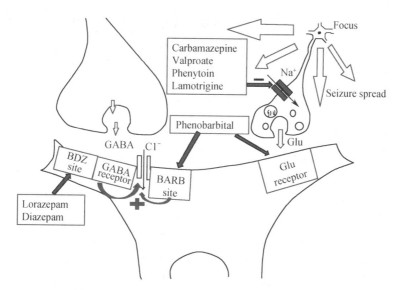

Figure 13-1　The mechanism of antiepileptic drugs

GABA, γ-aminobutyric acid; Glu, glutamic acid; BDZ, benzodiazepines; BARB, barbiturates (Michael J. Neal. Medical pharmacology at a glance. 4th ed.)

3. Antiepileptic agents

Phenytoin sodium (苯妥英钠)

【Pharmacokinetics】Phenytoin has slow and irregular oral absorptions and its bioavailability is approximately 95%, and the peak level after oral administration is reached in approximately 4-12 hours. It is 70%-95% bound to plasma protein, and is metabolized in the liver by the hepatic P450 mixed oxidase system and discharged by the kidney.

【Pharmacodynamics】Phenytoin blocks inward Na^+ current during propagation of the action potential, and therefore prevents post tetanic potentiation (强直后增强), limits development of maximal seizure activity, and reduces the spread of seizures. Phenytoin also shows an inhibitory effect on calcium channels and the sequestration of Ca^{2+} in nerve terminals, thereby inhibiting voltage-dependent neurotransmission at the level of the synapse.

【Clinical indications】Phenytoin is one of the most commonly used first-line drug or adjunctive treatments for most types of seizures (grand mal and psychomotor epilepsy), except absence seizures (petit mal). It exerts antiepileptic activity without causing general depression of the central nervous system.

Phenytoin can be used for some trigeminal neuralgia (三叉神经痛), glossopharyngeal neuralgia (舌咽神经痛)and sciatic neuralgia(坐骨神经痛), but carbamazepine(卡马西平) may be preferable.

The use of phenytoin in the treatment of cardiac arrhythmias (心律失常) is discussed in relative Chapters.

【Adverse reactions】Dose-relative adverse effects caused by phenytoin are nausea and vomiting, rash, blood dyscrasias (血性恶病质), headaches, vitamin K and folate deficiencies (叶酸缺乏), loss of libido (性欲减退), hormonal dysfunction, and bone marrow hypoplasia(骨髓抑制). Gingival hyperplasia (thickening of the gums, 齿龈增生) is the main concern associated with this drug.

Carbamazepine (卡马西平)

【Pharmacokinetics】Carbamazepine is a crystalline substance that is insoluble in water, which limits the route to oral administration. The absorption of carbamazepine was slow and irregular, reaching the peak of blood concentration in about 2-4 hours. Approximately 75%-85% of the drug is plasma protein bound, and it has a free fraction of 20%-24% of the total plasma concentration. The elimination half-life ranges from 5 to 26 hours and is shortened after repeated treatment in healthy volunteers and patients with epilepsy because of induction of hepatic cytochrome P450 system activity.

【Pharmacodynamics】Carbamazepine is similar to that of phenytoin. Carbamazepine blocks sodium channels at therapeutic concentrations and inhibits the high frequency discharge of epileptic focus. Postsynaptic transmission (突触后传递) action of GABA can be enhanced by carbamazepine.

【Clinical indications】Carbamazepine is a broad-spectrum antiepileptic drug, which has different degrees of efficacy for various types of epilepsy. It has good efficacy for psychomotor seizures and grand mal, and is less effective in the treatment of petit mal (absence seizures).

【Adverse reactions】Carbamazepine can produce dose-related adverse effects, which include dizziness, diplopia, nausea, ataxia, and blurred vision. Rare idiosyncratic adverse effects include aplastic anemia (再生障碍性贫血), agranulocytosis (粒细胞缺乏), and thrombocytopenia (血小板减少).

Phenobarbital (苯巴比妥)

【Pharmacokinetics】Phenobarbital is a powerful inducer of the hepatic microsomal enzymes. It has an oral or intramuscular bioavailability of 80%-100% in adults. Time to peak plasma level is 1-3 hours, but it may be delayed after oral administration in patients with poor gastrointestinal motility.

【Pharmacodynamics】Phenobarbital has a direct action on $GABA_A$ receptors by binding to the barbiturate-binding site that prolongs the duration of chloride channel opening. It also reduces sodium and potassium conductance and calcium influx and depresses glutamate excitability. In all, it can inhibit not only the abnormal discharge of the focus, but also the diffusion of abnormal discharge.

【Clinical indications】Phenobarbital has the similar effects to phenytoin and carbamazepine in the treatment of partial and secondarily generalized seizures. Phenobarbital is effective in a wide variety of seizures and is a second-line drug because of its adverse effects such as sedation and cognitive slowing. Nevertheless, phenobarbital is not indicated in the treatment of absence seizures.

【Adverse reactions】Sedation is prominent, particularly at the beginning of therapy. Psychomotor slowing, poor concentration, depression, irritability, ataxia (共济失调), and decreased libido are adverse reactions. Long-term use of phenobarbital may be associated with tolerance. Occasionally, megaloblastic anemia (巨幼红细胞性贫血), leukopenia (白细胞减少) and thrombocytopenia (血小板减少) may occur.

Primidone (扑米酮)

Primidone is a slight variant of the phenobarbital molecule. In the body, it is biotransformed into phenobarbital, and much of its therapeutic effect probably depends on the phenobarbital produced, although the parent compound may have some therapeutic effects of its own. Its disadvantages are like phenobarbital, including sedating, etc.

Sodium valproate (丙戊酸钠)

【Pharmacodynamics】Sodium valproate is a broad-spectrum antiepileptic drug and effective for all types of epilepsy. It has multiple mechanisms of action, including enhancing GABA-ergic tone in the substantial nigra (黑质), limiting sustained repetitive firing, or modulate excitatory amino acid neurotransmission. It may have a great effect on inhibiting GABA transaminase at very high concentrations, thus increasing levels of GABA by inhibiting GABA metabolism. It could inactivate voltage-dependent Na^+ channel, reduce T-type Ca^{2+} current, and inhibit abnormal firing originated from thalamus (丘脑).

【Clinical indications】Valproate is a broad-spectrum anti-seizure drug effective in the treatment of absence, myoclonic, partial, and tonic-clonic seizuers. Similar to phenytoin and carbamazepine, valproate inhibits tonic hind limb extension in maximal electroshock seizures and kindled extension in maximal electroshock seizures and kindled seizures at nontoxic doses. Valproate is very effective against absence seizures. Although ethosuximide is the drug of choice when absence seizure occurs alone, valproate is preferred if the patient has concomitant generalized tonic-clonic attacts.

【Adverse reactions】The most common side effects are transient gastrointestinal symptoms, including anorexia (食欲缺乏), nausea, and vomiting. Other effects include sedation, ataxia and tremor. The primary risk of fatal hepatic dysfunction occurs in children under 2 years of age that are receiving this drug. Neural tube defects may occur in the offspring of woman who took valproate during pregnancy.

Benzodiazepines (苯二氮䓬类)

The benzodiazepines are used primarily as sedative and anti-anxiety drugs, and a large number of benzodiazepines have broad anti-seizure properties. Diazepam (地西泮) and lorazepam (劳拉西泮) administered intravenously are used for all varieties of status epilepticus, but they are not recommended for chronic usage, because of its rapid development of tolerance.

Clonazepam (氯硝西泮) has higher affinity for the GABA receptor site than diazepam and have some action on Na^+ channel conductance. Clonazepam is a potent drug for myoclonic seizures and subcortical myoclonus, It is also effective in generalized convulsions and, to a lesser extent, in partial epilepsies. It is very effective in the emergency treatment of status epilepticus, like diazepam, and can be given intravenously or rectally.

Ethosuximide (乙琥胺)

Ethosuximide is particularly effective on absence seizures. It can reduce the T-type Ca^{2+} currents in thalamic neurons responsible for generating the rhythmic discharge of an absence attack. Ethosuximide was absorbed rapidly by oral administration, and the concentration of ethosuximide reached the peak 3 hours later. *In vivo*, the binding rate with plasma protein is low, about 1/4 of ethosuximide is excreted in prototype, and the rest is metabolized by liver and excreted by kidney.

Lamotrigine (拉莫三嗪)

Lamotrigine is a benzotriazine compound that is chemically unrelated to any of the other antiepileptic drugs. Its major Pharmacodynamics is to block voltage-dependent sodium-channel conductance by inhibiting depolarization of the glutaminergic presynaptic membrane (谷氨酸能神经突触前膜), thus inhibiting release of glutamate.

Lamotrigine is effective in partial onset and secondarily generalized tonic-clonic seizures, primary generalized seizures, atypical absence seizures, and tonic/atonic seizures.

Severe rash may develop and occasionally lead to Stevens-Johnson syndrome, which may be fatal. Other commonly reported adverse reactions are blood dyscrasias, ataxia, diplopia, psychosis, tremor, somnolence, and insomnia.

4. Rational use of antiepileptic drugs and general principles for the therapy of the epilepsies

4.1 Definite diagnosis before treating commence

Before starting therapy, it is important to rule out pseudo-seizures (假性癫痫发作) (not uncommon), poisoning, or primary disease. If a primary disease is present (e.g., a tumor, an infection), this should be treated, not the seizures. In addition, before initiating therapy, it is important to make sure that the seizure problem is chronic. Occasionally people have a single seizure that is never repeated. Before therapy is started, the type of seizure must be carefully established.

4.2 Choice of medication

Different types need different drugs. Early diagnosis and treatment of seizure disorders with a single appropriate agent offers the best prospect of achieving prolonged seizure-free periods with the lowest risk of toxicity.

4.3 Determination of increase dosage or combine medication

Treatment is begin with a single drug. If the drug of choice is not effective, another single drug is tried. Eventually, if the patient has very resistant seizures, or more than one seizure type, polypharmacy may be attempted.

4.4 Determining whether to stop or reduce the dosage

If a patient has had no seizures for several years, drugs may be slowly withdrawn according to the seizure threshold being normalized. Patients outgrow some types of childhood attacks and even adults occasionally cease to have seizures. Antiseizure drugs should not be withdrawn quickly because rebound exacerbation of seizure may occur.

4.5 Monitoring of medicine use

Measurement of plasma drug concentration at appropriate intervals greatly facilitates the initial adjustment of dosage to minimize dose-related adverse effects without sacrificing seizure control. If toxicity occurs, monitoring helps to identify the particular drugs responsible and can guide adjustment of dosage.

重 点 小 结

药物	药理作用	临床应用	不良反应
苯妥英钠	阻断钠通道、钙通道，抑制病灶高频放电的扩散	癫痫大发作、神经疼痛、心律失常	胃肠道反应、巨幼红细胞性贫血、齿龈增生
卡马西平	膜稳定作用，抑制病灶放电	广谱抗癫痫，用于精神运动性发作、抗躁狂	眩晕、视物模糊、骨髓抑制、肝损伤
丙戊酸钠	抑制 GABA 代谢，抑制钠通道、钙通道	广谱抗癫痫，用于肌阵挛性发作	肝损伤
乙琥胺	抑制钙通道	小发作首选	头痛、头晕、粒细胞减少

目 标 检 测

题库

一、单项选择题

1. 用于癫痫持续状态的首选药是（ ）
   A. 硫喷妥钠静脉注射　　　　　B. 苯妥英钠肌内注射　　　　C. 地西泮静脉注射
   D. 戊巴比妥钠肌内注射　　　　E. 水合氯醛灌肠
2. 治疗癫痫大发作及部分性发作最有效的药物是（ ）
   A. 地西泮　　B. 苯巴比妥　　C. 苯妥英钠　　D. 乙琥胺　　E. 乙酰唑胺
3. 治疗癫痫小发作的首选药是（ ）
   A. 乙琥胺　　B. 苯妥英钠　　C. 苯巴比妥钠　　D. 扑米酮　　E. 地西泮
4. 对癫痫失神小发作疗效最好的药物是（ ）
   A. 乙琥胺　　B. 卡马西平　　C. 扑米酮　　D. 丙戊酸钠　　E. 苯妥英钠
5. 对各种类型的癫痫发作均有效的药物是（ ）
   A. 苯巴比妥　　B. 苯妥英钠　　C. 丙戊酸钠　　D. 乙琥胺　　E. 地西泮
6. 对癫痫大发作或小发作均无效,且可诱发癫痫的药物是（ ）
   A. 苯妥英钠　　B. 地西泮　　C. 苯巴比妥　　D. 氯丙嗪　　E. 水合氯醛

二、思考题

简述抗癫痫药的临床应用原则。

（徐志立）

Chapter 14　Opioid analgesics

 学习目标

　　1. **掌握**　镇痛药的概念、分类；吗啡、哌替啶的药理作用及机制、临床应用和不良反应。

　　2. **熟悉**　可待因、美沙酮、喷他佐辛、曲马多、罗通定、纳洛酮、纳曲酮的主要药理作用和临床应用。

　　3. **了解**　吗啡衍生物的构效关系。

1. Overview

Pain (疼痛), a subjective experience, is defined as an unpleasant sensory and emotional experience associated with actual or potential tissue damage. The treatment plan of pain depends on the classes and the states of pain. Analgesics (镇痛药) is a class of agents that relieve pain. Opioids (阿片样物质) are a mainstay of pain treatment, they are natural, semisynthetic, or synthetic compounds that produce morphine-like effects. An opioid is any agent, regardless of structure, that has the functional and pharmacological properties of an opiate (阿片制剂). Because they work on the central nervous system and induce narcosis (麻醉) or sleep, opioid analgesics also are called narcotic analgesics (麻醉性镇痛药).

1.1　Opioids and opioid receptors

Opiates refer to compounds related to the structure of products in opium (阿片). Opiates include natural plant alkaloids, such as morphine, codeine, and many semisynthetic derivatives. Endogenic opioid peptides are called endogenous opioid peptides (内阿片肽) or endorphin (内啡肽) because many of them are peptides. They are natural ligands for opioid receptors.

Three subfamilies (亚家族) of opioid receptors, μ, δ, κ receptors, are widely distributed (Table 14-1). Their profound and diverse effects on the function of the CNS are consistent with the density and distribution of receptors. In addition, these receptors are expressed in periphery. μ, δ, and κ receptors are members of G protein-coupled family of receptors (G-蛋白偶联受体) and inhibit adenylyl cyclase (腺苷酸环化酶).

Table 14-1　Summary of opioid receptors

Receptor	Effects						
	Analgesia sites	Depress respiratory	Miosis	Gut	Euphoria	Sedation	Addiction
μ	Brain cord periphery	+++	++	++	+++	++	+++
δ	Cord	++	−	++	−	−	−
κ	Periphery cord	+	+	+	−	++ Dysphoria	+

The analgesic properties of opioids are mainly related to μ receptors, which can effectively regulate the response to various nociception (伤害性刺激), including thermal stimulus, mechanical or chemical stimulus. By controlling responses to chemical and thermal injury, κ receptors that located in the dorsal horn (背角) also contribute to analgesia. In the periphery, δ receptors has high selectivity to a endorphin which called encephalin (脑啡肽). Since opioids may act as full agonists, moderate agonists, partial agonists or mixed agonists in a receptor or its subtypes, it is not surprising that opioids analgesics have different pharmacological effects.

1.2　Mechanism of analgesia

1.2.1　Nociception

Acute activation of small high threshold sensory nerve afferents (传入神经) produces temporary input to the spinal cord (脊髓), which in turn activates neurons projected contralaterally to the thalamus (丘脑) and somatosensory cortex (躯体感觉皮质). A parallel spin fugal projection (投射) is the medial thalamus (丘脑内侧), which activates the anterior cingulate cortex (前扣带皮质) of the limbic system (边缘系统). The output generated by violently activating the ascending system (上行系统) is enough to evoke a painful reports.

1.2.2　Mechanism of analgesia

Opioids produce analgesia (镇痛作用) similar to that of endogenous opioid peptides by binding to opioid receptors. Opioid receptors, as a member of the membrane receptor family, are related to ion channels on the membrane, increase K^+ efflux (钾离子外流) (hyperpolarization, 超极化) and reduce presynaptic (突触前膜) Ca^{2+} influx (钙离子内流), regulate intracellular concentration of K^+ and Ca^{2+}. Then the membrane potential (细胞膜电位) of neurons is changed to inhibit the release of neurotransmitters (神经递质) such as glutamate (谷氨酸), norepinephrine (去甲肾上腺素), serotonin (5-羟色胺) and substance P (P物质), and to inhibit the transfer of pain (Figure 14-1).

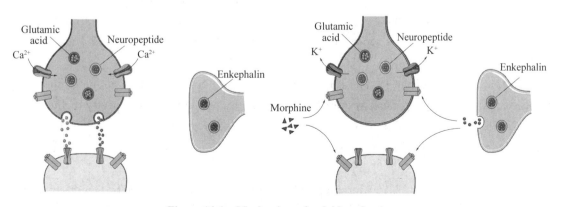

Figure 14-1　Mechanism of opioid analgesics

2. Full opioid agonists

Morphine (吗啡)

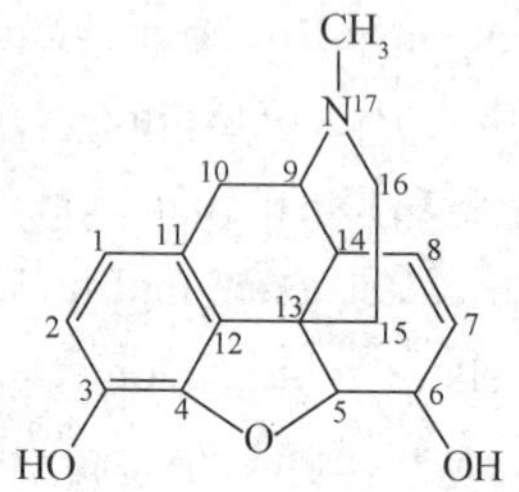

Since the early 19th century, morphine has been obtained from immature seed capsules of the poppy plant Papaver somniferum (罂粟). It is a typical opioid agonist named after Morpheus, the Greek god of the dreams. The structure of morphine is shown in Figure 14-2.

【Pharmacokinetics】 Generally speaking, opioids are well absorbed through subcutaneous or intramuscular pathways and moderately absorbed from the gastrointestinal tract (胃肠道). Morphine is available in suppositories (肛门栓) because it is sufficient to be absorbed through the rectal (直肠) mucosa. Morphine is also widely used in spinal

Figure 14-2 Chemical structure of morphine

cord delivery in order to produce analgesia. Although morphine has a significant effect on the CNS, it passes through the blood-brain barrier at a lower rate. Because of an important first metabolism (首过消除)in the liver, its oral bioavailability is only about 25%. The main pathway of morphine metabolism is conjugation with glucuronic acid (葡糖醛酸). Morphine is mainly eliminated by glomerular filtration (肾小球滤过), while very little morphine is unchanged in bile and feces. It passes through the blood placental barrier and secretes in breast milk.

【Pharmacodynamics】

(1) Central nervous system

1) Analgesia and sedation (镇痛和镇静) Morphine causes analgesia and relieves pain by raising the pain threshold at the spinal cord level, and more importantly, by changing the brain's perception of pain. It relieves pain without losing consciousness. Morphine produces a strong sense of satisfaction and happiness, known as euphoria (欣快感). The excitement may be caused by the release of dopamine neurons (多巴胺能神经元) in the ventral tegmental area(中脑腹侧被盖区). However, dysphoria (烦躁) sometimes may occur, an unpleasant state characterized by unease and discomfort. As a phenanthrene derivative (菲类衍生物), morphine causes obvious sedation, such as lethargy (嗜睡) or sleep. If used in conjunction with other central inhibitors (中枢抑制剂), morphine can lead to very deep sleep. Morphine is reported to disrupt normal REM sleep (快动眼睡眠) and non-REM sleep (非快动眼睡眠).

2) Respiratory inhibition (抑制呼吸) Morphine binds to opioid receptors in the brain stem and respiratory center, which can cause respiratory inhibition by reducing the sensitivity of the center to carbon dioxide (二氧化碳). This may occur in normal doses of morphine and is related to the doses. Respiratory inhibition is the most common cause of death in acute opioid overdose (吗啡过量).

3) Antitussive effect (镇咳) Morphine and codeine have antitussive effects. Generally speaking, the receptors involved in antitussive action are different from those involved in analgesia. The inhibition of morphine on cough may accumulate airway secretion, resulting in airway obstruction (气道阻塞).

4) Miosis (缩瞳)　Although morphine suppresses respiration, which can lead to pupil, the pinpoint pupil (针尖样瞳孔) is characteristic of morphine poisoning. This symptom is of great value in the diagnosis of morphine overdose. Pinpoint pupil is the result of stimulation of μ and κ receptors. There is a weak tolerance to this effect, and all morphine abusers may show pinpoint pupils.

5) Others　Morphine can directly stimulate the chemoreceptor trigger zone (催吐化学感受区) in the area postrema (延髓极后区) to cause nausea and vomiting.

(2) Smooth muscle

1) Gastrointestinal tract　Opioid receptors exist in the gastrointestinal tract with high density. Morphine activates the receptors, and reduces the movement of intestinal smooth muscle (胃肠道蠕动) and increases the tension of smooth muscle, resulting in constipation (便秘).

2) Biliary tract (胆道)　Due to contracting the gallbladder and constriction of the Odd's sphincter (奥迪括约肌), morphine can increase biliary tract pressure, which may result in biliary colic (胆绞痛).

(3) Cardiovascular system　Like most opioids, low doses of morphine has no significant effect on blood pressure or heart rate. High dose morphine is associated with respiratory inhibition (呼吸抑制) and carbon dioxide retention (二氧化碳潴留), which can induce hypotension and bradycardia (心动过缓). Morphine dilates cerebral blood vessels and increases cerebrospinal fluid pressure (颅内压). Therefore, it is usually prohibited in people with brain injury or head trauma.

(4) Others　Morphine increases the release of histamine from mast cells (肥大细胞), resulting in urticaria (荨麻疹), sweating and vasodilation. Because morphine contracts the bronchus, it should be used carefully in patients with asthma. Morphine can promote the release and secretion of growth hormone (生长激素) and prolactin (催乳素). It increases antidiuretic hormones (抗利尿激素) and leads to urinary retention.

【Clinical indications】

(1) Pain (疼痛)　Morphine has a significant analgesic effect and is used to treat pain, especially severe pain and advanced cancer (晚期癌症) pain. Morphine combined with muscarinic receptor blocker atropine can be used in the treatment of biliary or renal colic (胆、肾绞痛). Morphine can not only relieve pain, but also relieve nociceptive sensations or anxiety caused by emergencies.

(2) Cardiac asthma (心源性哮喘)　Although bronchial asthma is a contraindication (禁忌证) of morphine, it is an appropriate drug for patients with cardiac asthma. These effects may include reducing anxiety, improving tidal volume (潮气量) and pulmonary edema (肺水肿), and reducing cardiac preload and afterload.

(3) Diarrhea (腹泻)　Raw opiates can treat chronic unknown diarrhea. If diarrhea is associated with infection, chemotherapeutic drugs should be used.

(4) Cough (咳嗽)　Although certain opioid analgesics including morphine are effective antitussive agents, especially to dry cough, but for the addiction and drug abuse, they are not often used in recent years.

【Adverse reactions】

(1) Common adverse reactions　For opioids, many side-effects are common. In most μ agonists, severe respiratory inhibition may occur, and acute opioid overdose may lead to death. Respiratory motility (呼吸运动) may be suppressed in patients with emphysema (肺气肿)or corpulmonale (肺源性心

脏病). If opioids are used, breathing must be closely monitored. Especially in patients with head injury (颅脑损伤), serious elevated intracranial pressure may occur. Morphine should be used carefully in patients with asthma, liver disease or renal dysfunction.

(2) Tolerance and physical dependence   Repeated use can produce tolerance to respiratory inhibition, analgesia, excitement, and sedation of morphine. However, tolerance usually does not develop the drug effect of pupil contraction and constipation. Physical and psychological dependence can be controlled by morphine. Withdrawal can lead to a series of autonomous exercise and psychological responses, incapacitating people to work and causing serious symptoms, but these effects rarely leads to death.

(3) Others   The interaction between other drugs and morphine is rare. Although the depressant actions of morphine are enhanced by phenothiazines (吩噻嗪类), monoamine oxidase inhibitors (MAOIs, 单胺氧化酶抑制剂), and tricyclic antidepressants (三环类抗抑郁药).

Pethidine (哌替啶)

Pethidine, a κ agonist, has certain μ agonist activity and is a kind of low efficiency synthetic opioid independent of morphine structure. It is used for short-term treatment of acute pain, and pethidine is easier to pass through the blood brain barrier (血脑屏障) than morphine because of high lipophilicity (亲脂性), and then sometimes causes excitement in the CNS and even neurotoxicity. Peperidine can be absorbed by all administration routes, with the exception of intramuscular injection. Pethidine has an active metabolite, normeperidine (去甲哌替啶) which is renally excreted. Normeperidine can induce a toxicity of the central nervous system, such as mental disorder (精神障碍), hyperreflexia (反射亢进), myoclonus (肌阵挛), and may also lead to seizures (癫痫). Pethidine should not be used in elderly patients with renal insufficiency (肾功能不全), liver function insufficiency (肝功能不全) and respiratory disorder. Serotonin syndrome has also been reported in patients receiving both meperidine and certain serotonin reuptake inhibitors (5-羟色胺再摄取抑制剂).

Methadone (美沙酮)

Methadone is a synthetic, very lipophilic, oral effective, and long-acting opioid. The effect of methadone is mediated by μ receptor, so it is effective in the treatment of both nociceptive and neuropathic pain. Methadone has a similar analgesic effect compared with morphine. Methadone is also used to control the withdrawal of opioid and heroin addicts. Methadone is administrated parenterally or orally. It is easily absorbed after oral administration, is bio-transformed in the liver, and is excreted almost entirely in feces. Methadone increases bile pressure and leads to constipation, but less than what morphine does. During long-term use, it can produce lighter physical dependence, which is more persistent than other opioids.

Fentanyl (芬太尼)

Fentanyl is a synthetic opioid related to phenylpiperidines (苯基哌啶). It is highly lipophilic and shows characteristics of a rapid onset and short duration (维持时间短). In the liver, fentanyl is metabolized to inactivated metabolite (无活性代谢产物). Both the prototype drug and the inactive metabolites are removed through urine. Fentanyl is usually intravenously injected, epidurally, or intrathecal. Oral mucous membrane preparations and aseptic patches are also available. In addition to playing an important role in anesthesia, fentanyl is also used for the management of severe pain (剧痛). Adverse reactions include nausea, vomiting, excitement, addiction and muscle stiffness.

3.　Moderate opioid agonists

Codeine (可待因)

Codeine, also known as methylmorphine (甲基吗啡), is a natural opioid, compared with morphine, it is a weak analgesia. It is used only in mild to moderate pain and is usually used in combination with acetaminophen (对乙酰氨基酚). Codeine has good antitussive activity and the dose is less than that cause analgesia. It can be used as a central active antitussive drug (中枢性镇咳药) in dry cough patients. Compared with complete opioid agonists, codeine has similar ADRs, tolerance and dependence, which is slightly than that of morphine.

4.　Mixed opioid agonist-antagonists

Pentazocine (喷他佐辛)

Pentazocine acts as an agonist on κ receptor and is a weak antagonist of μ and δ receptors. It is used to relieve moderate to severe pain with mild or no abuse potential, and can also be used as a supplement to preoperative drugs and anesthesia. Pentazocine induces withdrawal syndrome in morphine abusers. It may be administered either orally or parenterally. At high doses, pentazocine can cause respiratory inhibition and reduce GI activity. High doses of pentazocine can increase blood pressure and cause hallucinations, nightmares, anxiety disorders, dizziness and tachycardia. Due to recent adverse reactions, it should be used cautiously in patients with angina pectoris or coronary artery disease.

5.　Other analgesics

Tramadol (曲马多)

Tramadol, central analgesic, a synthetic codeine analog (类似物) that binds to μ opioid receptors and has a higher affinity metabolite to μ receptors than the parent form (原型). Tramadol, administered orally or intramuscularly, experiences extensive liver metabolism and subsequent kidney excretion, in addition to its weak inhibition of norepinephrine and serotonin reuptake. Its respiratory inhibitory activity is lower than that of morphine, and used to treat moderate to severe pain. Common side effects of tramadol include nausea, vomiting, dizziness, dry mouth, sedation and headache. Anaphylactoid reactions (过敏反应) have been reported. Excessive or drug interaction with certain drugs can lead to excitement in the CNS and toxicity to seizures. Tramadol, like other drugs that bind to μ opioid receptors, is associated with misuse and abuse.

Rotundine (罗通定)

Rotundine, also named l-tetrahydropalmatine (左旋四氢巴马汀), acts as a selective dopamine D_1 receptor antagonist, and is valid for both acute and chronic pain. Although, its analgesic effect is weaker than the peperidine, it has higher efficacy than the NSAIDs (非甾体抗炎药). Rotundine inhibits the CNS, then produces sedation and hypnosis. The drug is usually administered orally or intramuscularly. Nausea or vomiting is seldom reported. Rotundine is no potential of addiction. At large doses, rotundine depresses the respiratory center.

6. Opioid antagonists

Opioid antagonists have high affinity with opioid receptors, but cannot activate receptor-mediated reactions. Opioid antagonists have no significant effect on normal individuals. However, in patients who are dependent on opioids, antagonists quickly reverse the effects of agonists, such as morphine or any complete μ agonist, and accelerate withdrawal symptoms of opioids.

Naloxone (纳洛酮)

Naloxone is a competitive antagonist for μ, κ, and δ receptors, and the unlimited value of μ receptor is ten times higher than that of κ receptor. It quickly replaces all receptor-bound opioid molecules. Naloxone is used to reverse opioid overdose coma and respiratory inhibition, which can lead to withdrawal syndrome for morphine abusers. Although naloxone is easily absorbed from the gastrointestinal tract, intravenous injection is commonly used. Naloxone is mainly metabolized in the liver and the half life time is about one hour.

Naltrexone (纳曲酮)

The effect of naltrexone is similar to that of naloxone. Naltrexone retains more efficacy by oral administration and has a longer duration of action than naloxone. Combined with other drugs, naltrexone is used for rapid detoxification of opioids. Naltrexone can cause hepatotoxicity.

重 点 小 结

药物	药理作用	临床应用	不良反应
阿片受体激动药：吗啡	激动阿片受体，镇痛、镇静，抑制呼吸，抑制胃肠蠕动	剧痛、中度疼痛、重度疼痛，心源性哮喘	成瘾性、呼吸抑制、便秘、诱发癫痫
阿片受体部分激动药：喷他佐辛	激动 κ 受体，部分激动 μ 受体	慢性剧痛、术后镇痛	剂量过大可引起呼吸抑制、心血管反应
阿片受体拮抗药：纳洛酮	竞争性阻断阿片受体	阿片类药物急性中毒、酒精中毒	诱发戒断症状

题库

目 标 检 测

一、选择题

（一）单项选择题

1. 与脑内阿片受体无关的镇痛药是（　　　）
　　A. 罗通定　　　B. 吗啡　　　　　C. 喷他佐辛　　　D. 哌替啶　　　E. 美沙酮
2. 胆绞痛或肾绞痛时宜选用（　　　）
　　A. 哌替啶　　　B. 对乙酰氨基酚　C. 阿托品　　　　D. 普萘洛尔　　E. 哌替啶＋阿托品
3. 吗啡不能用于下列何种疼痛（　　　）
　　A. 癌症重度疼痛　　　　　B. 急性锐痛　　　C. 分娩疼痛
　　D. 胆绞痛　　　　　　　　E. 心绞痛
4. 可用于吗啡和海洛因脱毒治疗的药物是（　　　）
　　A. 芬太尼　　　B. 可待因　　　　C. 喷他佐辛　　　D. 美沙酮　　　E. 哌替啶

（二）多项选择题

5. 下列药物中能与阿片受体结合的有（　　　）
　　A. 罗通定　　　B. 纳洛酮　　　　C. 可待因　　　　D. 喷他佐辛　　E. 哌替啶
6. 吗啡可用于治疗心源性哮喘是因为其具有下列哪些作用（　　　）
　　A. 镇静　　　　　　　　　B. 增加心输出量　　　　　C. 松弛支气管
　　D. 降低外周阻力　　　　　　　　　　　　E. 抑制呼吸中枢
7. 吗啡与哌替啶的共同特点有（　　　）
　　A. 激动阿片受体　　　　　B. 成瘾性　　　C. 提高胃肠道平滑肌张力
　　D. 用于人工冬眠　　　　　E. 缩瞳

二、思考题

从哌替啶、阿托品、阿司匹林镇痛的作用机制解释其镇痛作用的临床应用与特点。

PPT

Chapter 15　Nonsteroidal anti-inflammatory drugs

 学习目标

> **1. 掌握**　解热镇痛抗炎药的概念、药理作用、作用机制；阿司匹林的药理作用及作用机制、临床应用和不良反应。
>
> **2. 熟悉**　对乙酰氨基酚、吲哚美辛、双氯芬酸、布洛芬、吡罗昔康、塞来昔布的药理作用、作用机制、临床应用和不良反应。
>
> **3. 了解**　尼美舒利、美洛昔康的临床应用。

Antipyretic, analgesic and anti-inflammatory drugs are a kind of drugs with antipyretic and analgesic effects. Many drugs also have anti-inflammatory and anti rheumatic effects. Because their mechanism is different from glucocorticoids, they are often called non-steroidal anti-inflammatory drugs (NSAIDs, 非甾体抗炎药). NSAIDs are the competitive inhibitors of cyclooxygenase (COX, 环氧合酶), the enzyme which mediates the bioconversion of arachidonic acid (花生四烯酸) to inflammatory prostaglandins (PGs, 前列腺素) (Figure15-1). NSAIDs work by reducing the production of prostaglandins. Prostaglandlins are chemicals that promote inflammation,pain and fever.

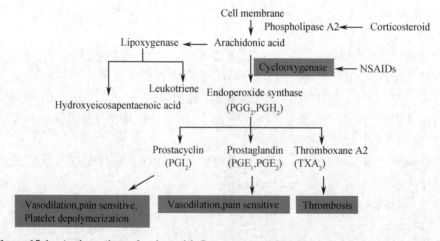

Figure 15-1　Antipyretic analgesic anti-inflammatory action site and pharmacological action

医药大学堂
WWW.YIYAODXT.COM

1. Pharmacodynamics

According to the different chemical structure, they are classified as salicylic acid, aniline, indole derivative, aryl acetic acid, enolic acid, pyrazolone derivative, alkanone and isobutyric acid. According to the selectivity to COX, there are non-selective COX inhibitors and selective COX-2 inhibitors. These drugs have three main effects: antipyretic (解热), analgesic (镇痛), and anti-inflammatory (抗炎).

1.1　Anti-inflammatory effect

NSAIDs are drugs that help reduce inflammation. They work by inhibiting the enzyme COXs, thus inhibiting biosynthesis of prostaglandin, an important mediator in the local inflammatory injures. COXs exist in at least two isoforms, COX-1 and COX-2. COX-1 is constitutive and makes PGs that protect the stomach and kidney from damage. COX-2 is induced by inflammatory stimuli, such as cytokines (e.g., IL-1, IL-6, IL-8, TNF, etc.), and produces PGs that contribute to the pain and swelling of inflammation. Most NSAIDs are non-selective COX inhibitors (非选择性环氧化酶抑制剂), which means that they block both COX-1 and COX-2. The efficacy of COX-2 selective drugs equals to that of non-COX-selective inhibitor, while the gastrointestinal (GI, 胃肠) safety may be improved.

1.2　Analgesic effect

NSAIDs block the production of certain body chemicals that cause inflammation. NSAIDs are good at treating pain caused by slow tissue damage, such as arthritis pain (关节痛). NSAIDs also work well fighting back pain (背痛), menstrual cramps (痛经) and headaches (头痛). NSAIDs exert their analgesic effect not only through peripheral inhibition of prostaglandin synthesis but also through a variety of other peripheral and central mechanisms. There is increasing evidence that NSAIDs have a central mechanism of action that augments the peripheral mechanism. This effect may be the result of interference with the formation of prostaglandins within the CNS. Alternatively, the central action may be mediated by endogenous opioid peptides (内源性阿片肽) or blockade of the release of serotonin (5-羟色胺). A mechanism involving inhibition of excitatory amino acids (兴奋性氨基酸) or N-methyl-D-aspartate receptor (N-甲基-D-天冬氨酸受体) activation has also been proposed.

1.3　Antipyretic effect

Antipyretics such as acetaminophen, aspirin, and related NSAIDs reduce fever by depressing inflammatory messages at both peripheral sites of tissue inflammation and within central nervous system thermoregulatory sites. Peripherally, aspirin and other NSAIDs suppress production of pyrogenic cytokines such as tumor necrosis factor (肿瘤坏死因子) and interleukin-1β (白细胞介素-1β) and block endothelial cell (内皮细胞) /leukocyte (白细胞) interactions through effects on adhesion molecule expression. These agents also promote the creation of anti-inflammatory molecules such as adenosine (腺苷) and aspirin-triggered lipoxins (脂氧素). Centrally, antipyretics lower the thermoregulatory set point primarily by blocking cyclooxygenase production of prostaglandin E_2 (PGE_2). Additional effects may stem from provoking the release of endogenous antipyretic compounds such as arginine vasopressin (精氨酸加压素). Acetaminophen differs from other antipyretic agents by its inability to reduce peripheral inflammation and its lack of effect on endogenous antipyretics.

1.4　Other effects

NSAIDs have a powerful and irreversible inhibitory effect on platelet aggregation by inhibiting cyclooxygenase. NSAIDs may inhibit the occurrence, development and metastasis of tumor.

2.　Non-selective cyclooxygenase inhibitors

Aspirin is a non-selective cyclooxygenase inhibitors(非选择性环氧化酶抑制药), which leads to reduced production of prostaglandins, and thromboxanes (血栓素), but not leukotrienes (白细胞三烯). There are a group of non-selective inhibitors of COXs, including aspirin, acetaminophen, ibuprofen, and indomethacin.

2.1　Salicylic acid

Aspirin (阿司匹林)

Aspirin is a medication used for pain, fever, and inflammation. It is also a blood thinner.

【Pharmacokinetics】Aspirin is available in oral forms. When taken, it is absorbed in the gastrointestinal tract. It is distributed to all tissues of the body. In pregnant women, it does cross the placenta (胎盘) to the fetus. It is also passed through breast milk to a nursing infant. In the body, it quickly breaks down into salicylic acid, and the liver changes it into metabolites. It is excreted by the kidneys. The half-life of aspirin is only 15-20 minutes. In higher doses, the half-life increases, and in toxic doses it may exceed 20 hours.

【Pharmacodynamics】

(1) **Analgesic action**　Aspirin produces analgesia by an ill-defined effect on the hypothalamus (central action) and by blocking generation of pain impulses (peripheral action). The peripheral action may involve blocking of prostaglandin synthesis via inhibition of cyclooxygenase enzyme.

(2) **Anti-inflammatory action**　Although the exact mechanism is unknown, aspirin can inhibit prostaglandin biosynthesis; it may also inhibit the synthesis or action of other mediators of inflammation.

(3) **Antipyretic action**　Aspirin relieves fever by acting on the hypothalamic (下丘脑) heat-regulating center to produce peripheral vasodilation (外周血管舒张). This increases peripheral blood supply and promotes sweating, which leads to loss of heat and to cooling by evaporation.

(4) Anticoagulant action　At low doses, aspirin appears to impede clotting by blocking prostaglandin biosynthesis, which prevents formation of the platelet-aggregating substance thromboxane A_2 (血栓素A_2). This interference with platelet activity is irreversible and can prolong bleeding time. However, at high doses, aspirin interferes with prostacyclin (前列环素) production, a potent vasoconstrictor and inhibitor of platelet aggregation (血小板聚集), possibly negating its anticlotting properties.

【 Clinical indications 】

(1) Headache, toothache, muscle pain, dysmenorrhea (痛经), cold and fever　Aspirin has strong antipyretic and analgesic effect.

(2) Rheumatoid arthritis (类风湿关节炎)　Aspirin can reduce the redness, swelling, heat, and pain caused by inflammation, and provide rapid relief from osteoarthritis symptoms with a high dose.

(3) Prevent recurrence of myocardial infarction (预防心肌梗死复发), cerebral ischemia (脑缺血), angina pectoris (心绞痛), postoperative deep vein thrombosis and pulmonary embolism (术后深静脉血栓形成和肺栓塞)　Low dose aspirin inactivates PG synthetase, inhibits platelet cyclooxygenase and reduces the production of thromboxane A2 in platelets, which in turn affects platelet aggregation and thrombosis(血栓症). High doses of aspirin directly inhibit PG synthetase, reduce prostacyclin synthesis, and promote thrombosis. Low dose aspirin is clinically used to treat coronary artery disease (冠状动脉疾病), cerebral ischemia, atrial fibrillation (心房纤颤), artificial heart valves (人工心脏瓣膜), arteriovenous fistulas (动静脉瘘) or other postoperative thrombosis (术后血栓形成).

【 Adverse reactions 】

(1) Gastrointestinal reaction (胃肠道反应)　Oral Administration can directly stimulate the gastric mucosa, causing epigastric discomfort, nausea, vomiting, sodium salicylate is particularly prone to occur. When the concentration of blood drug is high, it stimulates the chemoreceptor area of medulla oblongata, which can cause nausea and vomiting. Large dose (anti-rheumatism treatment) can cause gastric ulcer and painless gastric bleeding, aggravate gastric ulcer. Taking medicine after meals or taking antacids can reduce gastrointestinal reactions. The gastrointestinal reaction induced by aspirin is related to the direct stimulation of local gastric mucosal cells and the inhibition of COX-1, reduction of the production of prostaglandins such as PGE_2 and PGI_2 in gastric parietal tissues. Combined use of prostaglandin E_1 derivative misoprostol (米索前列醇) can reduce the incidence of ulcer.

(2) Bleeding　Aspirin slows the ability of the blood to form clots, which means it can reduce the chances of dangerous blood clots causing heart attacks and strokes. However, the same action means it increases the risk of serious bleeding, such as bleeding of blood vessels in the brain or gut. In some cases this type of bleeding can be as life-threatening as a heart attack or stroke. Serious liver disease, bleeding tendency of disease such as hemophilia, maternal, pregnant women are banned.

(3) Salicylic acid reaction (水杨酸反应)　Too large dose of aspirin cause headache, dizziness, nausea, vomiting, tinnitus and vision, hearing loss, which is known as salicylic acid poisoning performance.

(4) Allergic reaction　A few patients may present with urticaria (荨麻疹), angioedema (血管神经性水肿), and anaphylaxis (过敏性休克). Some asthma (哮喘) patients take aspirin or other antipyretic analgesics can induce asthma, known as " aspirin asthma". Because aspirin inhibits PG biosynthesis, the increase in leukotrienes and other lipoxygenase metabolites produced by arachidonic acid leads to bronchoconstriction and asthma. The condition can be treated by antihistamines and glucocorticoid. Aspirin could not be used in patients with asthma, nasal polyps (鼻息肉) or urticaria.

(5) Reye syndrome (瑞夷综合征) Children and adolescents who have a fever due to a viral infection treated by aspirin occasionally result in Reye syndrome. The symptoms are liver damage (肝损伤) and encephalopathy (脑病), which are lethal. Therefore, aspirin should be used with caution.

2.2　Anilines

Acetaminophen (对乙酰氨基酚)

【Pharmacokinetics】Acetaminophen has a high oral bioavailability (88%), it is well absorbed and reaches the peak blood concentrations within 90 minutes after ingestion. Acetaminophen is not widely bound to plasma proteins, and has a plasma half-life of 1.5-2.5 hours at the recommended doses. At the usual dose, acetaminophen is generally metabolized in the liver as inactive metabolites and excreted from the urine. However, long-term use or overuse can result in glutathione depletion and toxicity, resulting in necrosis of hepatocytes and renal tubules.

【Pharmacodynamics】Acetaminophen inhibits the synthesis of prostaglandins in the central nervous system, producing antipyretic and analgesic effects.

(1) Analgesic action Analgesic effect may be related to an elevation of the pain threshold.

(2) Antipyretic action Drug may exert antipyretic effect by direct action on hypothalamic heat-regulating center to block effects of endogenous pyrogen (致热原). This results in increased heat dissipation through sweating and vasodilation.

【Clinical indications】Headache and fever: the antipyretic and analgesic effects of acetaminophen are comparable to those of aspirin, but the anti-inflammatory effects are extremely weak. Acetaminophen is used for fever and pain relief. As acetaminophen has no gastrointestinal stimulation, it is suitable for the patients, in whom aspirin should not be used, with headache and fever.

【Adverse reactions】Acetaminophen poisoning can cause liver damage, long-term use of drugs at large dosage induces renal colic, acute or chronic renal failure, especilly in patients with renal dysfunction.

2.3　Indoles

Indomethacin (吲哚美辛)

【Pharmacodynamics】

(1) Analgesic, antipyretic, and anti-inflammatory actions Its anti-inflammatory effect is 10-40 times stronger than that of aspirin. Indomethacin is thought to produce its analgesic, antipyretic, and anti-inflammatory effects by inhibiting prostaglandin synthesis and possibly by inhibiting phosphodiesterase.

(2) Closure of patent ductusarteriosus Pharmacodynamics is believed to be through inhibition of prostaglandin synthesis.

【Clinical indications】Indomethacin is a nonsteroidal anti-inflammatory drug with potent antipyretic, analgesic, and anti-inflammatory activity that has been effectively used in the management of mild-to-moderate pain such as mandatory crista (强直性脊柱炎), osteoarthritis (骨关节炎) and in the treatment of cancerous and other uncontrollable fevers.

【Adverse reactions】

(1) Gastrointestinal reaction　Indomethacin causes loss of appetite (食欲减退), nausea (恶心), abdominal pain (腹痛), peptic ulcer (上消化道溃疡), occasional perforation (穿孔), bleeding, diarrhea (腹泻), and acute pancreatitis (急性胰腺炎).

(2) Central nervous system　20%-50% of patients have headache, dizziness (眩晕), occasionally mental disorder (精神失常).

(3) Hematopoietic System (造血系统)　Indomethacin may induce garanulocytopenia (粒细胞减少), thrombocytopenia (血小板减少), aplastic anemia (再生障碍性贫血).

(4) Allergic reaction　Indomethacin may induce rashes, asthma, angioedema, shock.

2.4　Aryl acetic acids

Diclofence (双氯芬酸)

【Pharmacodynamics】Diclofence is a powerful anti inflammatory and analgesic. The ED_{50} is many times lower than most anti-inflammatory NSAIDs and at least half that of indomethacin and naproxen. Diclofence is among the most effective inhibitor of PGE synthetase and markedly inhibites platelets aggregation in rats.

【Clinical indications】Diclofence is used for moderate pain, rheumatoid arthritis (类风湿关节炎),adhesive crest spondylitis (粘连性脊柱炎), non-inflammatory joint pain (非炎性关节痛), spondylitis (脊柱关节炎), and a variety of neuralgia (神经痛), surgery and post traumatic pain, as well as fever caused by a variety of pain.

【Adverse reactions】The side effects of diclofence are similar to those of aspirin, with occasional liver dysfunction and leukopenia.

2.5　Aryl propionic acids

Ibuprofen (布洛芬) and naproxen (萘普生)

【Pharmacokinetics】The oral absorption of these drugs is rapid and complete. The absorption amount is less affected by food and drugs. The plasma protein binding rate is high. They are mainly metabolized by the liver and excreted by the kidney.

【Pharmacodynamics】Ibuprofen inhibits the production of PG by inhibiting cyclooxygenase. Naproxen is a PG synthetase inhibitor.

【Clinical indications】Ibuprofen is used to treat rheumatoid arthritis, osteoarthritis (骨关节炎), mandatory arthritis, acute tendinitis (急性肌腱炎), synovial bursitis (滑膜囊炎), and dysmenorrheal (痛经).

【Adverse reactions】Gastrointestinal reactions are the most common adverse reactions. Long-term use of ibuprofen can cause stomach bleeding (胃出血), occasional headaches, tinnitus (耳鸣), dizziness and other central nervous system reactions. A small number of patients show skin and mucous membrane allergy, thrombocytopenia, headache, dizziness and visual impairment and other adverse reactions.

2.6　Enolates

Piroxicam (吡罗昔康) and meloxicam (美洛昔康)

Piroxicam and meloxicamare completely absorbed orally. These drugs have a rapid and long-lasting effect due to the circulation of the intestine and liver, but without accumulation in the blood. Most drugs are metabolized in the liver and excreted in urine and feces. Piroxicam relieves pain and inflammation but does not alter the progression of various arthritis diseases. Piroxicam also inhibits mucopolysaccharidase (黏多糖酶) and collagenase (胶原酶) activity in cartilage, reducing inflammation and cartilage (软骨) damage. Piroxicam mainly treats rheumatic and rheumatoid arthritis, acute gout (急性痛风), lumbar muscle strain (腰肌劳损), periarthritis of shoulder (肩周炎), and primary dysmenorrheal (原发性痛经). Long-term use of piroxicam may cause gastric ulcers and bleeding.

2.7　Pyrazolone

Butazone (保泰松) and oxyphenbutazone (羟布宗)

Butazone and oxyphenbutazone have strong anti-inflammatory, anti-rheumatic effect, but weak antipyretic effect. Long-term use of butazone produces cumulative toxicity. It is mainly used to treat rheumatism, rheumatoid arthritis and mandatory crista. Butazone had more side effects and were less used

3.　Selective cyclooxygenase-2 inhibitor

Most of the traditional NSAIDs are non-selective COX inhibitors, but COX-1 inhibition increases the risk of adverse events such as gastrointestinal, renal, and gastrointestinal bleeding reactions. COX-2 selective inhibitors (选择性环氧化酶–2抑制药) reduce these adverse events, but prospective studies have shown that COX-2 selective inhibitors increase the incidence of cardiovascular adverse events. Rofecoxib (罗非昔布) has been recalled worldwide due to adverse cardiovascular events. Nimesulide's oral formulation (尼美舒利) is banned in children under 12 years' old.

Celecoxib (塞来昔布)

【Pharmacokinetics】After oral administration, celecoxib is rapidly absorbed and achieves peak serum concentration in approximately 3 hours. It is mainly metabolized by CYP2C9 in the liver and excreted by urine and feces.

【Pharmacodynamics】Celecoxib exerts its anti-inflammatory and analgesic activities through blocking the synthesis of various inflammatory prostanoids. The prostanoids, which include PGs and thromboxane, are the end products of fatty acid (脂肪酸) metabolism produced by tissue-specific COX enzymatic activity. These products are important physiological and pathological mediators that are involved in a wide range of biological processes including inflammation (炎症), pain, cancer, glaucoma (青光眼), osteoporosiss (骨质疏松), cardiovascular diseases (心血管疾病), and asthma.

【Clinical indications】Celecoxib is used for the treatment of rheumatoid arthritis, osteodystrophy (骨营养不良) and osteoarthritis, as well as for postoperative analgesia, toothache, dysmenorrheal, and for the treatment of familial adenomatous polyps (腺瘤性息肉).

【Adverse reactions】

(1) Gastrointestinal reactionand renal damage (胃肠道反应及肾损伤) Low incidence of bleeding and ulceration, celecoxib may cause edema (水肿), polyuria (多尿), and renal damage (肾损伤).

(2) Cardiovascular system(心血管系统) Celecoxib increases the risk of severe cardiovascular thrombosis (心血管血栓), myocardial infarction (心肌梗死), and stroke (卒中).

重 点 小 结

类别	药物	药理作用	临床应用	不良反应
非选择性环氧化酶抑制药	水杨酸类药：阿司匹林	解热、镇痛、抗炎、抗风湿，抗血栓、抑制血小板聚集	慢性钝痛，缓解风湿性关节炎症状	胃肠道反应，出血，水杨酸反应，过敏反应，瑞夷综合征
	苯胺类药：对乙酰氨基酚	解热镇痛作用缓和持久，抗炎作用弱	感冒发热、头痛、牙痛、神经痛、肌肉痛、关节痛	急性中毒致肝坏死，长期使用肾损害
	芳基丙酸类药：布洛芬	抗炎镇痛作用强	风湿性及类风湿关节炎，一般疼痛发热	偶见血小板减少症、视物模糊
	吲哚类：吲哚美辛	解热、抗炎、抗风湿作用强	风湿性及类风湿关节炎、强直性脊柱炎、急性痛风，对癌性发热及其他不易控制的发热有效	胃肠道反应，头痛，眩晕，精神异常，造血功能抑制，过敏反应
	芳基乙酸类药：双氯酚酸	抗炎镇痛作用强	各种中等程度疼痛、类风湿关节炎、粘连性脊柱炎、非炎性关节痛	偶见肝功能异常，白细胞减少等
	烯醇酸类药：吡罗昔康	镇痛、解热、抗炎、抗痛风作用较强	风湿性、类风湿关节炎，急性痛风，腰肌劳损，肩周炎	长期服用致消化道出血、溃疡
选择性环氧化酶-2 抑制药	塞来昔布	抗炎、镇痛、解热	风湿性关节炎、类风湿关节炎和骨关节炎，术后镇痛、牙痛、痛经，家族性腺瘤性息肉	水肿、多尿、肾损害，心血管系统损伤

目 标 检 测

一、选择题

（一）单项选择题

1. 儿童出现病毒性疾病发热时，使用下列何药退热会引起肝衰竭合并脑病（　　）

　A. 阿司匹林　　B. 对乙酰氨基酚　C. 双氯芬酸　　　　D. 萘普生　　　　E. 美洛昔康

2. 解热镇痛抗炎药中，可用于治疗强直性脊柱炎的是（　　）

    A. 阿司匹林　　　　　　　　　B. 对乙酰氨基酚　　　　　　C. 吡罗昔康

    D. 塞来昔布　　　　　　　　　E. 吲哚美辛

3. 临床可用于治疗家族性腺瘤性息肉的是（　　）

    A. 吡罗昔康　　　　　　　　　B. 塞来昔布　　　　　　　　C. 布洛芬

    D. 对乙酰氨基酚　　　　　　　E. 吲哚美辛

4. 对癌性发热及其他不易控制的发热有效的是（　　）

    A. 吡罗昔康　　　　　　　　　B. 塞来昔布　　　　　　　　C. 布洛芬

    D. 对乙酰氨基酚　　　　　　　E. 吲哚美辛

5. 常用解热镇痛抗炎药主要是通过（　　）起作用

    A. 抑制体内 COX 的生物合成　　　B. 增加局部组织 PG 的生物合成

    C. 抑制中枢阿片受体　　　　　　　D. 激动中枢阿片受体

    E. 增加体内 COX 的生物合成

（二）多项选择题

6. 关于阿司匹林的作用及机制，下列哪些是正确的（　　）

    A. 抑制 COX-1　　　　　　　　B. 抑制 COX-2

    C. 减少血小板中 TXA_2 的生成　　D. 高浓度时直接抑制血管壁中 PG 合成酶

    E. 减少 PGI_2 合成

7. 阿司匹林的临床应用包括（　　）

    A. 头痛　　　　　　　　　　　B. 风湿性关节炎　　　　　　C. 缺血性心脏病

    D. 胃溃疡　　　　　　　　　　E. 哮喘

二、思考题

从阿司匹林的作用机制解释其药理作用和不良反应。

（朱星枚）

Chapter 16　Antihypertensive drugs

学习目标

1.掌握　抗高血压药的概念、分类及其代表药；利尿降压药、肾素－血管紧张素系统抑制药、钙通道阻滞剂、β受体阻断药的药理作用及机制、临床应用和不良反应。

2.熟悉　α₁受体阻断药、血管扩张药、中枢性神经抑制药的降压作用机制和临床应用。

3.了解　抗高血压药的治疗原则。

Hypertension (高血压) is a common and frequently-occurring disease, characterized by high systemic arterial blood pressure. Hypertension is defined as follows: systolic blood pressure/diastolic blood pressure ≥ 140/90 mmHg. It can be divided into two classes based on whether the pathology is clear or not. For most people, there's no clear cause of high blood pressure, and this type is called primary hypertension (原发性高血压), which tends to develop gradually. Some people have high blood pressure caused by an underlying condition, and this type is called secondary hypertension (继发性高血压), which tends to appear suddenly. The complications (并发症) of hypertension include stroke, kidney failure, heart failure, coronary heart disease, fundus lesions (眼底病变), etc. Most of these complications can lead to death or disability. Antihypertensive drugs (抗高血压药) can reduce blood pressure, ameliorate the injury of target organs, and prevent the complications.

1. Classification of antihypertensive drugs

Hypertension is a clinical feature caused by various reasons or diseases, and many factors can affect its pathological process, such as nerve dysfunction, the self-regulating function weakened, and abnormal hormone or locally active substance, etc. These factors keep the blood pressure steady mainly via modulating sympathetic nervous system (交感神经系统) and renin-angiotensin system (RAS, 肾素 – 血管紧张素系统). Antihypertensive drugs can exhibit hypotensive effect through directly or indirectly affecting these links (Figure 16-1).

Based on its position and pharmacodynamics, antihypertensive drugs can be divided into the following classes.

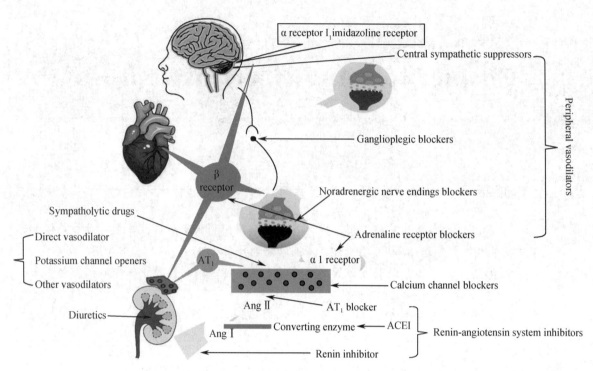

Figure 16-1   Schematic diagram of action site for antihypertensive drug

1.1   Diuretics

Hydrochlorothiazide (氢氯噻嗪).

1.2   Renin-angiotensin system inhibitors

(1) Angiotensin-converting enzyme inhibitor (ACEI)   captopril (卡托普利), enalapril (依那普利).

(2) Angiotensin Ⅱ receptor type 1 (AT1) blocker   losartan (氯沙坦), valsartan (缬沙坦).

(3) Renin inhibitor   remikiren (瑞米吉仑).

1.3   Calcium channel blockers

Nifedipine (硝苯地平), amlodipine (氨氯地平), felodipine (非洛地平).

1.4   Sympatholytic drugs

(1) Central nervous sympathetic depressant   clonidine (可乐定).

(2) Ganglionic blocker   mecamylamine (美卡拉明), trimetaphan.

(3) Noradrenergic nerve endings blocker   reserpine (利血平), guanethidine (胍乙啶).

(4) Adrenaline receptor blockers   propranolol and metoprolol (美托洛尔), prazosin (哌唑嗪), labetalol.

1.5　Peripheral vasodilators

(1) Direct vasodilator　hydrazine and sodium nitprusside (硝普钠).

(2) Potassium channel openers　pinacidil (吡那地尔), minoxidil (米诺地尔).

(3) Other vasodilators　ketanserin (酮色林), indapamide (吲达帕胺).

2. Commonly used antihypertensive drugs

2.1　Diuretics

Diuretics are commonly used as basic antihypertensive drugs, which can enhance efficacy and reduce water-sodium retention (水钠潴留) caused by other drugs when combined with other antihypertensive drugs. Thiazide diuretics are mainly used to treat hypertension in clinic.

Hydrochlorothiazide (氢氯噻嗪)

【Pharmacodynamics】 The antihypertensive effect of thiazide diuretics is mild, slow and lasting, and it can reduce postural blood pressure. The antihypertensive process is stable, and there is no obvious tolerance after long-term use, which generally does not cause orthostatic hypotension (体位性低血压). The antihypertensive effect of thiazide diuretics is weak when used alone, but synergistic or additive effects can be produced when combined with vasodilators and some sympathetic inhibitory drugs. Large-scale clinical trials have shown that long-term use of thiazide diuretics can reduce the incidence and mortality of cardiovascular and cerebrovascular complications, and improve the quality of life of patients with hypertension.

①The early use: it reduces blood pressure mainly through the discharge of sodium diuretic, decreasing blood volume and cardiac output. ②Long-term medication (3-4 weeks): due to Na^+ exclusion, the level of Na^+ in vascular smooth muscle is reduced. Through the Na^+-Ca^{2+} exchange mechanism, intracellular Ca^{2+} is also reduced, subsequently relaxing vascular smooth muscle. Meanwhile, the decreased intracellular Ca^{2+} causes that the vascular smooth muscle decreases its responsiveness to vasoconstrictor substances including norepinephrine (去甲肾上腺素), which makes the vascular tone and the blood pressure decreased. The arterial wall is induced to produce bradykinin (缓激肽), prostaglandin (前列腺素) and other vasodilators, which dilate the blood vessels and reduce the blood pressure.

【Clinical indications】 Thiazide diuretics are clinical treatment of hypertension, especially for patients with hypertension with heart failure.

【Adverse reactions】 Long-term use of large doses can lead to electrolyte disorders, adverse effects on glucose metabolism and lipid metabolism, compensatorily increased plasma renin activity and activation of RAS, which is not conducive to lower blood pressure.

2.2 Renin-angiotensin system inhibitors

RAS is composed of renin, angiotensin and its receptors. RAS can be classified into two groups: one is called circulating RAS, which exists in circulating system; the other one is called tissue RAS, which is distributed in heart, kidney, brain and vessel tissues. Renin is a proteolytic enzyme (蛋白水解酶) secreted by the glomerulus cells when blood volume is decreased or β receptors are activated, which can transform the angiotensin in the liver into angiotensin Ⅰ (Ang Ⅰ), and Ang Ⅰ can be further turned into angiotensin Ⅱ (Ang Ⅱ) under the action of angiotensin converting enzymes (ACE) in the plasma and tissues.

Ang Ⅱ can bind to angiotensin receptor in the membrane of the effectors to exert biological effect. According to the structure of receptor, pharmacological properties and different signal transduction processes, AT has AT_1, AT_2, AT_3 and AT_4 subtypes. The action of Ang Ⅱ is almost mediated by AT_1, which distributed in vessels, heart, kidney, adrenal cortex, brain, and lung tissues.

Ang Ⅱ can contract vascular smooth muscle, easily change the peripheral sympathetic nerve impulse transmission, and promote the release of catechol (儿茶酚) from the adrenalin medulla, resulting in increasing peripheral resistance and blood pressure via acting with AT; Ang Ⅱ acts on adrenocortical globules (肾上腺皮质球状带), promotes the release of aldosterone, and increases water-sodium retention and blood pressure; Ang Ⅱ can increase the rate of DNA and protein synthesis, enhance hypertrophy (心肌肥大) and proliferation of vascular smooth muscle cells, and reduce the compliance of vascular wall, causing vascular remodeling; Ang Ⅱ can increased DNA and protein synthesis in cardiomyocytes, promote gene recombination, fibroblast proliferation and cardiac remodeling.

RAS inhibitors contain: ①angiotensin-converting enzyme inhibitor (ACEI). ②Angiotensin Ⅱ receptor (AT_1) blocker. ③Renin inhibitor (Figure 16-2).

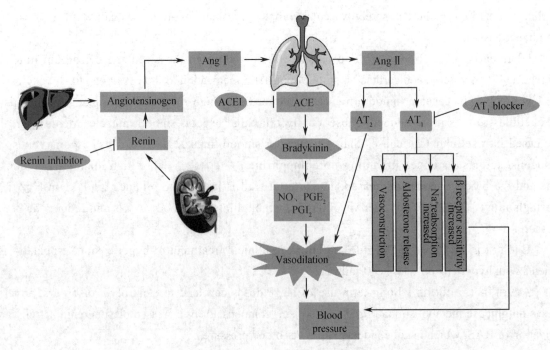

Figure 16-2   Renin-angiotensin system and its inhibitory component

2.2.1   Angiotensin Ⅰ converting enzyme inhibitor

【Pharmacodynamics】

(1) Antihypertensive effect   The antihypertensive effect of ACEI is accurate, effectively for the vast majority of hypertension. The antihypertensive characteristics of ACEI: ①hypertension is not accompanied by a reflex heart rate increase. ②It can prevent and reverse myocardial and vascular remodeling. ③It is not easy to cause lipid metabolism disorder and electrolyte disorder (电解质紊乱). ④Long use without tolerance and drug withdrawal rebound phenomenon (反跳现象).

(2) Effect on hemodynamics   ACEI can relax coronary arteries and large cerebral vessels, reduce the resistance of heart and cerebrovascular, and increase the blood flow of heart and brain. ACEI can significantly dilate bulbar arterioles and increase renal blood flow.

(3) Inhibit and reverse cardiovascular remodeling   ACEI inhibits and reverses cardiovascular remodeling via multiple ways: decrease heart load before and after in patients with high blood pressure and chronic cardiac dysfunction; reduce the production of Ang Ⅱ, and inhibit Ang Ⅱ-induced proliferation of cardiomyocytes and vascular smooth muscle cells; reduce myocardial fibrosis.

(4) Protect endothelial cells   ACEI can recovery endothelium-dependent vasodilator function through reducing ROS production and bradykinin degradation, promoting NO and PGI_2 production.

(5) Kidney protection   ACEI can block Ang Ⅱ production, subsequently reduce aldosterone synthesis. Therefore, it can reduce glomerular hypertension, hyperperfusion and hyperfiltration in terms of vascular resistance and blood volume.

(6) Anti-atherosclerosis effect   ACEI can reduce oxidation of LDL, suppress proliferation and migration of vascular smooth muscle cells, and inhibit functions of macrophages.

【Clinical indications】

(1) Hypertension   ACEI alone can control blood pressure in mild and moderate hypertension and has better effect on high renin hypertension.

(2) Chronic heart failure   ACEI can improve the prognosis of patients with chronic heart failure, prolong life and reduce mortality, and the effect is better than cardiotonic drugs.

(3) Acute myocardial infarction and prevention of stroke   ACEI can reduce the mortality of acute myocardial infarction with heart failure, improving systemic hemodynamics. Prophylactic drugs can reduce stroke.

(4) Diabetic nephropathy and other nephropathy   ACEI can stop kidney function from deteriorating.

【Adverse reactions】

(1) First dose hypotension   Oral absorption is fast and bioavailability is high. Thus, initial use should start at a small dose.

(2) Cough   Dry cough without phlegm is the most common.

(3) Angioedema (血管神经性水肿)   The symptom is acute edema of throat, lips and mouth.

(4) High potassium and low blood sugar   It can increase high potassium in blood, and enhance the sensitivity of insulin.

(5) The characteristic reaction with-SH structure   ACEI containing-SH structure can reduce blood zinc and cause taste and hair loss, etc.

(6) Others   It can cause acute renal failure.

Captopril (卡托普利)

【Pharmacokinetics】Captopril is rapidly absorbed orally, and its bioavailability is approximately 75%. The blood concentration reaches the peak at 1 hour, and $t_{1/2}$ is about 2 hours. Captopril is mainly metabolized in kidney. The plasma protein binding rate of captopril is 30%.

【Pharmacodynamics】Captopril has moderate intensity of hypotensive effect. It can reduce peripheral resistance, and increase renal blood flow, not accompanied by reflex heart rate. The antihypertensive mechanism of captopril is listed as: ①suppressing converting Ang Ⅰ into Ang Ⅱ via inhibiting ACE. ②Reducing aldosterone secretion.

【Clinical indications】

(1) Hypertension　Captopril is suitable for all kinds of hypertension.

(2) Chronic heart failure　Captopril can reduce the mortality of chronic heart failure.

(3) Myocardial infarction　Captopril has protection against myocardial ischemia, and reduce myocardial ischemia-reperfusion injury.

【Adverse reactions】Captopril can cause hypotension for initial use, thus should be started at a small dose. Long-term use can reduce blood zinc.

Characteristics of other ACEIs are shown in Table 16-1.

Table 16-1　Characteristics of other ACEIs

Drugs	Actions	Uses	Adverse reactions
Enalapril	Long-acting and efficient ACEI. Its inhibition is 10 times stronger than captopril	Various essential hypertension, renal hypertension, and congestive heart failure	Hypotension
Benazepril	Long-acting and efficient ACEI. Both prototype and metabolite have the effect of lowering blood pressure	Various essential hypertension and congestive heart failure	Hypotension
Cilazapril	It contains-SH, the maximum hypotensive effect occurs after 4-6 h of oral treatment	Various essential hypertension, renal hypertension	Embryonic toxicity

2.2.2　Angiotensin Ⅱ receptor(AT₁) blocker

AT₁ blockers have high selectivity on AT₁, which can directly block the effects caused by Ang Ⅱ via AT₁. The differences of pharmacological effects are shown in the following aspects: ①the antagonism to Ang Ⅱ is more complete and the antihypertensive effect is more stronger and lasting. ②It can not affect the degradation of bradykinin. ③It cancels the negative feedback regulation mechanism of renin release.

Losartan (氯沙坦)

【Pharmacodynamics】Losartan can be metabolized into EXP-3174. The latter has non-competitive AT₁ receptor blocking effect. Both of them can selectively bind to AT₁, blocking the pharmacological effects of Ang Ⅱ, subsequently decreasing blood pressure.

【Clinical Indications】Losartan is the first AT₁ receptor blocker for clinical use, which has a slow, stable and lasting antihypertensive effect. It can be used to treat various types of hypertension. Long-term use can inhibit left ventricular hypertrophy and increase of vessel wall in patients with chronic cardiac insufficiency.

【Adverse reactions】It has less adverse reactions, but occasionally causes dizziness, high blood potassium and upright hypotension. The initial dose should be reduced in cases of liver insufficiency or reduced circulating blood volume.

Valsartan (缬沙坦)

Oral absorption of valsartan is rapid, with plasma protein binding rate up to 94%-97%, mainly from bile excretion. It selectively blocks AT_1, which is 24 000 times stronger than AT_2. Long-term use can reverse myocardial hypertrophy and vascular remodeling. The incidence of adverse reactions is low, mainly headache, dizziness, fatigue and so on.

2.2.3　Renin inhibitor

Renin inhibitors decrease blood pressure via reducing renin activity, thereby inhibiting the formation of Ang Ⅰ. Renin inhibitors are divided into peptide and non-peptide types. The peptide renin inhibitors include Enalkiren (依那吉仑), which has low oral bioavailability and limited clinical use. Remikiren (瑞米吉仑) is a non-peptide renin inhibitor, which can increase renal blood flow when decreasing blood pressure.

2.3　Calcium channel blockers

Calcium channel blockers (CCBs) is one of antihypertensive drugs recommended by WHO. These drugs can selectively block voltage dependent calcium channel, suppress Ca^{2+} influx, and relax arterioles smooth muscle, resulting in reducing blood pressure. The major antihypertensive calcium channel blockers for clinical use are dihydropyridine drugs, including nifedipine, nitrendipine and amlodipine.

The antihypertensive characteristics of CCBs: ① activate baroreceptor-mediated sympathetic excitation, lowering blood pressure but increasing heart rate. ② Not reduce the blood flow to the heart, brain, kidney and other organs. ③ Long-term use can improve or reverse hypertrophy caused by hypertension and protect ischemic myocardium. ④ Inhibit platelet aggregation.

Nifedipine (硝苯地平)

【Pharmacodynamics】Nifedipine can inhibit Ca^{2+} influx to cause Ca^{2+} deficiency in vascular smooth muscle cells, leading to relaxation of arteriole smooth muscle, decrease of peripheral resistance and decrease of blood pressure.

【Clinical indications】Nifedipine is suitable for low renin hypertension (低肾素性高血压). It is also used for treating primary pulmonary hypertension, heart failure, Raynaud's disease (雷诺病), migraine and bronchial asthma in clinical.

【Adverse reactions】Facial flushing, headache, dizziness, palpitations, hypotension, and ankle edema commonly appear.

2.4　Adrenaline receptor blockers

2.4.1　β receptor blockers

Propranolol (普萘洛尔)

【Pharmacodynamics】The antihypertensive mechanism of propranolol is associated with blocking β receptors: ①block heart $β_1$ receptor, reduce myocardial contractility, and reduce cardiac output. ②Block β₁ receptor on the glomerulus cells and inhibit RAS. ③Block the β₂ receptor on the presynaptic membrane of the norepinephrine nerve and reduce the release of NA. ④Block β receptors in the vasomotor center. ⑤Increased synthesis of prostacyclin.

【Clinical indications】 It is better to treat hypertensive patients with high cardiac output or high plasma renin level, and it also has significantly therapeutic effect on hypertensive patients with tachycardia (心动过速), angina, migraine and anxiety disorder.

【Adverse reactions】 Long-term use of propranolol can affect lipid metabolism and increase blood lipid. It can delay the recovery speed of blood glucose, so hypertensive patients with diabetes should not use it. Do not suddenly stop the drug for long-term use, because it will cause withdrawal syndrome (停药综合征). Propranolol dosage varies greatly among individuals, and should be increased gradually from a small dose. The maximum dose not exceeding 300mg/d.

Characteristics of other β receptor blockers are shown in Table 16-2.

Table 16-2   Characteristics of other β receptor blockers

Drugs	Actions	Uses	Adverse reactions
Metoprolol	It is a selectively β receptor blocker, which acts on myocardial β₁ receptor and reduce contractile force and cardiac output	Various essential hypertension and angina pectoris	Fatigue, headache, bradycardia, gastrointestinal reactions
Atenolol	It has a high selection on myocardial β₁ receptor, but has less effect on β₂ receptor of vascular and bronchial smooth muscle	Various essential hypertension	Hypotension, bradycardia
Nadolol	It is a new long-acting β blocker, and reduce heart rate and cardiac output	Various essential hypertension, angina pectoris and arrhythmology	Similar to propranolol

2.4.2   α₁ receptor blockers

Prazosin (哌唑嗪)

【Pharmacodynamics】 Prazosin can selectively block α₁ receptor, dilate arterioles and venules, reducing blood pressure. It can not affect heart rate, cardiac output, and renal blood flow. Long-term use can reduce triglycerides, LDL, and increase HDL.

【Clinical indications】 Prazosin is suitable for all kinds of hypertension. It is more effective when used in combination with a β blocker. Prazosin can improve clinical symptoms of chronic cardiac insufficiency.

【Adverse reactions】 The first dose will occur. The symptoms are severe orthostatic hypotension and palpitations within 30-90min after administration of the drug.

2.4.3   α and β receptor blockers

Labetalol has β∶α antagonism at the ratio of 1∶3 after oral dosing. It can decrease blood pressure via reduction of systemic vascular resistance, not affecting heart rate or cardiac output. Labetalol has therapeutic effects on the hypertension of pheochromocytoma and hypertensive emergencies. It is recommended that oral daily doses of labetalol should be from 200 to 2400mg/d. Labetalol is administrated as repeated intravenous bolus injections of 20-80mg to treat hypertensive emergencies.

Carvedilol is used as a racemicmixture (外消旋混合物). The average half-life is 7-10 hours. The usual starting dosage of carvedilol for ordinary hypertension is 6. 25mg twice daily.

3. Other antihypertensive agents

3.1　Sympatholytic drugs

3.1.1　Central nervous sympathetic depressant

Clonidine (可乐定)

【Pharmacodynamics】The hypotensive effect of clonidine is moderate, and blood pressure increased briefly after intravenous infusion. Clonidine can inhibit the secretion and movement of gastrointestinal tract. It can also promote the release of endogenous opioid peptides, exhibiting sedative and analgesic effects.

【Clinical indications】Clonidine can be used to treat moderate hypertension, especially for hypertension with ulcers. Hypertensive crises (高血压危象) require intravenous drip administration.

【Adverse reactions】About 50% of the patients have dry mouth, constipation and other symptoms. Long-term use can cause water-sodium retention.

3.1.2　Ganglion-blocking agents

Ganglion-blocking agents are rarely used clinically, because they can block sympathetic and parasympathetic ganglia, and adverse reactions are numerous and severe. They are only used to treat hypertensive crises and hypertensive encephalopathy (高血压脑病). Mecamylamine and trimethaphan are two major Ganglion-blocking agents.

3.1.3　Noradrenergic nerve endings blocker

Noradrenergic nerve endings blockers mainly act on the nerve endings of norepinephrine and can reduce blood pressure by affecting the storage and release of catecholamines. Reserpine and guanethidine are used in clinical. Reserpine can bind to the amine pump on the vesicle membrane to inhibit the uptake of monoamine transmitters, so as to gradually reduce the synthesis and storage of the transmitters in the vesicle, leading to the depletion of blood pressure. Guanethidine blocks the release of norepinephrine from nerve endings, depleting the storage of norepinephrine. It can be used in severe or refractory hypertension.

3.2　Peripheral vasodilators

3.2.1　Direct vasodilator

This class of drugs can directly relax vascular smooth muscle, reduce peripheral resistance, and blood pressure. However, long-term application has a reflexive excitatory effect on the nerve-endocrine and sympathetic nervous system, and the plasma renin activity increases, causing water and sodium retention, which can partially offset the antihypertensive effect. Therefore, it is often used together with diuretics and β receptor blockers. Commonly used drugs are sodium nitroprusside, and hydrazine.

Sodium nitroprusside (硝普钠)

【Pharmacodynamics】Sodium nitroprusside can be metabolized into NO in vascular smooth muscle, activate guanylate cyclase (GC), and increase cGMP, then resulting in vascular smooth muscle relaxation.

【Clinical indications】Sodium nitroprusside can be used to treat hypertensive emergency and refractory chronic cardiac insufficiency.

【Adverse reactions】Silent drops can cause headaches, facial flushing, palpitations, nausea, and vomiting. Long-term or high dose use can cause thiocyanide accumulation poisoning. The drug is sensitive to light and should be avoided when used.

Hydralazine (肼屈嗪)

Hydralazine can directly relax arteriole smooth muscle, reduce peripheral resistance blood pressure quickly and strongly. It has no obvious relaxation effect on veins and does not cause orthostatic hypotension. The mechanism of reducing blood pressure may be: ① interference with Ca^{2+} influx of vascular smooth muscle cells. ② Promote the synthesis of intracellular NO and activate the release of cGMP in vascular smooth muscle. Common adverse reactions of hydrazine include headache, dizziness, flushing, palpitations and hypotension.

3.2.2　Potassium channel openers

Minoxidil (米诺地尔)

Minoxidil is an efficacious orally vasodilator. Its metabolite (minoxidil sulfate) can open potassium channels in smooth muscle membranes, which can stabilize the membrane at its resting potential and makes contraction less likely. Minoxidil dilates arterioles but not veins.

4. Application principles of antihypertensive drugs

The application principles of antihypertensive drugs show as follows.

4.1　Effective treatment and lifelong treatment

The effective treatment is to keep blood pressure under 140/90mmHg. Fewer than 10% of people with high blood pressure are under good control. In addition, the pathogenesis of hypertension is unknown, and there is no cure for hypertension. Therefore, lifelong treatment must be emphasized in the treatment of hypertension.

4.2　Protecting target organ

The target organ damages of hypertension include myocardial hypertrophy, glomerulosclerosis, and arteriole remodeling, etc. Reversing or suppressing the target organ damage should be considered in treating hypertension. ACEI, long-acting calcium channel blockers and AT_1 blockers have a better effect on protecting the target organ.

4.3 Stable reduction of blood pressure (平稳降压)

Studies show that unstable blood pressure can cause the organs damage. Spontaneous fluctuations of blood pressure within 24 hours are called blood pressure variability (BPV, 血压波动性). In hypertensive patients with the same blood pressure, patients with high BPV have severe damage to the target organs. The use of short-acting antihypertensive drugs increases the fluctuation of blood pressure, while the true 24-hour effective long-term inhibition is better.

4.4 Drug combination

Currently, any two classes of antihypertensive drugs combination are effective for hypertension therapy. Among them, β receptor blockers or RAS inhibitors plus calcium channel blockers exhibit the best effects.

重 点 小 结

药物	药理作用	临床应用	不良反应
氢氯噻嗪	排钠利尿，减少血容量、心输出量	高血压基础药	电解质紊乱，糖代谢、脂代谢异常
卡托普利	减轻或逆转高血压所致的血管壁增厚和心肌肥厚	各型高血压、慢性心功能不全、心肌梗死	首剂低血压、刺激性干咳、高血钾、低血锌
氯沙坦	选择性阻断 AT_1，拮抗 Ang II 作用，增加肾血流量和肾小球滤过率	各型高血压、慢性心功能不全	偶有头晕、高血钾、体位性低血压等
硝苯地平	抑制细胞外钙内流，小动脉扩张，血压下降	各型高血压	面部潮红、头痛、眩晕、心悸、踝部水肿等
普萘洛尔	阻断心肌 β_1 受体，减少心输出量；抑制肾素分泌；扩张血管	单用适合轻、中度高血压，合用适合中、重度高血压	升高血脂、反跳现象
哌唑嗪	选择性阻断 α_1 受体，扩张小动脉和小静脉	各型高血压	首剂现象、眩晕、疲乏、鼻塞、尿频
可乐定	激动突触前后 α_2 受体，抑制交感神经中枢的传出冲动和 NA 释放	高血压危象	镇静、嗜睡、口干、头痛以及便秘
硝普钠	扩张小动脉和小静脉；释放 NO	高血压急症	头痛、面部潮红、心悸、恶心

题库

目 标 检 测

一、选择题

（一）单项选择题

1. 氢氯噻嗪所具有的特点是（　　　）
    A. 降压作用温和、缓慢、持久　　　B. 能使正常血压降低　　　C. 保钾利尿
    D. 显著增高血浆肾素活性　　　E. 单用可治疗重度高血压

2. ACEI 不包括（　　　）
    A. 卡托普利　　　　　　　　　　B. 雷米普利　　　　　　　　C. 培哚普利
    D. 氯沙坦　　　　　　　　　　　E. 依那普利

3. ACEI 在降压时（　　　）
    A. 引起脂质代谢紊乱　　　　　　B. 引起哮喘　　　　　　　　C. 伴有反射性心率加快
    D. 改善心肌和动脉顺应性　　　　E. 有耐受性及停药的反跳现象

4. 首次给药可导致严重低血压药物是（　　　）
    A. 普萘洛尔　　　B. 硝苯地平　　　C. 哌唑嗪　　　D. 卡托普利　　　E. 氢氯噻嗪

5. 既有降压作用，又有抗心绞痛、抗心律失常作用的药物是（　　　）
    A. 利血平　　　B. 普萘洛尔　　　C. 硝普钠　　　D. 卡托普利　　　E. 氢氯噻嗪

6. 卡托普利的主要作用机制为（　　　）
    A. 使血管紧张素 II 生成减少　　　B. 直接扩张血管　　　　　　C. 抑制肾素的生成
    D. 竞争性对抗血管紧张素　　　　E. 抑制神经末梢释放去甲肾上腺素

7. 长期使用利尿药的降压机制主要是（　　　）
    A. 增加血浆肾素活性　　　　　　B. 抑制醛固酮分泌　　　　　C. 降低血浆肾素活性
    D. 排 Na^+ 利尿，降低血容量　　　E. 减少小动脉壁细胞内 Na^+

8. 可乐定的降压机制是（　　　）
    A. 激动中枢 α_2 受体　　　　　　B. 激动中枢 M 受体　　　　C. 阻断中枢的 α_2 受体
    D. 阻断中枢 α_2 受体　　　　　　E. 激动中枢的 I_1 咪唑啉受体

9. 关于 β 受体阻断药的降压机制，下列叙述哪项不正确（　　　）
    A. 抑制肾素释放　　　　　　　　B. 减少心输出量　　　　　　C. 具有中枢降压作用
    D. 减少交感递质释放　　　　　　E. 扩张肌肉血管

10. 高血压伴有糖尿病的患者不宜用（　　　）
    A. 噻嗪类　　　　　　　　　　　B. 中枢降压药　　　　　　　C. 血管扩张药
    D. 神经节阻断药　　　　　　　　E. 血管紧张素转化酶抑制剂

（二）多项选择题

11. 治疗高血压的基本原则的是（　　　）
    A. 有效治疗与终生治疗　　　　　B. 个体化治疗　　　　　　　C. 平稳降压
    D. 血压降至正常后停药　　　　　E. 保护靶器官

医药大学堂
WWW.YIYAODXT.COM

12. 关于米诺地尔正确的叙述是（　　）
    A. 引起水钠潴留　　　　　　　B. 开放钾通道
    C. 增加细胞内游离 Ca^{2+} 水平　　D. 反射性心率加快
    E. 主要用于严重的原发性高血压

二、思考题

抗高血压药为何常联合用药？举一实例并说明理由。

（程媛媛）

PPT

Chapter 17　Drugs used in heart failure

学习目标

1. **掌握**　治疗慢性心力衰竭药物的分类及代表药；强心苷类药的药理作用、作用机制、临床应用、不良反应及防治。

2. **熟悉**　血管紧张素Ⅰ转化酶抑制药、血管紧张素Ⅱ受体阻断药、β受体阻断药、利尿药的抗心力衰竭作用及临床应用。

3. **了解**　地高辛的药物代谢动力学特性；扩血管药、非强心苷类正性肌力药的抗心力衰竭作用特点及代表药。

Heart failure (HF, 心衰) occurs at the end stages of many heart diseases. It is a clinical syndrome in which the heart is unable to pump blood to meet the requirements of metabolizing tissues. The typical manifestations of left ventricular dysfunction are dyspnea (呼吸困难) and cough, while the symptoms of right ventricular dysfunction include jugular vein bloating, liver enlargement, and peripheral edema.

The reduced pumping function of the heart is a pathophysiologic sequence in response to an initial insult to myocardial dysfunction. The neuroendocrine (神经内分泌) compensatory regulation of the body plays an important role in the occurrence and development of HF (Figure 17-1). Briefly, a reduction in forward cardiac output leads to expanded activation of the sympathetic nervous system and the renin-angiotensin-aldosterone system (RAAS, 肾素–血管紧张素–醛固酮系统). Sympathetic nervous system activation is a fast-acting regulatory mechanism, which helps to maintain normal cardiac output and blood pressure. However, long-term sympathetic nerve activation down-regulates β_1 receptors and affects β_1 receptor-mediated signal transduction, which further reduces myocardial contractility, promotes cardiac remodeling (心脏重构), induces arrhythmias (心律失常), and even sudden death. On the other hand, RAAS activation increases the production of some physiologically active substances including plasma renin, angiotensin Ⅱ (Ang Ⅱ, 血管紧张素Ⅱ), and aldosterone, which in turn contract blood vessels, cause water and sodium retention, and promote cardiac remodeling.

The goal of pharmacotherapy is to relieve symptoms, improve quality of life, prevent or reverse cardiac remodeling, and prolong life of the patients. According to the pharmacodynamics, the anti-HF drugs are mainly divided into the following categories .

(1) Cardiac glycosides (强心苷类)　Digoxin (地高辛).

(2) Renin-angiotensin-aldosterone system inhibitors

1) Angiotensin Ⅰ converting enzyme inhibitors　Captopril (卡托普利).

2) Angiotensin Ⅱ receptor (AT$_1$) blockers　Losartan (氯沙坦).

3) Aldosterone antagonists　Spironolactone (螺内酯).

医药大学堂
WWW.YIYAODXT.COM

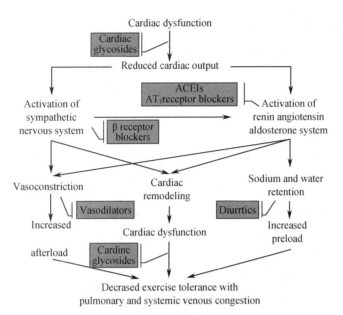

Figure 17-1 Pathophysiologic mechanisms of heart failure and major sites of drug action

ACEIs, angiotensin Ⅰ converting enzyme inhibitors; AT_1, type 1 angiotensin receptor

(3) β-receptor blockers   Carvedilol (卡维地洛), metoprolol (美托洛尔).

(4) Diuretics   Furosemide, hydrochlorothiazide.

(5) Others   ①Vasodilators. ②Other positive inotropic drugs.

1. Cardiac glycosides

Cardiac glycosides (强心苷类), also called digitalis, are mainly derived from medicinal plants such as *Digitalis purpuea* L. (紫花洋地黄) and *Digitalis lanata* Ehrh. (毛花洋地黄). Digoxin, digitoxin (洋地黄毒苷), and lanatoside C (毛花苷C) are the clinically used cardiac glycosides. Among them, digoxin is the most commonly used.

【Pharmacokinetics】Digoxin has a high polarity, so its oral absorption is not good enough. In addition, the pharmaceutic techniques have significant effects on the intestinal absorption of digoxin. Overall, the bioavailability of digoxin varies from 60% to 80%, showing significant individual differences. The absorbed digoxin is mainly excreted by the kidney in its original form. The elimination half-life ($t_{1/2}$) of digoxin is about 36-48h, so it is a medium-acting cardiac glycoside.

【Pharmacodynamics】

(1) Pharmacological effects on the heart

1) Positive inotropic effect (正性肌力作用)   Cardiac glycosides selectively act on the heart and significantly enhance myocardial contractility, showing as increased myocardial tension and increased shortening rate of myocardial contraction. The former helps to directly increase stroke volume (每搏输出量), while the latter helps to shorten the systolic period of the cardiac cycle (心动周期) and relatively prolong the diastolic period, which is conducive to venous return and stroke volume.

Cardiac glycosides increase the cardiac output of failing heart but not normal heart. In addition, cardiac glycosides do not increase or even reduce the oxygen consumption of failing heart. Cardiac glycosides can increase the free Ca^{2+} concentration in cardiomyocytes by inhibiting Na^+-K^+-ATPase on the cell membrane of cardiomyocytes. Due to the severe inhibition of Na^+-K^+-ATPase, the poisoning amount of cardiac glycosides will have a serious effect on the electrolytes, and thus cause arrhythmias.

2) Negative chronotropic effect (负性频率作用) The therapeutic dose of cardiac glycosides has minimal effect on normal heart rate but significantly reduce the heart rate of patients with HF. The treatment of cardiac glycosides can indirectly restore the sympathetic tension and heart rate through activating the decompression reflexes (减压反射). Furthermore, cardiac glycosides can directly increase the response of cardiomyocytes to the vagus nerve (迷走神经).

3) Effect on myocardial electrophysiological characteristics The effect of cardiac glycosides on myocardial electrophysiology (Table 17-1) varies with the dosage of the drug, myocardial sites, and myocardial state, etc. The effect of cardiac glycosides on the electrophysiology above the ventricle is related to the excitation of the vagus nerve, which promotes the outflow of K^+ in the third stage of the action potential. The effect of cardiac glycosides on Purkinje fibers (浦肯野纤维) is related to significantly decreased intracellular K^+ caused by the inhibition of Na^+-K^+-ATPase.

Table 17-1　Effect of cardiac glycosides on myocardial electrophysiology

Electrophysiology	Sinoatrial node	Atrium	Atrioventricular node	Purkinje fibers
Automaticity	↓			↑
Conductivity		↑	↓	↓
Effective refractory period		↓		↓

(2) Other pharmacological effects

1) Effect on blood vessels Cardiac glycosides can directly contract blood vessels. However, stimulatory effects of cardiac glycosides on the vagus nerve counteract this vasoconstrictive effect. Overall, cardiac glycosides have no significant effects on the peripheral resistance and blood pressure.

2) Effect on kidney Cardiac glycosides show significant diuretic effects in patients with HF. The mechanism is due to: ①indirect diuretic effect of cardiac glycosides that increase renal blood flow via increasing cardiac output. ②Direct diuretic effect of cardiac glycosides that reduce the reabsorption of Na^+ via inhibiting Na^+-K^+-ATPase of renal tubular epithelial cells.

3) Effect on the nervous and endocrine systems The therapeutic dose of cardiac glycosides reduces the sympathetic nerve activity and enhances the vagus nerve activity. Cardiac glycosides also antagonizes RAAS that is over-activated during cardiac insufficiency by reducing the plasma renin activity and the content of Ang II and aldosterone in HF patients. The toxic dose of cardiac glycosides significantly enhances the activity of the central and peripheral sympathetic nerves, leading to tachyarrhythmias (快速型心律失常). In addition, they can excite the chemical region of the effervescent medullary region and induce vomiting. Furthermore, they also cause central nervous excitement symptoms such as behavioral disorders, mental disorders, delirium (谵妄), and convulsions.

【Clinical indications】

(1) Heart failure In general, cardiac glycosides can improve the ventricular function, hemodynamics, and exercise endurance of patients with HF. They definitely improve symptoms of HF and have long-lasting and intolerable effects. Therefore, they are still widely used for long-term outpatients. However, their clinical applications are limited due to their small therapeutic indexes and toxicity. In addition, long-term use of cardiac glycosides cannot reduce the mortality of patients with HF. In general, cardiac glycosides are mostly used in HF with systolic dysfunction as well as those with poor efficacy of diuretics, ACEI, and β blockers, but are less effective in HF with diastolic dysfunction. To be more specific, cardiac glycosides show: ①excellent effect on HF with atrial fibrillation or ventricular tachycardia (心动过速). ②Good effect on HF caused by heart valve diseases, congenital heart diseases, arteriosclerosis, and hypertension. ③Poor effect on HF secondary to diseases like hyperthyroidism (甲状腺功能亢进), severe anemia (贫血), and vitamin B_1 deficiency (due to the disorder of myocardial energy metabolism in these situations). ④Poor effect on HF with pulmonary heart diseases, active myocarditis (心肌炎), or active rheumatism (风湿病) (due to myocardial hypoxia and energy metabolism disorders in these cases). ⑤Ineffectiveness on HF with mechanical obstruction, such as constrictive pericarditis (缩窄性心包炎), severe mitral stenosis (二尖瓣狭窄) (because ventricular diastole and filling are disturbed in these cases).

(2) Supraventricular arrhythmias　Cardiac glycosides can be used to treat supraventricular arrhythmias such as atrial fibrillation (心房颤动), atrial flutter (心房扑动), and paroxysmal supraventricular tachycardia (阵发性室上性心动过速). The use of cardiac glycosides should be avoided in ventricular arrhythmias. Cardiac glycosides may cause ventricular fibrillation in this case.

【Adverse reactions】Cardiac glycosides have small therapeutic indexes. The therapeutic dose is close to 60% of the toxicity dose. In addition, various factors, such as hypokalemia, hypomagnesemia, hypercalcemia, myocardial ischemia and hypoxia, renal insufficiency, and drug-drug interactions, can induce cardiac glycoside poisoning. Therefore, the incidence of cardiac glycoside poisoning is relatively high. In addition, the symptoms of cardiac glycoside poisoning and the symptoms of cardiac insufficiency are easily confused, which makes the identification of cardiac glycoside poisoning more difficult.

(1) Gastrointestinal toxicity　Gastrointestinal toxicity, manifested as loss of appetite, nausea, diarrhea, and vomiting, is a relatively common and early onset toxic reaction caused by cardiac glycosides.

(2) Central nervous system toxicity　Dizziness, headache, fatigue, insomnia, delirium (谵妄), and visual disturbances (视觉障碍) such as yellow vision, green vision, blurred vision could occur.

(3) Cardiotoxicity　Almost all arrhythmias seen in the clinic may occur. Ventricular premature beats (室性期前收缩) occur early and are most common, while ventricular tachycardia (室性心动过速) and ventricular fibrillation (室颤) are the most serious.

In order to prevent the occurrence of cardiac glycoside poisoning, the use of diuretics that induces hypokalemia should be stopped and potassium should be supplied. Poisoning precursors should be carefully alerted. When a certain number of premature ventricular contractions, sinus bradycardia (心动过缓) (less than 60 times per minute), and visual disturbances are observed, cardiac glycosides should be reduced or discontinued in time. Blood concentrations of cardiac glycosides should be monitored to ensure the safety. Poisoning can be diagnosed when the local drug concentration of digoxin exceeds 3ng/ml and digitoxin exceeds 45ng/ml.

Once poisoning occurs, the use of cardiac glycosides should be stopped immediately. For cardiac glycoside caused tachyarrhythmia, appropriate oral or intravenous drip of potassium chloride may be used according to the severity of the poisoning. For severe tachyarrhythmia, phenytoin sodium (苯妥英钠) or lidocaine (利多卡因) should also be used. Phenytoin sodium not only has the antiarrhythmic effect, but also can compete with cardiac glycosides for Na^+-K^+-ATPase and recover its activity. Therefore, phenytoin sodium should be used as the first choice for severe tachyarrhythmia. For cardiac glycoside caused bradyarrhythmia (缓慢型心律失常), potassium salt cannot be supplemented. Otherwise cardiac arrest can be caused. In this case, atropine (an M receptor blocker) can be given intravenously. The Fab fragment of digoxin antibody should be injected intravenously to the patients with life-threatening serious poisoning. The Fab fragment of digoxin antibody has high selectivity and strong affinity for cardiac glycoside. It can dissociate cardiac glycosides from Na^+-K^+-ATPase.

2. Renin-angiotensin-aldosterone system inhibitors

2.1 Angiotensin Ⅰ converting enzyme inhibitor (ACEIs, 血管紧张素转化酶抑制剂)

ACEIs, such as captopril (卡托普利), enalapril (依那普利), lisinopril (赖诺普利), and ramipril (雷米普利), are commonly used to treat HF. Clinical trials have shown that ACEIs can not only improve the symptoms and quality of life of patients with HF, but also significantly reduce their mortality.

【Pharmacodynamics】ACEIs reduce the conversion of Ang Ⅰ into Ang Ⅱ via inhibiting the angiotensin Ⅰ converting enzyme (ACE). Inhibition of the production of Ang Ⅱ can in turn inhibit aldosterone production. In addition, ACEIs show inhibitory effects on kininase Ⅱ (激肽酶Ⅱ) and hence increase the levels of bradykinin (缓激肽), PGI_2, and nitric oxide (NO) that have vasodilating effects. Based on these basic activities, the following anti-HF effects of ACEIs are produced.

(1) **Improve hemodynamics** ACEIs reduce cardiac afterload and finally increase cardiac output by reducing systemic vascular resistance (dilating arteries more than veins), which helps to improve ischemic symptoms in arterial system; ACEIs reduce cardio-muscular tension and improve diastolic function via decreasing the end-diastolic volume and filling pressure of left ventricular; ACEIs increase coronary blood flow via dilating coronary arteries, thereby improving myocardial ischemia and reducing tachycardia in HF; ACEIs improve edema via increasing urine output, which is caused by increased renal blood flow due to reduced renal vascular resistance.

(2) **Prevent and reverse myocardial hypertrophy and cardiovascular remodeling** Binding of Ang Ⅱ to the AT_1 receptor stimulates myocardial cells to synthesize proteins, promotes interstitial cell proliferation and protein synthesis, and ultimately causes myocardial cell hypertrophy (肥大), myocardial interstitial collagen deposition, and cardiac remodeling. Through inhibiting the production of Ang Ⅱ and increasing the levels of bradykinin, PGI_2, and NO, ACEIs prevent and reverse cardiomyocyte hypertrophy and cardiac remodeling. ACEIs also effectively prevent vascular remodeling and improve vascular compliance.

(3) **Inhibit the activity of sympathetic nerve** The inhibitory effect of ACEIs on the production

of Ang Ⅱ in turn diminishes the activation of the presynaptic membrane AT receptors in sympathetic nerve endings, which helps to reduce the release of norepinephrine and inhibit sympathetic nerve activity. Thereby, ACEIs help to improve cardiac function and significantly reduce tachyarrhythmias in HF through inhibiting the activity of sympathetic nerve.

(4) Others   ACEIs protect vascular endothelial cells due to their anti-oxidant effect. In addition, ACEIs increase the responsivity of diabetes patients to insulin. Therefore, ACEIs are beneficial for the treatment of concomitant diabetes in HF patients.

【 Clinical indications 】 As first-line drugs, ACEIs are widely used in clinic for the treatment of HF at all stages. ACEIs can not only relieve symptoms, improve exercise tolerance, improve quality of life, prevent and reverse cardiac hypertrophy, reduce mortality, but also delay the progress of early cardiac insufficiency and the occurrence of HF in patients without clinical symptoms.

2.2   Angiotension Ⅱ receptor blockers

The commonly used drugs include losartan (氯沙坦), valsartan (缬沙坦). The effect of this class of drugs on HF is similar to that of ACEIs. This class of drugs can directly block the binding of Ang Ⅱ to its AT_1 receptor. They do not cause the "escape" of Ang Ⅱ. Compared with ACEIs, Ang Ⅱ receptor blockers are less likely to cause cough and angioedema because they do not affect bradykinin metabolism. Clinically, such drugs are often used as the substitutes of ACEIs in HF patients.

2.3   Aldosterone antagonists

Aldosterone causes water and sodium retention and edema, increases ventricular filling pressure, promotes myocardial fibrosis, and induces arrhythmia and sudden death. Spironolactone (螺内酯, 即安体舒通) is a aldosterone antagonist, mainly used in severe HF with ascites. It is often used in combination with ACEIs and Ang Ⅱ receptor blockers.

3. β receptor blockers

Commonly used drugs include carvedilol (卡维地洛), metoprolol (美托洛尔), and bisoprolol (比索洛尔).

【 Pharmacodynamics 】 β receptor blockers play an important role in the treatment of HF by antagonizing the over-activated sympathetic nerves.

(1) Improve ventricular function and hemodynamics   Long-term use of β receptor blockers can increase the expression of myocardial β_1 receptors and restore its signal transduction, thereby improving the response of cardiomyocytes to catecholamines (儿茶酚胺类). In addition, β receptor blockers can inhibit RAAS by reducing renin release. Inhibition of RAAS helps to dilate blood vessels, reduce water and sodium retention, and reduce the anterior and posterior load of the heart, finally improve hemodynamics.

(2) Improve myocardial ischemia and anti-arrhythmias The use of β receptor blockers can reduce myocardial oxygen consumption by slowing the heart rate. Additionally, β receptor blockers help to prolong the left ventricular filling time, which is helpful to improve myocardial ischemia. β receptor blockers also have significant antiarrhythmic effects, which are important for reducing mortality and sudden death of HF patients.

(3) Improve cardiac remodeling β receptor blockers can block β receptor and antagonize the toxic effect of excessive catecholamine on the heart. They prevent the large amount of Ca^{2+} influx caused by excessive catecholamine, reduce the large amount of energy consumption and mitochondrial damage, and avoid the necrosis of cardiac cells, so as to improve the cardiac remodeling. β receptor blockers can also inhibit RAAS via reducing renin release, and thus diminish the promoting effects of both Ang Ⅱ and aldosterone in cardiac hypertrophy and remodeling.

【Clinical indications】For patients with an ejection fraction of less than 35% and grades Ⅱ to Ⅲ (NYHA classification) cardiac function, β receptor blockers can be routinely used. However, the following issues should be noted. ①β receptor blockers have the best effect on the patients whose HF is basically caused by dilated cardiomyopathy. ②They should be started with a small dose and be gradually increased to a dose that the patient can tolerate. ③They should be combined with other anti-HF drugs including diuretics, ACEIs, and digoxin. ④β receptor blockers have a slow onset and should be used for a long time. The average effective time in terms of cardiac function improvement is about 3 months, and the improvement of cardiac function is positively correlated with the treatment time. ⑤They should be used with caution or forbidden in patients with severe bradycardia, severe left ventricular dysfunction, obvious atrioventricular block, hypotension, and bronchial asthma.

4. Diuretics

Diuretics(利尿药) are traditionally used to treat HF, and they are still the current standard auxiliary drugs. Diuretics are mainly used to relieve water and sodium retention in HF. But diuretics alone do not reduce the mortality of HF patients.

The first choice is thiazide diuretics. However, for the patients with glomerular filtration rate less than 30ml/min and the elderly patients with renal dysfunction, the effect of thiazide diuretics is weak, and loop diuretics can be used. For patients with severe HF and ascites, spironolactone can be used.

Hypokalemia caused by thiazide and loop diuretics is prone to induce arrhythmias. Potassium salts should be supplemented when necessary. In addition, thiazide and loop diuretics are usually combined with potassium-sparing diuretics. But potassium-sparing diuretics, such as triamterene (氨苯蝶啶) and amiloride (阿米洛利), should not be used in combination with ACEIs because they can increase blood potassium.

5. Other drugs for heart failure

5.1   Vasodilators (扩血管药)

Vasodilators can reduce the preload and relieve the congestion symptoms of the lung by reducing venous return via dilating the vein (volume vessels). Vasodilators can also reduce peripheral resistance by dilating arterioles (resistance vessels) so as to reduce afterload and improve cardiac function, and finally increase cardiac output and relieve the symptoms of tissue ischemia. Vasodilators are easy to develop tolerance and cannot prevent the development of HF. In general, vasodilators are clinically used as auxiliary drugs. Commonly used drugs include nitrates (硝酸酯类) [such as nitroglycerin (硝酸甘油) and isosorbide nitrate (硝酸异山梨酯)], hydralazine (肼屈嗪), sodium nitroprusside (硝普钠), and prazosin (哌唑嗪).

5.2   Other positive inotropic drugs (其他正性肌力药)

These positive inotropic drugs include catecholamines and phosphodiesterase inhibitors (磷酸二酯酶抑制药). Because this kind of drugs may increase the mortality of HF patients, they are not suitable for routine treatment.

Catecholamines increase cardiac contractility by activating cardiac β_1 receptors, and dilate blood vessels by activating β_2 and dopamine receptors expressed on vascular smooth muscle. Therefore, short-term application of catecholamines can increase cardiac output and improve hemodynamics of HF patients. Commonly used drugs include dopamine (多巴胺), dobutamine (多巴酚丁胺), and ibopamine (异波帕胺).

Phosphodiesterase inhibitors have both positive inotropic and vasodilating effects. This kind of drugs, including amrinone (氨力农), milrinone (米力农), and vesnarinone (维司力农), can improve symptoms and exercise tolerance.

重 点 小 结

药物	药理作用	临床应用	不良反应
强心苷类药	正性肌力作用、负性频率作用	收缩功能障碍为主的 HF，以及对利尿药、ACEI、β 受体阻断药疗效欠佳者；室上性心律失常	各种心律失常、中枢神经系统及胃肠道反应
RAAS 抑制药	改善血流动力学、防止和逆转心血管重构	各阶段 HF	刺激性干咳、血管神经性水肿等
β 受体阻断药	改善心室功能和血流动力学、改善心肌缺血和抗心律失常、改善心脏重构	轻、中度且病情稳定的 HF	心脏抑制、诱发或加重哮喘等

续表

药物	药理作用	临床应用	不良反应
利尿药	缓解水钠潴留	伴有水钠潴留、明显肺充血和外周水肿的 HF	水、电解质紊乱
扩血管药	扩张血管、降低心脏前负荷及后负荷	辅助用药	耐受、体位性低血压等
非强心苷类正性肌力药	正性肌力作用	缓解症状，非常规治疗用药	增加 HF 患者的病死率

题库

目 标 检 测

一、选择题

（一）单项选择题

1. 强心苷加强心肌收缩力是通过（　　　）
   A. 阻断心脏 M 受体　　　　　　B. 兴奋心脏 β 受体　　　　　C. 抑制心肌细胞 Na^+-K^+-ATP 酶
   D. 促进交感神经递质释放　　　E. 抑制迷走神经递质释放

2. 治疗强心苷导致的室性心动过速，应首选（　　　）
   A. 利多卡因　　　B. 苯妥英钠　　　C. 维拉帕米　　　D. 普萘洛尔　　　E. 阿托品

3. 强心苷中毒引起房室传导阻滞时，除停用强心苷外，最好选用（　　　）
   A. 阿托品　　　B. 利多卡因　　　C. 苯妥英钠　　　D. 氢氯噻嗪　　　E. 奎尼丁

4. 易诱发强心苷心脏毒性的药物是（　　　）
   A. 普萘洛尔　　　B. 氢氯噻嗪　　　C. 螺内酯　　　D. 卡托普利　　　E. 氯沙坦

5. 下列尤其适用于伴有糖尿病的心力衰竭的是（　　　）
   A. 地高辛　　　B. 氢氯噻嗪　　　C. 卡托普利　　　D. 卡维地洛　　　E. 普萘诺尔

（二）多项选择题

6. 下列药物中长期使用后既能改善心力衰竭症状又能降低病死率的是（　　　）
   A. 地高辛　　　B. 美托洛尔　　　C. 卡托普利　　　D. 卡维地洛　　　E. 米力农

7. 为解救地高辛中毒应该（　　　）
   A. 立即停用地高辛
   B. 引起缓慢型心律失常时应及时补钾
   C. 使用苯妥英钠等抗心律失常药
   D. 使用地高辛抗体 Fab 片断
   E. 引起快速型心律失常时须及时停用排钾利尿药

二、思考题

为何 β 受体阻断药可用于治疗轻、中度心力衰竭而禁用于严重心力衰竭？

（马秉亮）

Chapter 18　Antiarrhythmic drugs

PPT

学习目标

1. **掌握**　抗心律失常药的分类及代表药物；奎尼丁、利多卡因、苯妥英钠、普萘洛尔、胺碘酮、维拉帕米的药理作用、临床应用、主要不良反应及禁忌证。

2. **熟悉**　抗心律失常药的基本作用机制和体内过程。

3. **了解**　心律失常发生的电生理机制；奎尼丁、利多卡因、苯妥英钠、普萘洛尔、腺苷的用药方法；奎尼丁晕厥的急救与处理。

Arrhythmias are due to problems with the electrical conduction system of the heart. It also known as heart arrhythmia or cardiac arrhythmia, a group of conditions in which the heartbeat is irregular, too fast, or too slow. The heart rate that is too fast—above 100 beats per minute in adults—is called tachycardia (心动过速), and a heart rate that is too slow—below 60 beats per minute—is called bradycardia (心动过缓). There are four main groups of arrhythmias: extra beats, supraventricular tachycardia (室上性心动过速), ventricular arrhythmia (室性心律失常) and bradycardia. Extra beats include premature atrial contractions (房性期前收缩), premature ventricular contractions (室性期前收缩) and premature junctional contractions (交界性期前收缩).

1. Mechanisms of arrhythmias

A cardiac arrhythmia is simply defined a variation from the normal rhythm that is not physiologically justified. The mechanisms responsible for cardiac arrhythmias are generally divided into 3 major categories: ①enhanced or abnormal impulse formation. ②Depolarization and triggered activity. ③Conduction disturbances. The irregular heartbeats may be due to intermittent premature contractions or to sustained arrhythmias such as atrial fibrillation (which results in irregular ventricular rate).

1.1　Abnormal impulse formation

Abnormal impulse formation can result in abnormal frequency, as in symptomatic sinus bradycardia (心动过缓), but abnormal location of impulse formation is more often, which can cause an ectopic pacemaker (异

医药大学堂

位起搏).

1.1.1 Abnormal automaticity(节律异常)

Abnormal automaticity includes both reduced automaticity, which causes bradycardia, and increased automaticity, which causes tachycardia. Arrhythmias caused by abnormal automaticity can result from diverse mechanisms. Such as, β Adrenergic stimulation, hypokalemia, and mechanical stretch of cardiac muscle cells increase phase 4 slope and so accelerate pacemaker rate, whereas acetylcholine reduces pacemaker rate both by decreasing phase 4 slope and through hyperpolarization. Alterations in sinus heart rate (窦性心律) can be accompanied by shifts of the origin of the dominant pacemaker within the sinoartrial (SA) node (窦房结) or to subsidiary pacemaker sites (起搏点) elsewhere in the atria. Impulse conduction out of the SA node can be impaired or blocked as a result of disease or increased vagal activity thus leads to bradycardia. AV junctional (房室交界) rhythms occur when AV junctional pacemakers located either in the AV node (房室结) or in the His bundle (希氏束) accelerate to exceed the rate of SA node, or when the SA nodal activation rate was too slow to suppress the AV junctional pacemaker. Bradycardia can also occur in structurally normal hearts. Enhanced automaticity may occur in cells that normally display spontaneous diastolic depolarization—the sinus and AV nodes and the His-Purkinje system.

1.1.2 Secondary SA node dysfunction(窦房结功能障碍)

Because of malfunction of both membrane voltage and Ca^{2+} clocks, common diseases, such as heart failure and atrial fibrillation, may be associated with significant SA node dysfunction, which thus lead to sinus bradycardia.

1.2 Depolarization (去极化) and triggered activity (触发活动)

1.2.1 EAD(早后除极)

Most pharmacologic interventions or pathophysiological conditions associated with EADs can be categorized as acting predominantly through one of four different mechanisms: ①a reduction of repolarizing potassium currents I_{Kr}, class I_A and III antiarrhythmic agents. ②An increase in the availability of calcium current. ③An increase in the sodium-calcium exchange current caused by augmentation of Cai activity or upregulation of the INCx. ④ An increase in late sodium current. Combinations of these interventions or pathophysiological states can act synergistically to facilitate the development of EADs.

1.2.2 Role of delayed afterdepolarization-induced triggered activity(迟后除极和触发活动)

DADs and DAD-induced triggered activity are observed under conditions that augment intracellular calcium. This activity is also manifest in hypertrophied and failing hearts as well as in Purkinje fibers surviving myocardial infarction. In contrast to EADs, DADs are always induced at relatively rapid rates. DAD-induced arrhythmia is the catecholaminergic polymorphic ventricular tachycardia, which may be caused by the mutation of either the type 2 ryanodine receptor or the calsequestrin. The principal mechanism underlying these arrhythmias is the "leaky" ryanodine receptor, which is aggravated during catecholamine stimulation. "Late phase 3 EAD", which combines properties of both EAD and DAD, but has its own unique character. Late phase 3 EAD-induced triggered extrasystoles represent a new concept of arrhythmogenesis in which abbreviated repolarization permits "normal SR calcium release" to induce an EAD-mediated closely coupled triggered response, particularly under conditions permitting intracellular calcium loading. These EADs are distinguished by the fact that they interrupt the final phase of repolarization of the action potential. In contrast to previously described DAD or Cai-dependent EAD, it is normal, not spontaneous SR calcium release that is responsible for the generation of the EAD. Two principal conditions are required for the appearance of late phase 3 EAD: an APD abbreviation and a strong SR calcium release. Such conditions may occur when both parasympathetic and sympathetic (交感神经) influences are combined. Simultaneous sympathovagal activation is also known to be the primary trigger of paroxysmal atrial tachycardia (阵发性房性心动过速) and AF episodes in dogs with intermittent rapid pacing.

1.3   A return relationship with impulse and rhythm of the heart

1.3.1   Functionally defined re-entry

Re-entry is a common cause of arrhythmias (心律失常). Ventricular tachycardia and AV-nodal re-entry are typical examples. Re-entry can occur when a conduction path is partly slowed down. As a result of this, the signal is conducted by both a fast and a slow pathway. During normal sinus rhythm this generally does not cause problems, but when an extrasystole (期外收缩) follows rapidly upon the previous beat, the fast pathway is sometimes still refractory and cannot conduct the signal.

1.3.2   Reentrant activation

Two fundamental conditions necessary for the initiation and maintenance of circus movement excitation: unidirectional block—the impulse initiating the circulating wave must travel in one direction only; and for the circus movement to continue, the circuit must be long enough to allow each site in the circuit to recover before the return of the circulating wave. Although the basic beats elicited by stimuli applied near the center of the tissue spread normally throughout the preparation, premature impulses propagate only in the direction of shorter refractory periods. An arc of block thus develops around which the impulse is able to circulate and reexcite its site of origin. Recordings near the center of the circus movement showed only subthreshold responses. The investigators proposed the term "leading circle" to explain their observation. The functionally refractory region develops at the vortex of the circulating wavefront prevents the centripetal waves from short circuiting the circus movement and thus serves to maintain the reentry. Because the head of the circulating wavefront (波前) usually travels on relatively refractory tissue, a fully excitable gap of tissue may not be present; unlike other forms of reentry, the leading circle model may not be readily influenced by extraneous impulses initiated in areas outside the reentrant circuit and thus may not be easily entrained (Figure 18-1).

2. Mechanisms of antiarrhythmic drug

Anti-arrhythmic drugs almost invariably have multiple effects in patients, and their effects on arrhythmias can be complex. A single arrhythmia may result from multiple underlying mechanisms can result either from increased Na^+ channel late currents or decreased inward rectifier currents (内向整流电流). Thus, anti-arrhythmic therapy should be tailored to target the most relevant

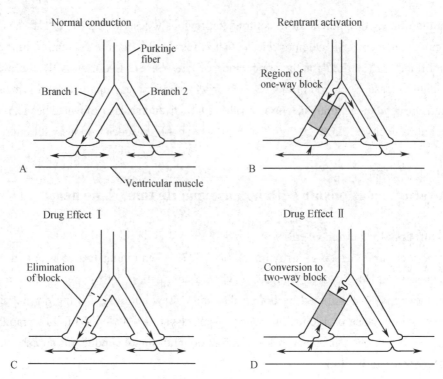

Figure 18-1   Reentrant activation: mechanism and drug effects

(A) In normal conduction, impulses from the branched Purkinje fiber stimulate the strip of ventricular muscle in two places. Within the muscle, waves of excitation spread from both points of excitation, meet between the Purkinje fibers, and cease further travel.(B) In the presence of one-way block, the strip of muscle is excited at only one location. Impulses spreading from this area meet no impulses coming from the left and, therefore, can travel far enough to stimulate branch 1 of the Purkinje fiber. This stimulation passes back up the fiber, past the region of one-way block, and then stimulates branch 2, causing reentrant activation.(C) Elimination of reentry by a drug that improves conduction in the sick branch of the Purkinje fiber.(D) Elimination of reentry by a drug that further suppresses conduction in the sick branch, thereby converting one-way block into two-way block

underlying arrhythmia mechanism. Drugs may slow automatic rhythms by altering any of the four determinants of spontaneous pacemaker discharge: ①decrease phase 4 slope. ②Increase threshold potential. ③Increase maximum diastolic potential. ④Increase APD. Anti-arrhythmic drugs may block arrhythmias owing to DADs or EADs by two major mechanisms: ①inhibition of the development of afterdepolarizations. ②Interference with the inward current, which is responsible for the upstroke. Recent advances have elucidated the structural and molecular determinants of ion channel permeation and drug block.

2.1   Na$^+$ channel block

Sodium channel blockers are drugs which impair the conduction of sodium ions through sodium channels.

Quinidine (奎尼丁)

Quinidine belongs to class Ⅰ antiarrhythmic agent (Ⅰa). It is originally derived from the bark of the cinchona tree. The drug causes increased action potential duration, as well as a prolonged QT interval.

【Pharmacokinetics】Quinidine is well absorbed and is 80% bound to plasma proteins (血浆蛋白). Quinidine undergoes extensive hepatic oxidative metabolism, and about 20% is excreted unchanged by the kidney. One metabolite, 3-hydroxyquinidine, is nearly as potent as quinidine. Concentrations of unbound 3-hydroxyquinidine equal to or exceeding those of quinidine are tolerated by some patients. There is substantial individual variability in the range of dosages required to achieve therapeutic plasma concentrations of 2-5g/ml. Some of this variability may be assay dependent because not all assays exclude quinidine metabolites. The elimination half-life of oral quinidine is 6 to 8 hours, and it is eliminated by the cytochrome P450 system in the liver. About 20% is excreted unchanged via the kidneys.

【Pharmacodynamics】Quinidine's effect on I_{Na} is known as a 'use dependent block', which means at higher heart rates, the blockade increases, while at lower heart rates, the blockade decreases. By blocking the fast inward sodium current, quinidine decreases the phase 0 depolarization of the cardiac action potential. By binding to the same receptor sites, quinidine inhibits Na^+-K^+-ATPase. The effect of quinidine on the ion channels leads to prolong the cardiac action potential, thereby prolonging the QT interval on the ECG. Quinidine actually tends to shorten the PR interval largely as a result of its vagolytic properties. Action potential duration either is unaffected or shortened by Na^+ channel block, but some Na^+ channel-blocking drugs do prolong cardiac action potentials by other mechanisms, usually blocking K^+ channel.

【Clinical indications】Quinidine is occasionally used to prevent ventricular arrhythmias (室性心律失常), particularly in Brugada syndrome, although its safety in this indication is uncertain. It reduces the recurrence of atrial fibrillation after patients undergo cardioversion, but it has proarrhythmic effects (致心律失常作用) and trials suggest that it may lead to an overall increased mortality in these patients. Quinidine is also used to treat short QT syndrome.

【Adverse reactions】Quinidine can cause thrombocytopenia, granulomatous hepatitis, myasthenia gravis, and torsades de pointes, so is not used much today. Torsades can occur after the first dose. Diarrhea (腹泻) is the most common adverse effect during quinidine therapy, occurring in 30%-50% of patients. Quinidine-induced thrombocytopenia is mediated by the immune system, and may lead to thrombocytic purpura. Quinidine intoxication is known as cinchonism, with tinnitus being among the most characteristic and common symptoms of this toxicity syndrome. A high dosage of quinidine is used to try to convert atrial fibrillation to normal rhythm, this aggressive approach to quinidine dosing has been abandoned, and quinidine induced ventricular tachycardia is unusual.

Lidocaine (利多卡因)

Lidocaine, also known as lignocaine, is a medication used to numb tissue in local anesthetic.

【Pharmacokinetics】Lidocaine is about 95% metabolized in the liver mainly by CYP3A4 to the pharmacologically active metabolites monoethylglycinexylidide and then subsequently to the inactive glycine xylidide. About 60% to 80% circulates bound to the protein alpha acid glycoprotein. The oral bioavailability (口服生物利用度) is 35% and the topical bioavailability is 3%. The elimination half-life of lidocaine is biphasic and around 90 to 120min in most patients.

【Pharmacodynamics】Lidocaine alters signal conduction in neurons by prolonging the inactivation of the fast voltage-gated Na^+ channels in the neuronal cell membrane responsible for action potential propagation. With sufficient blockage, the voltage-gated (电压门控) sodium channels will not open and an action potential will not be generated. Careful titration allows for a high degree of selectivity in the blockage of sensory neurons, whereas higher concentrations also affect other types of neurons.

【Clinical indications】

(1) Ventricular tachycardia　Lidocaine induced block reflects an increased likelihood that the Na^+ channel protein assumes a nonconducting conformation in the presence of drug. Recovery from block is very rapid, so lidocaine exerts greater effects in depolarized or rapidly driven tissues. Lidocaine is not useful in atrial arrhythmias possibly because atrial action potentials are so short that the Na^+ channel is in the inactivated state only briefly compared with diastolic times (舒张期), which are relatively long. Lidocaine increased current through inward rectifier channels.

(2) Chronic pain　Intravenous lidocaine infusions are also used to treat chronic pain and acute surgical pain as an opiate sparing technique. Inhaled lidocaine can be used as a cough suppressor acting peripherally to reduce the cough reflex. This application can be implemented as a safety and comfort measure for patients who have to be intubated, as it reduces the incidence of coughing and any tracheal damage it might cause when emerging from anaesthesia (麻醉). Lidocaine, along with ethanol, ammonia, and acetic acid, may also help in treating jellyfish stings, both numbing the affected area and preventing further nematocyst discharge.

【Adverse reactions】Adverse drug reactions are rare when lidocaine is used as a local anesthetic and is administered correctly. In addition, there are some side effect. ① CNS excitation, nervousness,agitation, anxiety, apprehension, tingling around the mouth and so on. ② CNS depression with increasingly heavier exposure. ③ Cardiovascular, hypotension, bradycardia, arrhythmias, flushing, and cardiac arrest some of which may be due to hypoxemia secondary to respiratory depression. ④Respiratory, bronchospasm, dyspnea, respiratory depression or arrest. ⑤ Gastrointestinal, metallic taste, nausea, vomiting and so on.

2.2　Action potential prolongation (延长动作电位)

Most drugs that prolong the action potential do so by blocking K^+ channels, although enhanced inward Na^+ current also can cause prolongation. Enhanced inward current may underlie QT prolongation by ibutilide. Block of cardiac K^+ channels increases APD and reduces normal automaticity. Increased APD, seen as an increase in QT interval, increases refractoriness and therefore should be an effective way of treating re-entry.

Amiodarone (胺碘酮)

Amiodarone exerts a multiplicity of pharmacologic effects, none of which is clearly linked to its arrhythmia-suppressing properties.

【Pharmacokinetics】Amiodarone's oral bioavailability is about 22%-65%, presumably because of poor absorption. This incomplete bioavailability is important in calculating equivalent dosing regimens when converting from intravenous to oral therapy. After the initiation of amiodarone therapy, increases in refractoriness, a marker of pharmacologic effect, require several weeks to develop. Excretion is primarily hepatic and biliary (胆道) with almost no elimination via the renal route and it is not dialyzable. Elimination half-life average of 58 days for amiodarone and 36 days for the active metabolite, desethylamiodarone.

【Pharmacodynamics】Amiodarone is categorized as a class III antiarrhythmic agent, and prolongs phase 3 of the cardiac action potential, the repolarization phase where there is normally decreased calcium permeability and increased potassium permeability. It has numerous other effects, however, including actions that are similar to those of antiarrhythmic classes Ⅰa, Ⅱ, and Ⅳ. Amiodarone is a blocker of voltage gated potassium and voltage gated calcium channels. Amiodarone slows conduction rate and prolongs the refractory period of the SA and AV nodes. Amiodarone shows β blocker-like and calcium channel blocker-like actions on the SA and AV nodes, increases the refractory period via sodium-channel and potassium-channel effects, and slows intra-cardiac conduction of the cardiac action potential, via sodium-channel effects.

【Clinical indications 】

(1) Ventricular tachycardia (室性心动过速)　Amiodarone may be used in the treatment of ventricular tachycardia in certain instances. Individuals with hemodynamically unstable ventricular tachycardia should not initially receive amiodarone. Amiodarone can be used in individuals with hemodynamically stable ventricular tachycardia.

(2) Atrial fibrillation (心房颤动)　Intravenous amiodarone has been shown to reduce the incidence of atrial fibrillation after open heart surgery when compared to placebo. It is a commonly prescribed off-label treatment due to the lack of equally effective treatment alternatives. The benefit of amiodarone in the treatment of atrial fibrillation in the critical care population has yet to be determined but it may prove to be the agent of choice where the patient is hemodynamically unstable and unsuitable for DC cardioversion.

【Adverse reactions 】A therapeutic plasma amiodarone concentration range of 0.5-2g/ml has been proposed. Because of amiodarone's slow accumulation in tissue, a high-dose oral loading regimen usually is administered for several weeks before maintenance therapy is started.

(1) Arrhythmia (心律失常)　Maintenance dose is adjusted based on adverse effects and the arrhythmias being treated. If the presenting arrhythmia is life-threatening, dosages of 300mg/d normally are used unless unequivocal toxicity occurs. On the other hand, maintenance doses of 200mg/d are used if recurrence of an arrhythmia would be tolerated, as in patients with atrial fibrillation.

(2) Pulmonary fibrosis (肺纤维化)　The most serious adverse effect during chronic amiodarone therapy is pulmonary fibrosis, which can be rapidly progressive and fatal. Underlying lung disease, doses of 400mg/d or more, and recent pulmonary insults such as pneumonia appear to be risk factors. With low doses, such as 200mg/d or less used in atrial fibrillation, pulmonary toxicity is unusual.

(3) Thyroid (甲状腺)　Induced abnormalities in thyroid function are common. Both under and overactivity of the thyroid may occur. Amiodarone is structurally similar to thyroxine and also contains iodine. Both of these contribute to the effects of amiodarone on thyroid function.

(4) Whorl keratopathy (轮状角膜病变)　Corneal micro-deposits are almost universally present (over 90%) in individuals taking amiodarone longer than 6 months, especially doses greater than 400mg/d. These deposits typically do not cause any symptoms. About 1 in 10 individuals may complain of a bluish halo. Anterior subcapsular lens deposits are relatively common (50%) in higher doses (greater than 600mg/d) after 6 months of treatment.

(5) Other　Abnormal liver enzyme results are common in patients on amiodarone. Long-term administration of amiodarone is associated with a light-sensitive blue-grey discoloration of the skin; such patients should avoid exposure to the sun and use sunscreen that protects against ultraviolet-A and ultraviolet-B. Use during pregnancy may result in a number of problems in the baby including thyroid problems, heart problems, neurological problems, and preterm birth.

2.3 Ca²⁺ channel block

The major electrophysiologic effects resulting from block of cardiac Ca^{2+} channels are in nodal tissues.

Verapamil (维拉帕米)

Verapamil's mechanism in all cases is to block voltage-dependent calcium channels.

【Pharmacodynamics】Calcium channel blockers are considered class Ⅳ antiarrhythmic agents. Since calcium channels are especially concentrated in the sinoatrial and atrioventricular nodes, these agents can be used to decrease impulse conduction through the AV node, thus protecting the ventricles from atrial tachyarrhythmias.

【Clinical indications】

Supraventricular tachycardia (室上性心动过速) Verapamil is used for controlling ventricular rate in supraventricular tachycardia and migraine headache prevention. It is a class Ⅳ antiarrhythmic and more effective than digoxin in controlling ventricular rate.

【Adverse reactions】The most common side effect of verapamil is constipation (便秘) (7.3%). Other side effects include dizziness (3.3%), nausea (2.7%), low blood pressure (2.5%), and headache (2.2%). Along with other calcium channel blockers, verapamil is known to induce gingival enlargement. Acute overdose is often manifested by nausea, weakness, slow heart rate, dizziness, low blood pressure, and abnormal heart rhythms.

2.4 Blockade of β adrenergic receptors

β adrenergic stimulation increases the magnitude of the Ca^{2+} current and slows its inactivation, increases the magnitude of repolarizing K^+ and Cl^- currents , increases pacemaker current thereby increasing sinus rate, increases the Ca^{2+} stored in the sarcoplasmic reticulum thereby increasing likelihood of spontaneous Ca^{2+} release and DADs, and under pathophysiologic conditions, can increase both DAD and EAD-mediated arrhythmias.

Propranolol (普萘洛尔)

Propranolol is a medication of the β blocker class. It is used to treat high blood pressure, a number of types of irregular heart rate, thyrotoxicosis, capillary hemangiomas, performance anxiety, and essential tremors. It is used to prevent migraine headaches, and to prevent further heart problems in those with angina or previous heart attacks.

【Pharmacodynamics】Propranolol is a competitive antagonist of β_1 adrenergic receptors in the heart. It competes with sympathomimetic neurotransmitters for binding to receptors, which inhibits sympathetic stimulation of the heart. Blockage of neurotransmitter binding β_1 receptors on cardiac myocytes inhibits activation of adenylate cyclase, which in turn inhibits cAMP synthesis leading to reduced PKA activation. Since propranolol blocks β adrenoceptors, the increase in synaptic norepinephrine only results in α adrenoceptor activation, with the α_1 adrenoceptor being particularly important for effects observed in animal models. In addition to its effects on the adrenergic system (肾上腺素系统), there is evidence that indicates that propranolol may act as a weak antagonist of certain serotonin receptors, namely the 5-HT$_{1A}$, 5-HT$_{1B}$, and 5-HT$_{2B}$ receptors.

【Clinical indications】Hypertension, angina pectoris, myocardial infarction, tachycardia associated with various conditions, including anxiety, panic, hyperthyroidism, and lithium therapy, portal hypertension, to lower portal vein pressure, prevention of esophageal variceal bleeding and ascites, anxiety, hypertrophic cardiomyopathy.

【Adverse reactions】Propranolol should be used with caution in people with diabetes (糖尿病) mellitus or hyperthyroidism (甲状腺功能亢进), since signs and symptoms of hypoglycaemia may be masked. Peripheral artery disease and Raynaud's syndrome, which may be exacerbated. Phaeochromocytoma, as hypertension may be aggravated without prior alpha blocker therapy. Myasthenia gravis, which may be worsened. Other drugs with bradycardic effects.

2.5   Other drugs

Adenosine (腺苷)

Adenosine is a naturally occurring nucleoside that is administered as a rapid intravenous bolus for the acute termination of re-entrant supraventricular arrhythmias.

【Pharmacodynamics】The effects of adenosine are mediated by its interaction with specific G protein-coupled adenosine receptors (G蛋白偶联腺苷受体). When it is administered intravenously, adenosine causes transient heart block in the atrioventricular (AV) node. This is mediated via the A$_1$ receptor, inhibiting adenylyl cyclase, reducing cAMP and so causing cell hyperpolarization (超极化) by increasing K$^+$ efflux via inward rectifier K$^+$ channels, subsequently inhibiting Ca^{2+} current. It also causes endothelial-dependent (内皮依赖性) relaxation of smooth muscle as is found inside the artery walls. This causes dilation of the "normal" segments of arteries, i.e., where the endothelium is not separated from the tunica media by atherosclerotic plaque.

【Clinical indications】

Acute re-entrant supraventricular arrhythmias   Adenosine activates acetylcholine-sensitive K$^+$ current in the atrium and sinus and AV nodes, resulting in shortening of APD, hyperpolarization, and slowing of normal automaticity. Adenosine also inhibits the electrophysiologic effects of increased intracellular cyclic AMP that occur with sympathetic stimulation. Because adenosine thereby reduces Ca^{2+} currents, it can be anti-arrhythmic by increasing AV nodal refractoriness and by inhibiting DADs elicited by sympathetic stimulation. Administration of an intravenous bolus of adenosine to humans transiently slows sinus rate and AV nodal conduction velocity and increases AV nodal refractoriness. Adenosine is an endogenous purine nucleoside that modulates many physiological processes, and is administered as a rapid intravenous bolus for the acute termination of re-entrant supraventricular arrhythmias.

【Pharmacokinetics】Adenosine is eliminated with a $t_{1/2}$ of seconds by carrier-mediated uptake, which occurs in most cell types, including the endothelium, and subsequent metabolism by adenosine deaminase. Adenosine probably is the only drug whose efficacy requires a rapid bolus dose, preferably through a large central intravenous line; slow administration results in elimination of the drug prior to its arrival at the heart.

【Adverse reactions】A major advantage of adenosine therapy is that adverse effects are short lived because the drug is transported into cells and deaminated so rapidly. Transient asystole is common but usually lasts less than 5 seconds and is in fact the therapeutic goal. Most patients feel a sense of chest fullness and dyspnea when therapeutic doses (6-12mg) of adenosine are administered. Rarely, an adenosine bolus can precipitate bronchospasm or atrial fibrillation presumably by heterogeneously shortening atrial action potentials.

重 点 小 结

类别	药物	药理作用	临床应用	不良反应
Ⅰ类钠通道阻滞药	Ⅰa适度钠通道阻滞药：奎尼丁、普鲁卡因胺	适度阻滞钠通道，降低0相上升速度，抑制心肌细胞膜，延长ERP显著	心房纤颤、心房扑动、室上性和室性心动过速的转复与预防	心脏毒性严重，Q-T间期延长和尖端扭转型室速
	Ⅰb轻度钠通道阻滞药：利多卡因、苯妥英钠	轻度阻滞钠通道，减少动作电位4相除极斜率，降低自律性	室性心律失常，心肌梗死或强心苷中毒所致的室性心动过速	剂量过大引起心率减慢、房室传导阻滞和低血压
	Ⅰc明显钠通道阻滞药：普罗帕酮	明显阻滞钠通道，减慢传导性的作用最为明显	室上性和室性期前收缩，室上性和室性心动过速	消化道不良反应，房室传导阻滞、加重心力衰竭
Ⅱ类β肾上腺素受体阻断药	普萘洛尔	降低窦房结、心房和浦肯野纤维自律性	室上性心律失常，窦性心动过速	窦性心动过缓，房室传导阻滞诱发心力衰竭和哮喘
Ⅲ类延长APD药（钾通道阻滞药）	胺碘酮	对心脏多种离子通道均有抑制作用，明显延长APD和ERP	心房扑动，心房颤动，室上性心动过速和室性心动过速	窦性心动过缓，房室传导阻滞及Q-T间期延长
Ⅳ类钙通道阻滞药	维拉帕米	降低窦房结自律性，减慢房室结传导，延长窦房结、房室结ERP	治疗阵发性室上性心动过速首选，房室结折返引起的心律失常	便秘、腹胀、腹泻、头痛，血压降低、窦性停搏
其他	腺苷	缩短APD，降低自律性	室上性心律失常	胸闷，心脏骤停

目 标 检 测

题库

一、单项选择题

1. 关于抗心律失常药物取消折返的机制，下列何项叙述错误（　　　　）

   A. 减弱膜反应性，变单向传导阻滞为双向传导阻滞

   B. 增强膜反应性，取消单向传导阻滞

   C. 绝对延长ERP

   D. 相对延长ERP

   E. 使邻近细胞ERP不均一

医药大学堂
WWW.YIYAODXT.COM

2. 可消除迟后除极所引起的触发活动的药物是（　　　）
　　A. 毒毛花苷 K　　　　　　　B. 维拉帕米　　　　　　C. 阿托品
　　D. 异丙肾上腺素　　　　　　E. 以上都不是

3. 兼具抗胆碱和阻滞 α 受体作用的抗心律失常药物是（　　　）
　　A. 利多卡因　　　　　　　　B. 普萘洛尔　　　　　　C. 奎尼丁
　　D. 胺碘酮　　　　　　　　　E. 美西律

4. 奎尼丁不具有下列哪项药理作用（　　　）
　　A. 拟胆碱　　　　　　　　　B. 降低自律性　　　　　C. 减慢传导
　　D. 阻断 α 受体　　　　　　　E. 延长 ERP

二、多项选择题

5. 缓慢型心律失常宜选用下列哪些药物治疗（　　　）
　　A. 奎尼丁　　　　　　　　　B. 利多卡因　　　　　　C. 阿托品
　　D. 异丙肾上腺素　　　　　　E. 维拉帕米

6. 抗心律失常药物减慢自动起搏的方式有（　　　）
　　A. 增加最大舒张电位　　　　B. 减慢 4 期自动除极速率　　C. 上移阈电位
　　D. 延长 APD　　　　　　　　E. 增加最大舒张电位与阈电位距离

7. 苯妥英钠作为治疗强心苷中毒所致心律失常的首选药物，其原因是（　　　）
　　A. 与强心苷竞争 Na^+-K^+-ATP 酶
　　B. 降低蒲肯野纤维的自律性
　　C. 抑制强心苷中毒所致的迟后除极及触发活动
　　D. 恢复因强心苷中毒而受抑制的房室传导
　　E. 增加窦房结自律性

8. 关于腺苷的叙述，正确的是（　　　）
　　A. 激活钾通道，降低窦房结、房室结自律性
　　B. 减慢房室结传导
　　C. 抑制迟后除极
　　D. 主要用于迅速终止折返性室上性心动过速
　　E. 使用时无须静脉快速给药

（王宏婷）

Chapter 19　Antianginal drugs

 学习目标

1. 掌握　抗心绞痛药的概念、分类、药理作用及机制、临床应用和不良反应。
2. 熟悉　硝酸甘油、普萘洛尔、硝苯地平的临床应用。
3. 了解　硝酸异山梨酯、亚硝酸异戊酯、维拉帕米、地尔硫䓬的临床应用。

Angina pectoris (心绞痛), the primary symptom of ischemic heart disease, is caused by transient episodes of myocardial ischemia that are due to an imbalance between the myocardial oxygen supply and demand. This imbalance may be caused by an increase in myocardial oxygen demand (which is determined by heart rate, ventricular contractility, and ventricular wall tension) or by a decrease in myocardial oxygen supply (primarily determined by coronary blood flow, but occasionally modified by the oxygen carrying capacity of the blood) or sometimes by both situations (Figure 19-1). Because blood flow is inversely proportional to the fourth power of the artery's luminal radius, the progressive decrease in vessel radius that characterizes coronary atherosclerosis can impair coronary blood flow and lead to symptoms of angina when myocardial O_2 demand increases, as with exertion (so called typical angina pectoris). There are three types of angina as the followings. ①Stable angina (稳定型心绞痛): stable angina occurs when the heart is working harder than usual, for instance, during exercises. It has a regular pattern and can be predicted to happen over months or even years. Rest or medication relieves symptoms. ②Unstable angina (不稳定型心绞痛): unstable angina does not follow a regular pattern. It can occur at rest and is considered less common and more serious because rest and medication do not relieve it. This version can signal a future heart attack within a short time-hours or weeks. ③Variant of angina (变异型心绞痛): variant of angina is rare and can occur at rest without any underlying coronary artery disease. This angina is usually due to abnormal narrowing or relaxation of the blood vessels, reducing blood flow to the heart. It can be relieved by medicine.

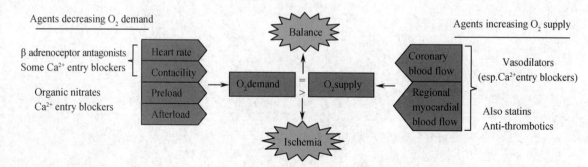
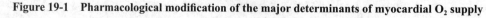

Figure 19-1　Pharmacological modification of the major determinants of myocardial O_2 supply

1. Organic nitrates

All therapeutically active agents in the nitrate group have identical mechanisms of action and similar toxicities. Therefore, pharmacokinetic factors govern the choice of agent and mode of therapy (Figure 19-2).

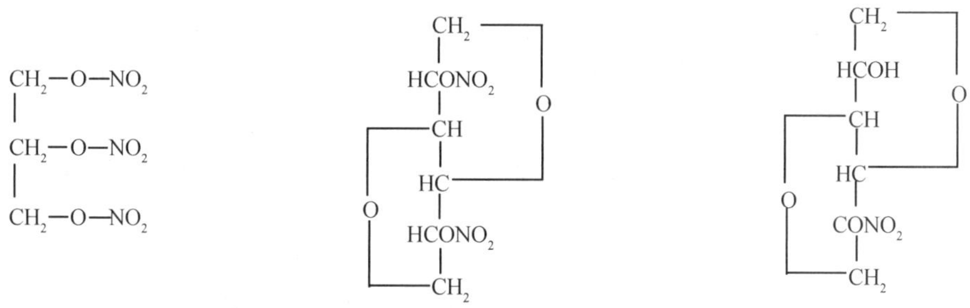

CH$_2$—O—NO$_2$
|
CH$_2$—O—NO$_2$
|
CH$_2$—O—NO$_2$

Nitroglycerin
（硝酸甘油）

Isosorbide dinitrate
（硝酸异山梨酸）

Isosorbide-mononitrate
（单硝酸异山梨酸）

Figure 19-2　The structures of organic nitrates

Nitroglycerin (硝酸甘油)

Nitroglycerin was first synthesized in 1846 by Sobrero, who observed that a small quantity placed on the tongue elicited a severe headache. It is still the most commonly used drug to prevent angina pectoris, due to its advantages of quick onset, definite curative effect, convenient use and economy.

【Pharmacokinetics】The concentrations of nitroglycerin in plasma reach the peak within 4 minutes after sublingual administration; the drug has a $t_{1/2}$ of 1-3 minutes. The onset of action of nitroglycerin may be even more rapid if it is delivered as a sublingual spray rather than as a sublingual tablet. Glyceryl dinitrate metabolites, which have about one-tenth the vasodilator potency, appear to have half-lives of about 40 minutes.

【Pharmacodynamics】Nitroglycerin relaxes all types of smooth muscle irrespective of the cause of the preexiting muscle tone. It has practically no direct effect on cardiac or skeletal muscle.

(1) Effects on myocardial O$_2$ requirements　By their effects on the systemic circulation, the organic nitrates also can reduce myocardial O$_2$ demand. The major determinants of myocardial O$_2$ consumption include left ventricular wall tension, heart rate, and myocardial contractility. Ventricular wall tension is affected by a number of factors that may be considered under the categories of preload and afterload. Preload is determined by the diastolic pressure that distends the ventricle (ventricular end diastolic pressure). Increasing end-diastolic volume augments the ventricular wall tension (by the law of Laplace, tension is proportional to pressure times radius). Increasing venous capacitance with nitrates decreases venous return to the heart, decreases ventricular end-diastolic volume, and thereby decreases O$_2$ consumption. An additional benefit of reducing preload is that it increases the pressure gradient for perfusion across the ventricular wall, which favors subendocardial perfusion. Afterload is the impedance against which the ventricle must eject. In the absence of aortic valvular disease, afterload is related to peripheral resistance. Decreasing peripheral arteriolar resistance reduces afterload and thus myocardial work and O_2 consumption. Organic nitrates decrease both preload and afterload as a result of respective dilation of venous capacitance and arteriolar resistance vessels.

(2) Effects on total and regional coronary blood flow Myocardial ischemia is a powerful stimulus to coronary vasodilation, and regional blood flow is adjusted by autoregulatory mechanisms. In the presence of atherosclerotic coronary artery narrowing, ischemia distal to the lesion stimulates vasodilation; if the stenosis is severe, much of the capacity to dilate is used to maintain resting blood flow. When demand increases, further dilation may not be possible. After demonstration of direct coronary artery vasodilation in experimental animals, it became generally accepted that nitrates relieved anginal pain by dilating coronary arteries and thereby increasing coronary blood flow. In the presence of significant coronary stenoses, there is a disproportionate reduction in blood flow to the subendocardial regions of the heart, which are subjected to the greatest extravascular compression during systole; organic nitrates tend to restore blood flow in these regions toward normal conditions (Figure 19-3).

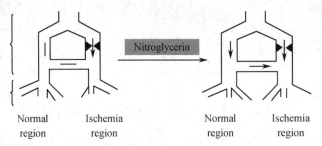

Figure 19-3   Nitroglycerin redistributes coronary flow and increases ischemic region perfusion

(3) Hemodynamic effects The nitrovasodilators promote relaxation of vascular smooth muscle. Low concentrations of nitroglycerin preferentially dilate veins more than arterioles. This venodilation decreases venous return, leading to a fall in left and right ventricular chamber size and end-diastolic pressures, but usually results in little change in systemic vascular resistance. Systemic arterial pressure may fall slightly, and heart rate is unchanged or may increase slightly in response to a decrease in blood pressure. Pulmonary vascular resistance and cardiac output are slightly reduced.

Higher doses of organic nitrates cause further venous pooling and may decrease arteriolar resistance as well, thereby decreasing systolic and diastolic blood pressure and cardiac output and causing pallor, weakness, dizziness, and activation of compensatory sympathetic reflexes. The reflex tachycardia and peripheral arteriolar vasoconstriction tend to restore systemic vascular resistance; this is superimposed on sustained venous pooling. Coronary blood flow may increase transiently as a result of coronary vasodilation but may decrease subsequently if cardiac output and blood pressure decrease sufficiently. In patients with autonomic dysfunction and an inability to increase sympathetic outflow (multiple-system atrophy and pure autonomic failure are the most common forms, much less commonly seen in the autonomic dysfunction associated with diabetes), the fall in blood pressure consequent to the venodilation produced by nitrates cannot be compensated. In these clinical contexts, nitrates may reduce arterial pressure and coronary perfusion pressure significantly, producing potentially life-threatening hypotension and even aggravating angina. The appropriate therapy in patients with orthostatic angina and normal coronary arteries is to correct the orthostatic hypotension by expanding volume (fludrocortisone and a high-sodium diet), to prevent venous pooling with fitted support garments, and to carefully titrate use of oral vasopressors. Because patients with autonomic dysfunction occasionally may have coexisting coronary artery disease, the coronary anatomy should be defined before therapy is undertaken.

(4) Protect myocardial ischema and reperfusion injury   Nitrites, organic nitrates, nitroso compounds, and a variety of other nitrogen oxide containing substances (including nitroprusside; see later in the chapter) lead to the formation of the reactive gaseous free radical NO and related NO-containing compounds. Nitric oxide gas also may be administered by inhalation. The exact mechanisms of denitration of the organic nitrates to liberate NO remains an active area of investigation. Phosphorylation of the myosin light chain regulates the maintenance of the contractile state in smooth muscle. NO can activate guanylyl cyclase, increase the cellular level of cyclic GMP, activate PKG, and modulate the activities of cyclic nucleotide phosphodiesterases (PDEs 2, 3 and 5) in a variety of cell types. In smooth muscle, the net result is reduced phosphorylation of myosin light chain, reduced Ca^{2+} concentration in the cytosol, and relaxation. One important consequence of the NO mediated increase in intracellular cyclic GMP is the activation of PKG, which catalyzes the phosphorylation of various proteins in smooth muscle. Another important target of this kinase is the myosin light-chain phosphatase, which is activated on binding PKG and leads to dephosphorylation of the myosin light chain and thereby promotes vasorelaxation and smooth muscle relaxation in many other tissues. The pharmacological and biochemical effects of the nitrovasodilators appear to be identical to those of an endothelium-derived relaxing factor now known to be NO. Although the soluble isoform of guanylyl cyclase remains the most extensively characterized molecular "receptor" for NO, it is increasingly clear that NO also forms specific adducts with thiol groups in proteins and with reduced glutathione to form nitrosothiol compounds with distinctive biological properties. Mitochondrial aldehyde dehydrogenase has been shown to catalyze the reduction of nitroglycerin to yield bioactive NO metabolites, providing a potentially important clue to the biotransformation of organic nitrates in intact tissues. The regulation and pharmacology of eNOS have been reviewed (Figure 19-4).

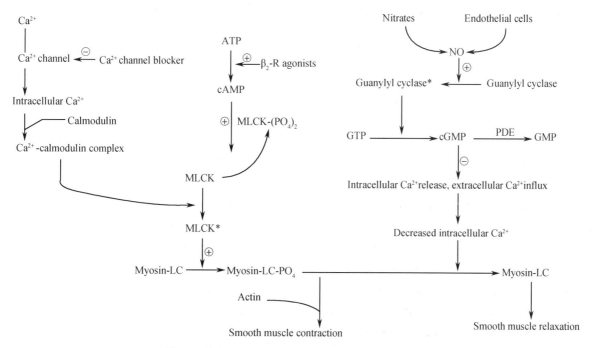

Figure 19-4   Pharmacodynamics of organic nitrates
* Active type; MLCK(myosin light chain kinase); PDE(phosphodiesterase)

【Adverse reactions】Untoward responses to the therapeutic use of organic nitrates are almost all secondary to actions on the cardiovascular system. Headache is common and can be severe. Transient episodes of dizziness, weakness, and other manifestations associated with postural hypotension may develop, particularly if the patient is standing immobile, and may progress occasionally to loss of consciousness, a reaction that appears to be accentuated by alcohol. It also may be seen with very low doses of nitrates in patients with autonomic dysfunction. Even in severe nitrate syncope, positioning and other measures that facilitate venous return are the only therapeutic measures required. All the organic nitrates occasionally can produce drug rash. Intracranial hypertension and glaucoma are prohibited.

Isosorbide dinitrate (硝酸异山梨酯)

Isosorbide dinitrate is a moderate to long acting oral organic nitrate used for the relief and prophylactic management of angina pectoris. It relaxes the vascular smooth muscle and consequent dilatation of peripheral arteries and veins, especially the latter. Dilatation of the veins promotes peripheral pooling of blood and decreases venous return to the heart, thereby reducing left ventricular end-diastolic pressure and pulmonary capillary wedge pressure. Arteriolar relaxation reduces systemic vascular resistance, systolic arterial pressure, and mean arterial pressure.

Isosorbide-mononitrate (单硝酸异山梨酯)

Isosorbide mononitrate is an organic nitrate with vasodilating properties. It is an antianginal agent that works by relaxing the smooth muscles of both arteries and veins, but predominantly veins to reduce cardiac preload. Isosorbide mononitrate is an active metabolite of isosorbide dinitrate.

2. β adrenoceptor antagonists

β adrenergic receptor antagonists are effective in reducing the severity and frequency of attacks of exertional angina and in improving survival in patients who have had an MI. Most β adrenergic receptor antagonists apparently are equally effective in the treatment of exertional angina. propranolol (普萘洛尔), atenolol (阿替洛尔), metoprolol (美托洛尔), nadolol (纳多洛尔), arteolol (卡替洛尔), bisoprolol (比索洛尔), labetalol (拉贝洛尔).

【Pharmacodynamics】

(1) **Decrease myocardial oxygen demand** The effectiveness of β adrenergic receptor antagonists in the treatment of exertional angina is attributable primarily to a fall in myocardial O_2 consumption at rest and during exertion, although there also is some tendency for increased flow toward ischemic regions. The decrease in myocardial O_2 consumption is due to a negative chronotropic effect (particularly during exercise), a negative inotropic effect, and a reduction in arterial blood pressure (particularly systolic pressure) during exercise. Not all of β adrenergic receptor antagonists are beneficial in all patients. The decreases in heart rate and contractility cause increases in the systolic ejection period and left ventricular end-diastolic volume; these alterations tend to increase O_2 consumption. However, the net effect of β receptor blockade usually is to decrease myocardial O_2 consumption, particularly during exercise.

(2) Increase blood supply to ischemic regions Myocardial oxygen consumption decrease self regulation to promote the blood supply to compensative dilating ischemic area.

Nitrates, β adrenoceptor antagonists and calcium antagonists in angina pectori are shown in Table 19-1.

Table 19-1 Nitrates, β adrenoceptor antagonists and calcium antagonists in angina pectoris

Myocardial oxygen demand	Nitrates	β-adrenoceptor antagonists	Calcium antagonists	
			Nifedipine	Verapamil
Preload	↓	↑	↓	None
Afterload	↓	None	↓	↓
Heat rate	Reflex ↑	↓	Reflex ↑	↓
Contractility	Reflex ↑	↓	Reflex ↑	↓

3. Calcium antagonists

The Ca^{2+} channel antagonists produce their effects by the L-type Ca^{2+} channels and reducing Ca^{2+} flux through the channel.

【 Pharmacodynamics 】Calcium antagonists can improve the blood supply to the ischemia dilated coronary artery, open collateral circulation and inhibit platelet aggregation. They can also increase the release of endogenous NO and enhance the direct vasodilator effect of calcium channel blockers. Calcium antagonists can protect mitochondria function and maintain energy supply via reduce Ca^{2+} overload. In addition, calcium antagonists decrease myocardial contractile force, which reduces myocardial oxygen requirements. They decrease O_2 demand (inhibit contractility, decrease peripheral resistance), improve work efficiency of myocardium.

Nifedipine (硝苯地平)

Nifedipine is an inhibitor of L-type voltage gated calcium channels that reduces blood pressure and increases oxygen supply to the heart. Immediate release nifedipine's duration of action requires dosing of 3 times daily. Nifedipine dosing is generally 10-120mg daily. Patients should be counselled regarding the risk of excessive hypotension, angina, and myocardial infarction.

Verapamil (维拉帕米)

Verapamil is indicated in the treatment of vasopastic angina, unstable angina, and chronic stable angina. It is also indicated to treat hypertension, for the prophylaxis of repetitive paroxysmal supraventricular tachycardia, and in combination with digoxin to control ventricular rate in patients with atrial fibrillation or atrial flutter. Given intravenously, it is indicated for the treatment of various supraventricular tachyarrhythmias, including rapid conversion to sinus rhythm in patients with supraventricular tachycardia and for temporary control of ventricular rate in patients with atrial fibrillation or atrial flutter.

Diltiazem (地尔硫草)

The decrease in intracellular calcium inhibits the contractile processes of the myocardial smooth muscle cells, causing dilation of the coronary and systemic arteries, increased oxygen delivery to the myocardial tissue, decreased total peripheral resistance, decreased systemic blood pressure, and decreased afterload. Diltiazem lowers myocardial oxygen demand through a reduction in heart rate, blood pressure, and cardiac contractility; this leads to a therapeutic effect in improving exercise tolerance in chronic stable angina.

重 点 小 结

药物	药理作用	临床应用	不良反应
硝酸酯类：硝酸甘油	降低心肌耗氧量，扩张冠状动脉、增加缺血区血液灌注，降低左室充盈压，增加心内膜供血，改善左室顺应性，保护缺血的心肌细胞、减轻缺血损伤	各种类型心绞痛	面颊部皮肤潮红、搏动性头痛、眼内压升高
β 受体阻断剂药：普萘洛尔	改善心肌缺血区供血、降低心肌耗氧量	硝酸酯类不敏感或疗效差的稳定型心绞痛、改善心肌缺血区供血	诱发或加重支气管哮喘、突然停药有反跳现象
钙通道阻滞药：硝苯地平	降低心肌耗氧量、舒张冠状血管、保护缺血心肌细胞、抑制血小板聚集	稳定型和不稳定型心绞痛	面颊部皮肤潮红、头痛、眩晕、心悸、恶心、便秘

目 标 检 测

一、选择题

（一）单项选择题

1. 硝酸酯类药舒张血管的机制是（　　　　）
   A. 直接作用于血管平滑肌　　　　B. 阻断 α 受体　　　　C. 促进前列环素生成
   D. 释放 NO　　　　E. 阻滞 Ca^{2+} 通道

2. 硝苯地平对稳定型心绞痛治疗受限的原因是（　　　　）
   A. 能增加心肌的耗氧量　　　　B. 此类患者对本药吸收差　　　　C. 可能导致心衰
   D. 能促进血小板聚集　　　　E. 能增加发作次数

3. 为克服硝酸酯类耐受性，可采取的措施不包括（　　　　）
   A. 采用最小剂量　　　　B. 补充含巯基药物　　　　C. 增加给药频率
   D. 采用间歇给药法　　　　E. 加用卡托普利

4. 硝酸甘油抗心绞痛的主要机制是（　　）

　　A. 选择性扩张冠脉，增加心肌耗氧量

　　B. 阻断 β 受体，降低心肌耗氧量

　　C. 减慢心率，降低心肌耗氧量

　　D. 扩张动脉和静脉，降低心肌耗氧量；扩张冠状动脉和侧支血管，改善局部缺血

　　E. 抑制心肌收缩力，降低心肌耗氧量

5. 硝酸甘油的不良反应主要为下列何项所致（　　）

　　A. 心输出量减少　　　　　　B. 消化道刺激　　　　　　C. 肝功能损害

　　D. 血管舒张　　　　　　　　E. 低血钾

6. 不宜用于变异型心绞痛的抗心绞痛药物是（　　）

　　A. 硝酸异山梨酯　　　　　　B. 普萘洛尔　　　　　　　C. 硝苯地平

　　D. 维拉帕米　　　　　　　　E. 硝酸甘油

7. 硝酸酯类药物临床应用时应注意（　　）

　　A. 对急性大发作应用超大剂量

　　B. 为预防发作，可采取经皮肤不间断给药

　　C. 为减少不良反应，应避免与含巯基药物合用

　　D. 应限制用量，以免降压过度

　　E. 因可降低心输出量，伴心衰患者禁用

（二）多项选择题

8. 硝酸酯类药与 β 受体阻断药联合应用抗心绞痛的药理依据是（　　）

　　A. 作用机制不同产生协同作用　　B. 消除反射性心率加快　　C. 降低室壁肌张力

　　D. 缩短射血时间

9. β 受体阻断药抗心绞痛作用机制包括（　　）

　　A. 降低心肌耗氧量　　　　　　B. 扩大心室容积　　　　　　C. 增加缺血区血供

　　D. 延长冠脉灌流时间　　　　　　E. 减慢心率，舒张期延长

二、思考题

从硝酸甘油的作用机制解释其抗心绞痛特点。

（乌仁图雅）

Chapter 20   Drugs for hyperlipidemia

 学习目标

1. **掌握** 抗高脂血症药的概念、分类；代表药物洛伐他汀、胆汁酸结合树脂、氯贝丁酯的药理作用及机制、临床应用和不良反应。

2. **熟悉** 瑞舒伐他汀、烟酸、考来烯胺的主要药理作用和临床应用。

3. **了解** 氟伐他汀的药理作用、临床应用。

Hyperlipidemia (高脂血症) is a major and primary cause of atherosclerosis and atherosclerosis-induced conditions, such as coronary heart disease (CHD), ischemic cerebrovascular disease, and peripheral vascular disease. Atherosclerosis is characterized by lipid deposition and a smooth muscle proliferation in the vascular system. Drugs that reduce the concentration of plasma lipoproteins generally decrease the levels of cholesterol and triglyceride, they affect either the circulation levels of low density lipoprotein (LDL) or very low density lipoprotein (VLDL). The commonly used drugs for reduction of plasma total cholesterol (TC) and LDL are 3-hydroxy-3-methylglutaryl coenzyme A (HMG-CoA) reductase inhibitors (statins) inculding lovastatin, bile acid binding resins such as cholestyramine. The mainly used drugs for reduction of plasma triglycerides and VLDL are fibrates such as gemfibrazil and niacins. Other drugs used in the prevention and treatment of atherosclerosis are antioxidants such as probucol and n-3 polyenoic fatty acids, n-6 polyenoic fatty acids, mucopolysccharides and polysccharides.

Blood lipids are lipids in the blood, either free or bound to other molecules, including total cholesterol, triglyceride (TG), phospholipid (PL), and free fatty acid.

Lipoproteins (脂蛋白) are macromolecular assemblies that contain lipids and proteins. The lipid constituents include free and esterified cholesterol, triglycerides, and phospholipids. The protein components, known as apolipoproteins or apoproteins, provide structural stability to the lipoproteins and also may function as ligands in lipoprotein-receptor interactions or as cofactors in enzymatic processes that regulate lipoprotein metabolism.

Chylomicrons (乳糜微粒) are synthesized from the fatty acids of dietary triglycerides and cholesterol absorbed from the small intestine by epithelial cells. Fat-soluble vitamins also are incorporated into chylomicrons after absorption.

1. Drugs for reducing elevated TG and LDL

The statins are the most effective and best-tolerated agents for treating dyslipidemia. These drugs are competitive inhibitors of HMG-CoA reductase(3-羟基-3-甲基戊二酸单酰辅酶A还原酶), which catalyzes an early, rate-limiting step in cholesterol biosynthesis.

Statins (他汀类)

Statins were isolated from a mold, penicillium citrinum, and identified as inhibitors of cholesterol biosynthesis in 1976 by Endo and his colleagues. Subsequent studies by Brown and Goldstein established that statins act by inhibiting HMG-CoA reductase. The first statin studied in humans was compactin, renamed mevastatin, which demonstrated the therapeutic potential of this class of drugs. Alberts and colleagues at Merck developed the first statin approved for use in humans, lovastatin (formerly known as mevinolin), which was isolated from Aspergillus terreus. Six other statins are also available. Pravastatin and simvastatin are chemically modified derivatives of lovastatin. Atorvastatin, fluvastatin, rosuvastatin, and pitavastatin are structurally distinct synthetic compounds.

【Pharmacodynamics】Statins (or HMG-CoA reductase inhibitors) are a class of drugs that reduce cholesterol in individuals who have dyslipidemia (abnormal fats in the blood) and thus are at risk for cardiovascular disease. Statins work by blocking the HMG-CoA reductase in the liver that is responsible for making cholesterol.

(1) **Effects on blood lipids**   Statin is indicated for the treatment of hyperlipidemia to reduce the level of total cholesterol, low-density lipoprotein cholesterol (LDL-C), apolipoprotein B (Apo B), and triglycerides, and to increase high-density lipoprotein cholesterol (HDL-C) level.

(2) **Other pharmacological effects**   Statin can improving endothelial function; affecting plaque stability, inhibiting inflammatory response, proliferation and migration of vascular smooth muscle cells (VSMCs), and reducing platelet aggregaion and the susceptibility of lipoproteins to oxidation.

【Adverse reactions】Initial post-marketing surveillance studies of the statins revealed an elevation in hepatic transaminase to three times greater than the upper limit of normal, with an incidence as great as 1%. The risk of myopathy and rhabdomyolysis increases in proportion to statin dose and plasma concentrations.

Pravastatin (普伐他汀)

Therapy is initiated with a 20 mg or 40 mg dose that may be increased to 80 mg. This drug should be taken at bedtime. Because pravastatin is a hydroxy acid, bile-acid sequestrants will bind it and reduce its absorption. Practically, this is rarely a problem because the resins should be taken before meals and pravastatin should be taken at bedtime. Pravastatin also is marketed in combination with buffered aspirin. The small advantage of combining these two drugs should be weighed against the disadvantages inherent in fixed-dose combinations.

Fluvastatin (氟伐他汀)

The starting dose of fluvastatin is 20 or 40 mg, and the maximum is 80 mg per day. Like pravastatin, it is administered as a hydroxy acid and should be taken at bedtime, several hours after ingesting a bile-acid sequestrant (if the combination is used).

Atorvastatin (阿伐他汀)

Atorvastatin has a long $t_{1/2}$, which allows administration of this statin at any time of the day. The starting dose is 10mg, and the maximum is 80mg/d. Atorvastatin is marketed in combination with the Ca^{2+} channel blocker amlodipine (氨氯地平) for patients with hypertension or angina as well as hypercholesterolemia. The physician should weigh any advantage of combination against the associated risks and disadvantages.

Rosuvastatin (瑞舒伐他汀)

Rosuvastatin is available in doses ranging between 5 and 40 mg. It has a $t_{1/2}$ of 20-30 hours and may be taken at any time of day. Because experience with rosuvastatin is limited, treatment should be initiated with 5-10 mg daily, increasing stepwise, if needed, until the incidence of myopathy is better defined. If the combination of gemfibrozil with rosuvastatin is used, the dose of rosuvastatin should not exceed 10 mg.

Cholestyramine (考来烯胺) and colestipol (考来替泊)

Cholestyramine and colestipol are among the oldest of the hypolipidemic drugs, and they are probably the safest, because they are not absorbed from the intestine. The resins are most often used as second agents if statin therapy does not lower LDL-C levels sufficiently.

【Pharmacodynamics】The bile-acid sequestrants are highly positively charged and bind negatively charged bile acids. Because of their large size, the resins are not absorbed, and the bound bile acids are excreted in the stool. Because more than 95% of bile acids are normally reabsorbed, interruption of this process depletes the pool of bile acids, and hepatic bile-acid synthesis increases. As a result, hepatic cholesterol content declines, stimulating the production of LDL receptors, an effect similar to that of statins. The increase in hepatic LDL receptors increases LDL clearance and lowers LDL-C levels, but this effect is partially offset by the enhanced cholesterol synthesis caused by upregulation of HMG-CoA reductase. Inhibition of reductase activity by a statin substantially increases the effectiveness of the resins.

【Adverse reactions】Severe hypertriglyceridemia (高甘油三酯血症)is a contraindication to the use of cholestyramine and colestipol because these resins increase triglyceride levels. Constipation may occur but sometimes can be prevented by adequate daily water intake and psyllium.

2. Drugs for reducing elevated TG and VLDL

Fibric acid derivatives (贝特类)

Clofibrate (氯贝丁酯), the prototype of the fibric acid derivatives, is the ethyl ester of p-chlorophenoxyisobutyrate. Gemfibrozil (吉非罗齐) is a nonhalogenated phenoxypentanoic acid and thus is distinct from the halogenated fibrates. A number of fibric acid analogs [e.g., fenofibrate (非诺贝特), bezafibrate (苯扎贝特), ciprofibrate (环丙贝特)] have been developed and are used in Europe and elsewhere.

【Pharmacodynamics】Despite extensive studies in humans, the mechanisms by which fibrates lower lipoprotein levels, or raise HDL levels, remain unclear. Recent studies suggest that many of the effects of these compounds on blood lipids are mediated by their interaction with peroxisome proliferator-activated receptors (PPARs).

Nicotinic acid (烟酸)

【Pharmacodynamics】Niacin is a water-soluble B-complex vitamin that functions as a vitamin only after its conversion to nicotinamide adenine dinucleotide (NAD) or nicotinamide adenine dinucleotide phosphate (NADP), in which it occurs as an amide. Both niacin and its amide may be given orally as a source of niacin for its functions as a vitamin, but only niacin affects lipid levels. The hypolipidemic effects of niacin require larger doses than are required for its vitamin effects. Niacin is the best agent available for increasing HDL-C; it also lowers triglycerides by 35%-45% and reduces LDL-C levels by 20%-30%. Niacin also is the only lipid-lowering drug that reduces lipoprotein(a) [(Lp(a)] levels significantly.

In adipose tissue, niacin inhibits the lipolysis of triglycerides by hormone-sensitive lipase, which reduces transport of free fatty acids to the liver and decreases hepatic triglyceride synthesis. Niacin and related compounds may exert their effects on lipolysis by inhibiting adipocyte adenylyl cyclase.

【Adverse reactions】Two of niacin's side effects, flushing and dyspepsia, limit patient's compliance. The cutaneous effects include flushing and pruritus of the face and upper trunk, skin rashes, and acanthosis nigricans.

重 点 小 结

药物	药理作用	临床应用	不良反应
他汀类降脂药：洛伐他汀	具有明显的调血脂作用，降低 LDL-C 的作用最强，TC 次之，降 TG 作用很弱，而 HDL-C 略有升高；改善血管内皮功能，抑制血管平滑肌细胞的增殖和迁移，抗氧化	调节血脂、预防心脑血管疾病	肌病和肝脏不良反应、胃肠反应、皮肤潮红、头痛
贝特类降脂药：非诺贝特	降低血浆 VLDL，因而降低 TG，伴有 LDL 水平的中度降低（降低10%左右），一定程度地增加 HDL 水平	混合型血脂异常及低 HDL 和高动脉粥样硬化性疾病风险的患者或以 TG 或 VLDV 升高为主的原发性高脂血症	横纹肌溶解症、腹痛、腹泻、恶心
烟酸类降脂药：维生素 B_3	降低血浆游离脂肪酸水平，增强对血浆乳糜微粒和甘油三酯的清除	防治糙皮病等烟酸缺乏病；扩张血管，治疗高脂血症	面部潮红、瘙痒、头痛、肝毒性
树脂类降脂药：考来烯胺	用药 1 周内 LDL-C 水平开始下降，2 周内达最大效应，可使血浆总胆固醇水平下降 20% 以上，LDL-C 水平下降 25%~35%，TG 水平可有所升高	Ⅱ 型高脂血症，动脉粥样硬化、肝硬化及胆石症引起的瘙痒	便秘、胃灼热、消化不良、恶心、呕吐、胃痛

目 标 检 测

一、单项选择题

1. 不属于贝特类降脂药的药理作用的是（　　　）
   A. 降低 VLDL
   B. 降低 TG
   C. 升高 VLDV
   D. 一定程度增加 HDL 水平
   E. LDL 水平中度降低

2. 关于高脂血症的治疗目标，叙述正确的是（　　　）
   A. 使血脂恢复正常标准
   B. 使血脂越低越好
   C. 使血脂持续下降
   D. 使血压恢复正常标准
   E. 使血脂升高

3. 现代高脂血症治疗的药物不包括（　　　）
   A. 他汀类降脂药
   B. 贝特类降脂药
   C. 烟酸类降脂药
   D. 头孢类消炎药
   E. 树脂类降脂药

4. 他汀类降脂药不包括（　　　）
   A. 非诺贝特
   B. 辛伐他汀
   C. 洛伐他汀
   D. 阿托伐他汀
   E. 瑞舒伐他汀

5. 有些降脂药服用后会出现副作用，如面色潮红，伴随皮肤瘙痒、头昏心悸、气短、出汗、畏寒等。这类降脂药是（　　　）
   A. 他汀类降脂药
   B. 贝特类降脂药
   C. 烟酸类降脂药
   D. 胆固醇吸收抑制剂
   E. 考来烯胺

二、多项选择题

6. 他汀类降脂药不能与下列哪些药联合使用（　　　）
   A. 烟酸类降脂药
   B. 贝特类降脂药
   C. 树脂类降脂药
   D. 胆固醇吸收抑制剂
   E. 抗氧化剂

（乌仁图雅）

Chapter 21 Drugs acting in blood system

 学习目标

1. **掌握** 肝素、双香豆素、抗血小板药的作用特点、作用机制、临床应用。
2. **熟悉** 维生素 K 的作用及临床应用。
3. **了解** 其他作用于血液系统药物的作用及临床机制。

Excessive bleeding and thrombosis may represent altered states of hemostasis. Impaired hemostasis results in spontaneous bleeding; stimulated hemostasis results in thrombus formation. The drugs used to arrest abnormal bleeding and inhibit thrombosis are subjects of this chapter.

1. Mechanisms of blood coagulation

Hemostasis (止血) is the spontaneous arrest of bleeding from a damaged blood vessel. The normal vascular endothelial cell is not thrombogenic, and the circulating blood platelets and clotting factors do not normally adhere to it to an appreciable extent. The immediate hemostatic response of a damaged vessel is vasospasm. Within seconds, platelets stick to the exposed collagen of the damaged endothelium (platelet adhesion, 血小板黏附) and to each other (platelet aggregation, 血小板聚集). Platelets then lose their individual membranes and form a gelatinous mass during viscous metamorphosis. This platelet plug quickly arrests bleeding but must be reinforced by fibrin for long-term effectiveness. Fibrin reinforcement results from local stimuli to blood coagulation: the exposed collagen of damaged vessels and the membranes and released contents of platelets. Prothrombin is bound by calcium to a platelet phospholipid (PL) surface, where activated factor X (X a), in the presence of factor V a, converts it into circulating thrombin. Several kinds of the blood clotting factors are targets for drug therapy. The main initiator of blood coagulation is the tissue factor (TF)/factor Vila pathway. The exposure of TF on damaged endothelium binds and activates circulating factor Ⅶ. Plasmin remodels the thrombus and limits the extension of thrombosis by proteolytic digestion of fibrin. Regulation of the fibrinolytic system is useful in therapeutics. Increased fibrinolysis is the effective therapy for thrombotic disease. Tissue plasminogen activator (t-PA), urokinase (尿激酶), and streptokinase all activate the fibrinolytic system.

2. Anticoagulants

2.1 Thrombin indirect inhibitors (间接凝血酶抑制剂)

Heparin (肝素)

【Chemistry and mechanism of action】Heparin is one kind of heterogeneous (异构) mixture of sulfated mucopolysaccharides (黏多糖). It binds to endothelial cell surfaces and a variety of plasma proteins. Its biologic activity is dependent upon the plasma protease inhibitor antithrombin. Antithrombin inhibits clotting factor proteases, especially thrombin (Ha), Ⅸ a, and Ⅹ a, by forming equimolar stable complexes with them. In the absence of heparin, these reactions are slow in the presence of heparin, they are accelerated 1000-fold. Only about a third of the molecules in commercial heparin preparations have an accelerating effect because the remainder lack the unique pentasaccharide sequence needed for high-affinity binding to antithrombin (Figure 21-1).

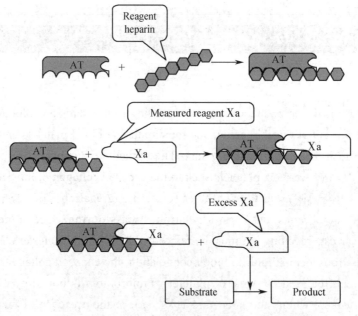

Figure 21-1   The mechanism of action of heparin

【Clinical indications】

(1) Thromboembolic disease   It is mainly used to prevent thrombosis and enlargement.

(2) Disseminated intravascular coagulation (DIC)   Used for various reasons of DIC, such as sepsis, early detachment of placenta, malignant tumor lysis leads to DIC.

(3) Ischemic heart disease   Such as unstable angina pectoris usually associated with intracoronary thrombosis, which is now believed that in addition to antianginal medications, anticoagulants and antiplatelet agents are also effective.

(4) Anticoagulant *in vitro* Cardiovascular surgery (心血管手术), hemodialysis and cardiopulmonary bypass.

【Adverse reactions】

(1) Bleeding Excessive anticoagulant action of heparin is treated by discontinuance of the drug. If bleeding occurs, administration of the specific antagonist such as protamine sulfate is suggested. Protamine is a highly basic peptide that combines with heparin as an ion pair to form a stable complex which is devoid of anticoagulant activity. Excess protamine must be avoided; it also has an anticoagulant effect. Protamine will not reverse the activity of fondaparinux (璜达肝素). Excessive danaparoid (达那肝素) can be removed by plasmapheresis.

(2) Thrombocytopenia Most of the cases occurred 7-10 days after administration, which is related to the immune response. Discontinued four days can be resumed. Therefore, platelet count should be measured during the administration of heparin

2.2　Direct thrombin inhibitors（直接凝血酶抑制剂）

The direct thrombin inhibitors (DTI) are a relatively new class of agents that exert their anticoagulant effect by directly binding to the active site of thrombin, thereby inhibiting thrombin's downstream effects. The DTIs bind thrombin without additional binding proteins, such as antithrombin (抗凝血酶), and they do not bind to other plasma proteins, argatroban and melagatran (两种药物名字，属于小分子抑制剂) are small molecules that bind only at the thrombin active site. Argatroban is a small molecule thrombin inhibitor that FDA has approved for use in patients with heparin-induced thrombocytopenia (HIT) with or without thrombosis and coronary angioplasty in patients with HIT. It, too, has a short half-life, which is given by continuous intravenous infusion, and monitoring is done by APTT. Its clearance is not affected by renal disease but is dependent on liver function. The drug requires dose reduction in patients with liver disease. Melagatran and its oral prodrug, ximelagatran, are under intensive study. Attractive features of ximelagatran include predictable pharmacokinetics and bioavailability-allowing for fixed closing and predictable anticoagulant response; no need for routine coagulation monitoring; lack of interaction with P450-interacting drugs; rapid onset and offset of action-allowing for immediate anticoagulation and thus no need for overlap with additional anticoagulant drugs. A published phase 3 trial in patients status post major orthopedic surgery found Ximelagatran is equivalent to warfarin in preventing postoperative.

Warfarin (华法林) and coumarin (香豆素)

【Pharmacokinetics】Pharmacokinetic mechanisms for drug interaction with oral anticoagulants are mainly enzyme induction, enzyme inhibition, and reduced plasma protein binding. Pharmacodynamic mechanisms for interactions with warfarin are synergism (impaired hemostasis, reduced clotting factor synthesis, as in hepatic disease), competitive antagonism (vitamin K), and an altered physiologic control loop for vitamin K (hereditary resistance to oral anticoagulants). The most serious interactions with warfarin are those that increase the anticoagulant effect and the risk of bleeding. The most dangerous one of these interactions are the pharmacokinetic interactions with the pyrazolones phenylbutazone and sulfinpyrazone. These drugs not only augment the hypoprothrom-binemia, but also inhibit platelet function and may induce peptic ulcer disease.

【Pharmacodynamics】Pharmacodynamics Coumarin anticoagulants block the 7-carboxylation of several glutamate residues in prothrombin and factors Ⅶ, Ⅸ, and Ⅹ as well as the endogenous anticoagulant proteins C and S. The blockade results in incomplete molecules that are biologically inactive in coagulation. This protein carboxylation is physiologically coupled with the oxidative deactivation of vitamin K. The anticoagulant prevents reductive metabolism of the inactive vitamin K epoxide back to its active hydroquinone form. Mutational change of the responsible enzyme and vitamin K epoxide reductase, can give rise to genetic resistance to warfarin in humans and especially in rats.

【Adverse reactions】Toxicity Warfarin crosses the placenta readily and can cause a hemorrhagic disorder in the fetus. Furthermore, fetal proteins with y-carboxyglutamate residues found in bone and blood may be affected by warfarin; the drug can cause serious birth defect characterized by abnormal bone formation. Thus, warfarin should never be administered during pregnancy. The pathologic lesion associated with the hemorrhagic infarction is venous thrombosis, suggesting that it is caused by warfarin-induced depression of protein C synthesis.

3. Antiplatelet drugs

3.1　Platelet metabolase inhibitors（血小板代谢酶抑制剂）

Aspirin (阿司匹林)

【Pharmacokinetics】Salicylic acid (水杨酸) is a simple organic acid with a pK_a of 3.0. Aspirin (acetylsalicylic acid, ASA) has a pK_a of 3.5. Sodium salicylate and aspirin are equally effective anti-inflammatory drugs, though aspirin may be more effective as the analgesic. The salicylates are rapidly absorbed from stomach and upper small intestine, yielding a peak plasma salicylate level within 1-2 hours. Aspirin is absorbed as such and is rapidly hydrolyzed (serum half-life 15minutes) to acetic acid and salicylate by esterases (酯酶) in tissue and blood. Salicylate is bound to albumin, but the binding is saturable (饱和) so that the unbound fraction increases as total concentration increases. Ingested salicylate and that generated by hydrolysis of aspirin may be excreted unchanged, but the metabolic pathways for salicylate disposition become saturated when the total body load of salicylate exceeds 600mg. Beyond this amount, increases in salicylate dosage increase salicylate concentration disproportionately. As doses of aspirin increase, salicylate elimination half-life increases from 3-5 hours (for 600mg/d dosage) to 12-16 hours (dosage > 3.6g/d). Alkalinization (碱化) of urine increases the rate of excretion of free salicylate and its water-soluble conjugates.

【Pharmacodynamics】Single low doses of aspirin (81mg daily) produce a slightly prolonged bleeding time, which doubles if administration is continuing for a week. The change is the clue to irreversible inhibition of platelet COX; so that aspirin's antiplatelet effect lasts 8 days (the life of the platelet).

【Clinical indications】Aspirin decreases the incidence of transient ischemic attacks, unstable angina, coronary artery thrombosis with myocardial infarction, and thrombosis after coronary artery bypass grafting. Epidemiologic studies suggest that the long-term use of aspirin at low dosage is associated with a lower incidence of colon cancer, which is possibly related to its COX-inhibiting effects.

【Adverse reactions】At the usual dosage, aspirin's main adverse effects are gastric upset (intolerance) and gastric and duodenal ulcers, while hepatotoxicity, asthma, rashes, and renal toxicity occur less frequently.

Upper gastrointestinal bleeding associated with aspirin use is usually related to erosive gastritis. A 3ml increase in fecal blood loss is routinely associated with aspirin administration; the blood loss is greater for higher closes. On the other hand, some mucosal adaptation occurs in many patients, so that the blood loss declines back to the baseline over 4-6 weeks; ulcers have been shown to heal while aspirin was taken concomitantly.

3.2　Platelet activation inhibitor（血小板活化抑制剂）

Clopidogrel (氯吡格雷) and ticlopidine (噻氯匹定)

Clopidogrel and ticlopidine reduce platelet aggregation by inhibiting the ADP pathway of platelets. These drugs are thienopyridine derivatives (衍生物) that achieve their antiplatelet effects by irreversibly blocking the ADP receptor on platelets. Unlike aspirin, these drugs have no effect to the prostaglandin metabolism. Randomized clinical trials with both drugs report efficacy in the prevention of vascular events among patients with transient ischemic attacks, completed strokes, and unstable angina pectoris. Use of Clopidogrel or Ticlopidine to prevent thrombosis is now considered as the standard practice in patients undergoing placement of a coronary stent. Adverse reactions of ticlopidine include nausea, dyspepsia, which are in up to 20% of patients, hemorrhage in 5%, and, most seriously, leukopenia in 1%, The leukopenia is detected by regular monitoring of the white blood cell count during the first 3 months of treatment. Development of thrombotic thrombocytopenic purpura (TTP) has also been associated with the ingestion of Ticlopidine. The dosage of Ticlopidine is 250mg twice daily. It is particularly useful in patients who cannot tolerate aspirin. Doses of Ticlopidine less than 500mg/d may be efficacious with fewer adverse reactions. Clopidogrel has fewer adverse reactions than ticlopidine and is rarely associated with neutropenia. Thrombotic thrombocytopenic purpura associated with Clopidogrel has recently been reported. Because of its superior side effect profile and dosing requirements, Clopidogrel is preferred over Ticlopidine. The antithrombotic effects of Clopidogrel are dose-dependent; within 5 hours after an oral loading dose of 300mg, 80% of platelet activity will be inhibited. The maintenance dose of Clopidogrel is 75mg/d, which achieves maximum platelet inhibition. The duration of the antiplatelet effect is 7-10 days.

3.3　Blockade of platelet GP II_b/III_a receptors（血小板受体阻断药）

The glycoprotein II_b/III_a inhibitors are used in patients with acute coronary syndromes. These drugs target the platelet II_b/III_a receptor complex. The II_b/Ha complex functions as a receptor mainly for fibrinogen and vitronectin but also for fibronectin and von Willebrand factor. Activation of this receptor complex is the "final common pathway" for platelet aggregation. There are approximately 50 000 copies of this complex on the platelet surface. Individuals lacking this receptor have a bleeding disorder called

Glanzmann's thrombasthenia. Abciximab, a humanized monoclonal antibody directed against the II_b/III_a complex including the vibronectin receptor, was the first agent approved in this class of drugs. It has been approved for use in per-cutaneous coronary intervention and in acute coronary syndromes. Eptifibatide is an analog of the sequence at the extreme carboxyl terminal of the delta chain of fibrinogen, which mediates the binding of fibrinogen to the receptor. Tirofiban is a smaller molecule with similar properties. eptifibatide (依替巴肽) and tirofiban (替罗非班) inhibit ligand.

4. Drugs used in bleeding disorders

Vitamin K (维生素K)

Vitamin K confers biologic activity upon prothrombin and factors IX, and X by participating in their postribosomal modification. Vitamin K is a fat-soluble substance found primarily in leafy green vegetables. The dietary requirement is low, because the vitamin is additionally synthesized by bacteria that colonize the human intestine. Two natural forms exist: vitamins K is found in food, vitamin K_2 (menaquinone, 甲基萘醌类) is found in human tissues and is synthesized by intestinal bacteria. vitamins K and K_2 require bile salts for absorption from the intestinal tract. Onset of effect is delayed for 6 hours but the effect is complete by 24 hours when treating depression of prothrombin activity by excessive warfarin or Vitamin K deficiency. Intravenous administration of Vitamin K, should be slow, because rapid infusion can produce dyspnea, chest and back pain, and even death. Vitamin K repletion is best achieved with intravenous or oral administration, because its bioavailability after subcutaneous administration is erratic. Vitamin K, is currently administered to all newborns to prevent the hemorrhagic disease of vitamin K deficiency, which is especially common in premature infants. The water-soluble salt of vitamin K_3 (menadione, 甲萘醌) should never be used in binding to the U b/ID receptor by occupancy of the receptor but do not block the vibronectin receptor. The three agents described above are administered parenterally. Oral formulations of U b/ID antagonists have been developed and are in various stages of development. However, lack of efficacy and significant thrombocytopenia has prevented progress with the oral analogs.

重 点 小 结

药物	药理作用	临床应用	不良反应
抗凝药：肝素	抗凝迅速、作用强、短效，体内外均有效	心血管手术，心导管术体外循环、血液透析，栓塞性疾病，弥散性血管内凝血	出血（缓慢静脉注射鱼精蛋白解救），血小板减少症，骨质疏松
阿司匹林	抑制血小板黏附、聚集及释放反应	防治血栓栓塞性疾病	胃肠道反应
维生素 K	参与凝血因子合成	维生素 K 缺乏性出血	较少

目 标 检 测

一、选择题

（一）单项选择题

1. 在体内外均有抗凝作用的抗凝血药是（　　）
   A. 肝素　　　　B. 双香豆素　　　C. 华法林　　　　D. 链激酶　　　　E. 双嘧达莫

2. 香豆素类药与下列哪种药合用作用减弱（　　）
   A. 广谱抗生素　　　　　　　B. 水杨酸盐　　　　　　　　　C. 血小板抑制剂
   D. 甲苯磺丁脲　　　　　　　E. 巴比妥类

3. 肝素抗凝血的作用机制是（　　）
   A. 抑制凝血因子Ⅱ、凝血因子Ⅶ、凝血因子Ⅸ、凝血因子Ⅹ的合成
   B. 抑制 ATA_2 合成酶
   C. 直接灭活多种凝血因子
   D. 与 Ca^{2+} 形成难解离的可溶性络合物
   E. 激活 AT Ⅲ，并加速灭活多种凝血因子

4. 治疗急性血栓栓塞性疾病如急性肺栓塞的药物是（　　）
   A. 尿激酶　　　B. 双香豆素　　　C. 肝素　　　　D. 右旋糖酐　　　E. 华法林

5. 治疗肝素过量引起的自发性出血，宜选用下列哪种药物（　　）
   A. 叶酸　　　B. 维生素 K　　　C. 氨甲环酸　　　D. 鱼精蛋白　　　E. 垂体后叶素

（二）多项选择题

6. 肝素可用于（　　）
   A. 细菌性脓毒血症所致的 DIC 早期　　　B. 血栓栓塞性疾病
   C. 心肌梗死　　　　　　　　　　　　　D. 预防心瓣膜修补术后血栓的形成
   E. 体外循环

7. 有关华法林叙述正确的是（　　）
   A. 抗凝血作用出现快　　　　　　　B. 体内外均有抗凝血作用
   C. 口服吸收完全　　　　　　　　　D. 西咪替丁可增强其作用
   E. 使用过量引起出血时可用维生素 K 对抗

8. 维生素 K 可用于（　　）
   A. 新生儿出血　　　　　　B. 双香豆素过量所致的出血　　　C. 胆瘘患者出血
   D. 梗阻性黄疸者出血　　　E. 继发性凝血酶原过低所致的出血

9. 用于防治血栓栓塞性疾病的药物有（　　）
   A. 阿司匹林　　　B. 肝素　　　C. 双香豆素　　　D. 维生素 K　　　E. 利多格雷

二、思考题

肝素与双香豆素在抗凝作用上有什么不同？

（吕　莹）

PPT

Chapter 22　Diuretic drugs

 学习目标

1. 掌握　利尿药的分类；代表药物呋塞米、氢氯噻嗪、螺内酯的药理作用、临床应用和不良反应。

2. 熟悉　乙酰唑胺、氨苯蝶啶、阿米洛利的主要药理作用和临床应用；渗透性利尿药的临床应用。

3. 了解　肾脏生理与利尿药的关系。

Diuretics (利尿药) increase the excretion of Na⁺ and water. They decrease the reabsorption of Na⁺ and (usually) Cl⁻ from the filtrate, increased water loss being secondary to the increased excretion of NaCl (natriuresis). The diuretics are used to adjust the volume and (or) composition of body fluids in a variety of clinical situations, including hypertension, heart failure, renal failure, nephrotic syndrome, and cirrhosis.

1. Renal physiology

The basic urine-forming unit of the kidney is the nephron, which consists of a filtering apparatus, the glomerulus, connected to a long tubular portion that reabsorbs and conditions the glomerular ultrafiltrate. Each human kidney is composed of approximately 1 million nephrons.Approximately 16%-20% of the blood plasma in the kidneys is filtered from the glomerular capillaries (肾小球毛细血管) into Bowman's capsule (肾小囊). The filtrate, although normally free of proteins and blood cells, does contain most low molecular weight (低分子质量) plasma components approximately in the same concentrations as found in the plasma. These include glucose, sodium bicarbonate (碳酸氢钠), amino acids, and other organic solutes, plus electrolytes, such as Na⁺, K⁻, And Cl⁻. The kidney regulates the ionic composition and volume of urine by the reabsorption or secretion of ions and (or) water at five functional zones along the nephron, namely the proximal convoluted tubule (近曲小管), the descending loop of Henle, the ascending loop of Henle (髓袢升支粗段), the distal convoluted tubule (远曲小管), and the collecting duct (Figure 22-1).

医药大学堂
WWW.YIYAODXT.COM

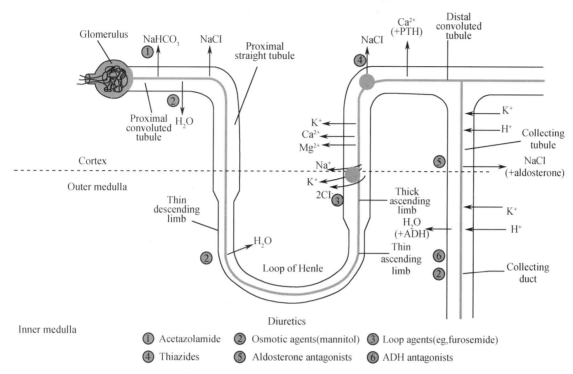

Figure 22-1 Anatomy and nomenclature of the nephron

1.1 Proximal convoluted tubule

In the extensively convoluted proximal tubule located in the cortex of the kidney, almost all of the glucose, bicarbonate, amino acids and other metabolites (代谢产物) are reabsorbed. Approximately two thirds of the Na^+ is also reabsorbed in the proximal tubule; chloride and water follow passively to maintain electrical and osmolar equality (保持电荷和渗透压的平衡).

Acid secretory system (酸分泌系统): In the proximal tubule, the free energy in the Na^+ gradient established by the basolateral Na^+ pump is used by a Na^+-H^+ antiporter (also referred to as a Na^+-H^+ exchanger or NHE) in the luminal membrane to transport H^+ into the tubular lumen in exchange for Na^+. In the lumen, H^+ reacts with filtered $HCO3^-$ to form H_2CO_3, which rapidly decomposes to CO_2 and water in the presence of carbonic anhydrase (碳酸酐酶)in the brush border (the actual reaction catalyzed by carbonic anhydrase is $OH^- + CO_2 \rightleftharpoons HCO_3^-$; however, $H_2O \rightleftharpoons OH^- + H^+$ and $HCO_3^- + H^+ \rightleftharpoons H_2CO_3$, so that the net reaction is $H_2O + CO_2 \rightleftharpoons H_2CO_3$).

Continued operation of the Na^+-H^+ antiporter maintains a low proton concentration in the cell, so that H_2CO_3 spontaneously ionizes to form H^+ and HCO_3^-, creating an electrochemical gradient for HCO_3^- across the basolateral membrane (Figure 22-2).

1.2 Descending loop of henle

The remaining filtrate, which is isotonic, next enters the descending limb of the loop of Henle and passes into the medulla of the kidney (肾髓质). The osmolarity increases along the descending portion of the loop Henle because of the countercurrent mechanism. This results in a tubular fluid with a three-fold increase in salt concentration.

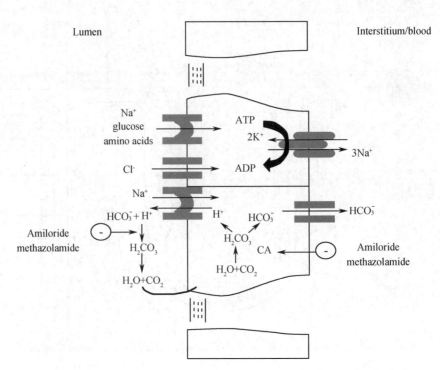

Figure 22-2   The bicarbonate (HCO$_3^-$) reabsorption in the proximal tubule

1.3   Ascending loop of henle

The ascending limb has very low permeability to water,enabling the build-up of a substantial concentration gradient across the wall of the tubule. It is here, in the thick ascending limb of the loop of Henle, that 20%-30% of filtered Na$^+$ is reabsorbed. There is active reabsorption of NaCl, unaccompanied by water, reducing the osmolarity of the tubular fluid and making the interstitial fluid of the medulla hypertonic. Ions move into the cell across the apical membrane by a Na$^+$/K$^+$/2Cl$^-$ symporter (Na$^+$/K$^+$/2Cl$^-$协同转运蛋白). The energy for this is derived from the electrochemical gradient for Na$^+$ produced by the Na$^+$-K$^+$ ATPase in the basolateral membrane. Chloride exits the cell into the circulation, partly by diffusion through chloride channels and partly by a symport mechanism with K$^+$. Most of the K$^+$ taken into the cell by the Na$^+$/K$^+$/2Cl$^-$ cotransporter returns to the lumen through apical potassium channels, but some K$^+$ is reabsorbed, along with Mg^{2+} and Ca^{2+}.

Reabsorption of salt from the thick ascending limb is not balanced by reabsorption of water, so tubular fluid is hypotonic with respect to plasma as it leaves the thick ascending limb and enters the distal convoluted tubule (Figure 22-3). Drugs affecting this site, such as loop diuretics (髓袢利尿药) are the most efficacious of all the diuretic classes.

1.4   Distal convoluted tub

The cells of the distal convoluted tubule are also impermeable to water. About 10% of the filtered sodium chloride is reabsorbed via Na$^+$/Cl$^-$ transporter, which is sensitive to thiazide diuretics (噻嗪类利尿药). Additionally, the Ca^{2+} excretion is regulated by parathyroid hormone (甲状旁腺素) in this portion of the tubule.

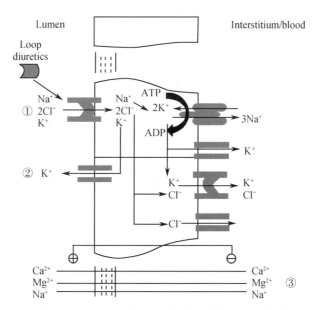

Figure 22-3 The transport mechanism in the thick ascending loop of Henle

①Loop diuretics block the Na^+ / K^+ / 2 Cl^- cotransporter. ②Increasing the excretion of Na^+ and Cl^-. These drugs also decrease the potential difference across indicates the tubule cell, which arises from the process of K^+. ③This leads to increased excretion of Ca^{2+} and Mg^{2+} by inhibiting paracellular coursing together

1.5 Collecting tubule and duct

The principal and intercalated cells (主细胞和闰细胞) of the collecting tubule are responsible for Na^+-K^+ exchange and for H^+ secretion and reabsorption K^+, respectively. Stimulation of aldosterone receptors (醛固酮受体) in the principal cells results in Na^+ reabsorption and K^+ secretion. Antidiuretic hormone (ADH, 抗利尿激素) receptors promote the reabsorption of water from the collecting tubules and ducts. This action is mediated by cAMP.

2. Drugs in common use

2.1 Carbonic anhydrase inhibitors (碳酸酐酶抑制剂)

Carbonic anhydrase is present in many nephron sites, but the predominant location of this enzyme is the luminal membrane of the proximal convoluted tubule, where it catalyzes the dehydration of H_2CO_3 as described above. By blocking carbonic anhydrase, inhibitors block $NaHCO_3$ reabsorption and cause diuresis. The prototypical carbonic anhydrase inhibitor is acetazolamide.

Acetazolamide (乙酰唑胺)

【Pharmacokinetics】Acetazolamide is well absorbed after oral administration. An increase in urine pH from the HCO_3^- diuresis is apparent within 30 minutes, maximal at 2 hours, and persists for 12 hours after a single dose. Excretion of the drug is by secretion in the proximal tubule S_2 segment. Therefore, dosing must be reduced in renal insufficiency.

【Pharmacodynamics】Acetazolamide inhibits carbonic anhydrase, located intracellularly and on the apical side of the proximal tubular epithelium [carbonic anhydrase catalyzes the reaction of CO_2 and H_2O leading to production of H^+ and HCO_3^- (bicarbonate)]. The decreased ability to exchange Na^+ for H^+ in the presence of acetazolamide results in a mild diuresis. Additionally, HCO_3^- is retained in the lumen with marked elevation in urinary pH. The loss of HCO_3^- causes a hyperchloremic metabolic acidosis and decreased diuretic efficacy following several days of therapy.

The ciliary body of the eye secretes HCO_3^- from the blood into the aqueous humor. Likewise, formation of cerebrospinal fluid in the choroid plexus involves HCO_3^- secretion. Although these processes remove HCO_3^- from the blood (the direction opposite to that in the proximal tubule), they are similarly inhibited by carbonic anhydrase inhibitors.

【Clinical indications】

(1) **Glaucoma (青光眼)** The most common use of acetazolamide is to reduce the elevated intraocular pressure of open angle glaucoma. Acetazolamide decreased the production of aqueous humor, probably by blocking carbonic anhydrase in the ciliary body of the eye.

(2) **Urinary alkalinization (碱化尿)** Uric acid, cystine, and other weak acids are most easily reabsorbed from acidic urine. Therefore, renal excretion of cystine (in cystinuria) and other weak acids can be enhanced by increasing urinary pH with carbonic anhydrase inhibitors. In the absence of continuous HCO_3^- administration, these effects of acetazolamide last only 2-3 days. Prolonged therapy requires HCO_3^- administration.

(3) **Epilepsy (癫痫)** Acetazolamide is sometimes used in the treatment of epilepsy-both generalized and partial. It reduces the severity and magnitude of the seizures.

(4) **Metabolic alkalosis (代谢性碱中毒)** Metabolic alkalosis is generally treated by correction of abnormalities in total body K^+, intravascular volume, or mineralocorticoid levels. However, when the alkalosis is due to excessive use of diuretics in patients with severe heart failure, replacement of intravascular volume may be contraindicated. In these cases, acetazolamide can be useful in correcting the alkalosis as well as producing a small additional diuresis for correction of volume overload. Acetazolamide can also be used to rapidly correct the metabolic alkalosis that may develop in the setting of respiratory acidosis.

(5) **Acute mountain sickness (高山病)** By decreasing cerebrospinal fluid formation and by decreasing the pH of the cerebrospinal fluid and brain, acetazolamide can increase ventilation and diminish symptoms of mountain sickness (weakness, dizziness, insomnia, headache, and nausea can occur in mountain travelers who rapidly ascend above 3000m. The symptoms are usually mild and last for a few days. In more serious cases, rapidly progressing pulmonary or cerebral edema can be life-threatening).

【Adverse reactions】

(1) **Hyperchloremic metabolic acidosis (高氯性代谢性酸中毒)** Acidosis predictably results from chronic reduction of body HCO_3^- stores by carbonic anhydrase inhibitors and limits the diuretic efficacy of these drugs to 2 or 3 days.

(2) **Renal stones (肾结石)** Phosphaturia and hypercalciuria occur during the bicarbonaturic response to inhibitors of carbonic anhydrase. Renal excretion of solubilizing factors (e.g., citrate) may also decline with chronic use. Calcium salts are relatively insoluble at alkaline pH, which means that the potential for

renal stone formation from these salts is enhanced.

(3) Renal potassium wasting (钾丢失)　Potassium wasting can occur because Na^+ presented to the collecting tubule is partially reabsorbed, increasing the lumen-negative electrical potential in that segment and enhancing K^+ secretion. This effect can be counteracted by simultaneous administration of potassium chloride.

(4) Other toxicities　Drowsiness and paresthesias (嗜睡和感觉异常) are common following large doses of acetazolamide. Carbonic anhydrase inhibitors may accumulate in patients with renal failure (肾衰竭), leading to nervous system toxicity. Hypersensitivity reactions (过敏反应) [such as fever, rashes, bone marrow suppression (骨髓抑制), and interstitial nephritis (间质性肾炎)]may also occur.

2.2　Loop or high-ceiling diuretics (袢利尿药或强效利尿药)

Furosemide (呋塞米), bumetanide (布美他尼), torsemide (托拉塞米), ethacrynic acid (依他尼酸)

【Pharmacokinetics】The loop diuretics are rapidly absorbed. They are eliminated by the kidney by glomerular filtration and tubular secretion. Absorption of oral torsemide is more rapid (1 hour) than that of furosemide (2-3 hours) and is nearly as complete as with intravenous administration. The duration of effect for furosemide is usually 2-3 hours and that of torsemide is 4-6 hours. Half-life depends on renal function. Since loop agents act on the luminal side of the tubule, their diuretic activity correlates with their secretion by the proximal tubule.

【Pharmacodynamics】Loop diuretics inhibit the $Na^+ / K^+ /2Cl^-$ cotransport of the luminal be in the ascending limb of the loop of Henle. Therefore, reabsorption of Na^+, K^+ and Cl^- is decreased. The loop diuretics are the most efficacious of the diuretic drugs, because the ascending limb accounts for the reabsorption of 25%-30% of filtered NaCl and downstream sites are not able to compensate for this increased Na^+ load.

The loop diuretics act promptly, even among patients who have poor renal function or who have not responded to thiazides or other diuretics (note: loop diuretics increase the Ca^{2+} content of urine, while thiazide diuretics decrease the Ca^{2+} concentration of the urine). The loop diuretics cause decreased renal vascular resistance and increased renal blood flow.

Loop diuretics induce synthesis of renal prostaglandins, which participate in the renal actions of these diuretics. In addition to their diuretic activity, loop agents have direct effects on blood flow through several vascular beds. Furosemide increases renal blood flow. Both furosemide and ethacrynic acid have also been shown to reduce pulmonary congestion and left ventricular filling pressures in heart failure before a measurable increase in urinary output occurs, and in anephric patients.

【Clinical indications】

(1) Acute pulmonary edema and other edematous (急性肺水肿和其他水肿)　A major use of loop diuretics is in the treatment of acute pulmonary edema. A rapid increase in venous capacitance in conjunction with a brisk natriuresis reduces left ventricular filling pressures and thereby rapidly relieves pulmonary edema. The edema of nephrotic syndrome often is refractory to other classes of diuretics, and loop diuretics often are the only drugs capable of reducing the massive edema associated with this renal disease. Loop diuretics also are employed in the treatment of edema and ascites of liver cirrhosis.

(2) Hyperkalemia (高钾血症)　In mild hyperkalemia or after acute management of severe hyperkalemia by other measures loop diuretics can significantly enhance urinary excretion of K^+.

(3) Hypercalcemia (高钙血症)　The loop diuretics (along with hydration) are also useful in treating hypercalcemia because they stimulate tubular Ca^{2+} secretion.

(4) Acute renal failure　Loop agents can increase the rate of urine flow and enhance K^+ excretion in acute renal failure. However, they do not shorten the duration of renal failure. If a large pigment load has precipitated acute renal failure (or threatens to), loop agents may help flush out intratubular casts and ameliorate intratubular obstruction.

(5) Anion overdose (阴离子药物过量)　Loop diuretics are useful in treating toxic ingestions (摄入中毒剂量) of bromide (溴化物), fluoride (氟化物), and iodide (碘化物) which are reabsorbed in the thick ascending limb. Saline solution must be administered to replace urinary losses of Na^+ and to provide Cl^-, so as to avoid extracellular fluid volume depletion.

【Adverse reactions】

(1) Acute hypovolemia (急性血容量减少)　Loop diuretics can cause a severe and rapid reduction in blood volume, with the possibility of hypotension and shock, and cardiac arrhythmias (心律失常).

(2) Ototoxicity (耳毒性)　Hearing can be affected adversely by the loop diuretics. Particularly when used in conjunction with the aminoglycoside antibiotics. Permanent damage may be elicited with continued treatment.

(3) Hyperuricemia (高尿酸血症)　Furosemide and ethacrynic acid compete with uric acid for the renal and biliary secretory systems, thus blocking its secretion and thereby causing the exacerbating gouty attacks (痛风发作).

(4) Potassium depletion (钾缺乏)　The heavy load of Na^+ presented to the collecting tubule results in increased exchange of tubular Na^+ for K^+, with the possibility of inducing hypokalemia. The loss of K^+ from cells in exchange for H^+ leads to hypokalemic alkalosis. Potassium depletion can be averted by the use of potassium-sparing diuretics or dietary supplementation with K^+.

(5) Allergic and other reactions　Except for ethacrynic acid, the loop diuretics are sulfonamides. Therefore skin rash, eosinophilia and, less often, interstitial nephritis are occasional side effects of these drugs. This toxicity usually resolves rapidly after drug withdrawal. Allergic reactions are much less common with ethacrynic acid.

2.3　The thiazides (噻嗪类) and related agents

The thiazides are the most widely used of the diuretic drugs. Chlorothiazide (氯噻嗪), the prototype thiazide diuretic, was the first modern diuretic that was active orally and was capable of affecting the severe edema of cirrhosis (肝硬化) and congestive heart failure with a minimum of side effects. Its properties are representative of the thiazide group, although newer derivatives such as hydrochlorothiazide (氢氯噻嗪) or chlorthalidone (氯噻酮) are now used more commonly.

Thiazides (噻嗪类)

【Pharmacokinetics】All of the thiazides can be administered orally, but there are differences in their metabolism. Chlorothiazide, the parent of the group, is not very lipid-soluble and must be given in relatively large doses. It is the only thiazide available for parenteral administration. All of the thiazides are secreted by the organic acid secretory system in the proximal tubule and compete with the secretion of uric acid by that system. As a result, thiazide use may blunt uric acid secretion and elevate serum uric acid level.

【Pharmacodynamics】The thiazide derivatives act is mainly in the distal tubule to decrease the reabsorption of Na^+ by inhibition of a Na^+/Cl^- cotransporter on the luminal membrane (Figure 22-4). They have a lesser effect in the proximal tubule. As a result, these drugs increase the concentration of Na^+ and Cl^- in the tubular fluid. The acid-base balance is not usually affected (note: because of the site of action of the thiazide derivatives is on the luminal membrane, these drugs must be excreted into the tubular lumen to be effective. Therefore, with decreased takes its function, thiazide diuretics lose efficacy).

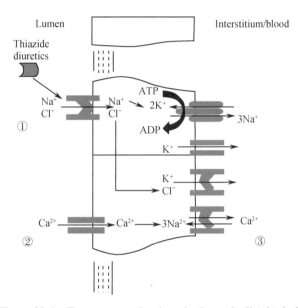

Figure 22-4   Transport mechanisms in the early distal tubule

Thiazide diuretics happens the excretion of Na^+ and Cl^- by inhibiting the Na^+/Cl^- cotransporter. ①The reabsorption of Ca^{2+}. ② It is increased by these drugs by a mechanism that may involve stimulation of Na^+/Ca^{2+} countertransport. ③Due to an increase in the concentration for Na^+ across the basolateral membrane

(1) **Increased excretion of Na^+ and Cl^-**   Chlorothiazide causes diuresis with increased Na^+ and Cl^- excretion, which can result in the excretion of a very hyperosmolar urine.

(2) **Loss of K^+**   Because thiazides increase the Na^+ in the filtrate arriving at the distal tubule, more K^+ is also exchanged for Na^+. Thus, prolonged use of these drugs results in continual loss K^+ from the body.

(3) **Decreased urinary calcium excretion (减少尿中钙的排泄)**   Thiazide diuretics decrease the Ca^{2+} content of urine by promoting the reabsorption of the Ca^{2+}. This contrasts with the loop diuretics which increase the Ca^{2+} concentration of the urine.

(4) **Reduced peripheral vascular resistance (降低外周血管阻力)**   An initial reduction in blood pressure results from a decrease in blood volume and therefore a decrease in cardiac output. With continued therapy, volume recovery occurs. However, there are continued hypotensive effects, resulting from reduced peripheral vascular resistance caused by relaxation of arteriolar smooth muscle.

【Clinical indications】

(1) **Hypertension (高血压)**   Clinically, the thiazides have long been the mainstay of antihypertensive medication, since they are inexpensive, convenient to be administered, and well tolerated. They are effective in reducing systolic and diastolic blood pressure for extended periods in the majority of patients

with mild to moderate essential hypertension.

(2) Congestive heart failure (充血性心力衰竭) Thiazides can be the diuretic of choice in reducing extracellular volume in mild to moderate congestive heart failure.

(3) Renal impairment (肾功能损伤) Patients with nephrotic syndrome accompanied by edema are initially treated with loop diuretics.

(4) Hypercalciuria (高尿钙症) The thiazides can be useful in treating idiopathic hypercalciuria because they inhibit urinary Ca^{2+} excretion. This is particularly beneficial for patients with calcium oxalate stones in the urinary tract.

(5) Diabetes insipidus (尿崩症) Thiazides has the unique ability to produce a hyperosmolar urine. Thiazides can substitute for the antidiuretic hormone in the treatment of nephrogenic diabetes insipidus. The urine volume of such individuals may drop from 11 L/d to about 3 L/d when treated with the drug.

【Adverse reactions】

(1) Potassium depletion (钾的丢失) Hypokalemia (低血钾) is the most frequent problem encountered with the thiazide diuretics and can predispose patients on digitalis to ventricular arrhythmias. The K^+ deficiency can be overcome by spironolactone, which interferes with aldosterone action, or by administering triamterene, which acts to retain K^+.

(2) Hyper uricemia (高尿酸血症) Thiazides happens serum uric acid by decreasing the amount of acid excreted by the organic acid secretory system. Being insoluble, the uric acid deposits in the joints, and a full-blown attack of gout may result in individuals predisposed to gouty attacks.

(3) Volume depletion (血容量不足) This can cause orthostatic hypotension or light-headedness.

(4) Hypercalcemia (高血钙) The thiazides inhibit the secretion of Ca^{2+}, sometimes leading to elevated levels of Ca^{2+} in the blood.

(5) Hyperglycemia (高血糖) and hyperlipidemia (高脂血症) Patients with diabetes mellitus, who are taking thiazides for hypertension, may become hyperglycemic and have difficulty in maintaining appropriate blood sugar levels. Thiazides causes a 5%-15% increase in total serum cholesterol and low-density lipoproteins (LDL). These levels may return toward baseline after prolonged use.

(6) Hypersensitivity (过敏反应) Photosensitivity or generalized dermatitis (光敏性或广泛性皮炎) occurs rarely. Serious allergic reactions are extremely rare but do include hemolytic anemia (溶血性贫血), thrombocytopenia (血小板减少), and acute necrotizing pancreatitis(急性坏死性胰腺炎).

(7) Other toxicities Weakness, fatigability, and paresthesias similar to those of carbonic anhydrase inhibitors may occur. Impotence (阳痿) has been reported but is probably related to volume depletion (体积消耗).

Chlorthalidone (氯噻酮)

Chlorthalidone is a thiazide derivative that behaves like hydrochlorothiazide. It has a very long duration of action and therefore is often used to treat hypertension. It is given once per day for this indication.

2.4 Potassium-sparing diuretics (保钾利尿药)

Spironolactone (螺内酯)

【Pharmacokinetics】 Spironolactone is a synthetic steroid that acts as a competitive antagonist to aldosterone. Spironolactone is well absorbed from the gut. Its plasma half-life is only 10 minutes, but its active metabolite, canrenone, has a plasma half-life of 16 hours.

【Pharmacodynamics】Spironolactone is a synthetic aldosterone antagonist (醛固酮拮抗剂) that competes with aldosterone for intracellular cytoplasmic receptor sites. The spironolactone receptor complex is inactive, that is, it prevents translocation of the receptor complex into the nucleus of the target cell, and thus does not bind to DNA. This results in a failure to produce proteins that are normally synthesized in response to aldosterone. These mediator proteins normally stimulate the Na^+-K^+ exchange sites of the collecting tubule. Thus, a lack of mediator proteins prevents Na^+ reabsorption and therefore K^+ and H^+ secretion. In most edematous states, blood levels of aldosterone are high, which is instrumental in retaining Na^+. When spironolactone is given to a patient with elevated circulating levels of aldosterone, the drug antagonizes the activity of the hormone, resulting in the retention of K^+ and excretion of Na^+ (Figure 22-5). Where there are no significant circulating levels of aldosterone, such as in Addison's diseases (艾迪生病) (primary adrenal insufficiency), no diuretic effect of the drug occurs.

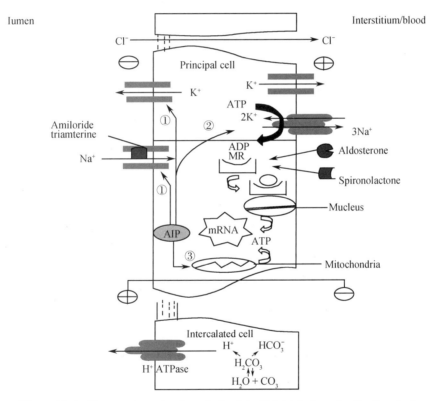

Figure 22-5   Transport mechanisms in the late distal tubule and collecting duct

【Clinical indications】

(1) **Diuretic (利尿)**   Although spironolactone has a low efficacy in mobilizing Na^+ from the body in comparison with the other drugs, it has the useful property of causing the retention of K^+. Because of this latter action, spironolactone is often given in conjunction with a thiazide or loop diuretic to prevent K^+ excretion that would otherwise occur with these drugs.

(2) **Secondary hyperaldosteronism (继发性醛固酮增多症)**   Spironolactone is the only potassium-sparing diuretic that is routinely used alone to induce net negative salt balance. It is particularly effective in clinical situations associated with secondary hyperaldosteronism.

【Adverse reactions】Because spironolactone chemically resembles some of sex steroids, it does have minimal hormonal activity and may induce gynecomastia in males (男子女性型乳房)and menstrual irregularities in females (女性月经不调). Because of this, the drug should not be given in high doses on a chronic basis. It is most effectively employed in mild edematous states. At low doses, spironolactone, informs chronically with few side effects: hyperkalemia, nausea (恶心) and lethargy (嗜睡), and mental confusion (精神错乱) can occur.

Triamterene (氨苯蝶啶) and amiloride (阿米洛利)

Triamterene and amiloride block Na⁺ transport channels resulting in a decrease in Na⁺-K⁺ exchange; they have K⁺-sparing diuretic actions similar to that of spironolactone. However, the ability of these drugs to block the K⁺- Na⁺ exchange site in the collecting tubule does not depend on the presence of aldosterone. Thus, they have diuretic activity even in individuals with Addison's disease. They, like spironolactone, are not very efficacious diuretics. Both triamterene and amiloride are frequently used in combination with other diuretics, usually for their potassium-sparing properties. For example, much like spironolactone, they prevent K⁺ loss that occurs with thiazides and furosemide. The side effects of triamterene are leg cramps and the possibility of increased blood urea nitrogen (尿素氮) as well as uric acid and K⁺ retention.

3. Dehydrant diuretics (osmotic diuretics)

Osmotic diuretics (渗透性利尿药) are pharmacologically inert substances [e.g., mannitol (D-甘露醇) and urea (尿素)] that are filtered in the glomerulus but not reabsorbed by the nephron. To cause a diuresis, they must constitute an appreciable fraction of the osmolarity of tubular fluid. Within the nephron, their main effect is exerted on those parts of the nephron that are freely permeable to water: the proximal tubule, descending limb of the loop, and (in the presence of ADH) the collecting tubules. Passive water reabsorption is reduced by the presence of non-reabsorbable solute within the tubule; consequently a larger volume of fluid remains within the proximal tubule. This has the secondary effect of reducing Na⁺ reabsorption.

Therefore, the main effect of osmotic diuretics is to increase the amount of water excreted, with a smaller increase in Na⁺ excretion. They are not useful in treating conditions such as heart failure associated with Na⁺ retention but have much more limited therapeutic indications, including emergency treatment of acutely raised intracranial or intraocular pressure (颅内压或眼内压). Such treatment has nothing to do with the kidney, but relies on the increase in plasma osmolarity (血浆渗透压) by solutes that do not enter the brain or eye; this results in extraction of water from these compartments.

In acute renal failure, which can occur as a result of haemorrhage (出血，尤指大出血), injury or systemic infections (全身感染), the glomerular filtration rate is reduced, and absorption of NaCl and water in the proximal tubule becomes almost complete, so that more distal parts of the nephron virtually "dry up", and urine flow ceases. Protein is deposited in the tubules and may impede the flow of fluid. Osmotic diuretics (e.g., mannitol in a dose of 12-15g) can limit these effects, at least if given in the earliest stages, albeit while increasing intravascular volume and risking left ventricular failure. Osmotic diuretics are given intravenously (静脉注射).

　　Adverse reactions include transient expansion of the extracellular fluid volume (with a risk of causing left ventricular failure) and hyponatraemia. Headache, nausea and vomiting can occur.

重 点 小 结

药物	药理作用	临床应用	不良反应
袢利尿药：呋塞米、布美他尼、托拉塞米、依他尼酸	利尿：特异性地抑制髓袢升支粗段皮质部和髓质部 Na^+- K^+-$2Cl^-$ 协同转运蛋白，干扰肾脏对尿液的稀释与浓缩功能	急性肺水肿、高钙血症、高钾血症、急性肾衰竭	耳毒性、高尿酸血症、急性血容量减少、钾丢失
噻嗪类利尿药：氯噻嗪、氢氯噻嗪	利尿：抑制远曲小管近端 Na^+-Cl^- 协同转运蛋白，抑制 Na^+ 和水的再吸收，使肾脏的尿液稀释功能降低；抗尿崩症；降压	高血压、充血性心力衰竭、肾功能损伤、高钙尿症、尿崩症	钾丢失、高尿酸血症、高血糖、高钙血症、过敏反应
保钾利尿药：螺内酯	可与醛固酮竞争醛固酮受体，间接抑制远曲小管远端和集合管 Na^+- K^+ 交换	利尿，用于继发性醛固酮增多症	高血钾、性激素样副作用

目 标 检 测

题库

一、选择题

（一）单项选择题

1. 下列哪个药有耳毒性（　　　）
　　A. 呋塞米　　　　B. 氢氯噻嗪　　　　C. 螺内酯　　　　D. 氨苯蝶啶　　　　E. 甘露醇

2. 利尿药中可用于治疗尿崩症的是（　　　）
　　A. 呋塞米　　　　　　　　B. 依他尼酸　　　　C. 螺内酯
　　D. 氨苯蝶啶　　　　　　　E. 氢氯噻嗪

3. 利尿药作用的强弱依赖于体内醛固酮水平的是（　　　）
　　A. 呋塞米　　　　B. 氢氯噻嗪　　　　C. 螺内酯　　　　D. 氨苯蝶啶　　　　E. 乙酰唑胺

4. 氢氯噻嗪的主要作用部位在（　　　）
　　A. 近曲小管　　　　　　　B. 集合管　　　　　　　C. 髓袢升支
　　D. 髓袢升支粗段　　　　　E. 远曲小管的近端

5. 常用利尿药主要通过（　　　）起作用
　　A. 降低肾血管阻力, 增加肾血流量
　　B. 提高肾小球滤过率
　　C. 抑制肾小管对电解质和水的重吸收
　　D. 对抗 ADH 的作用
　　E. 抑制肾素释放, 使醛固酮分泌减少

医药大学堂
WWW.YIYAODXT.COM

（二）多项选择题

6. 关于呋塞米的作用及机制的叙述，下列哪些是正确的（　　　）

   A. 作用部位主要在髓袢升支粗段

   B. 特异性地与 Cl^- 竞争 Na^+-K^+-$2Cl^-$ 协同转运蛋白 Cl^- 的结合部位

   C. 降低肾脏的浓缩功能和稀释功能

   D. 扩张肾血管，增加肾血流量

   E. 增加 PGE 释放

7. 螺内酯的特点是（　　　）

   A. Na^+ 和 Cl^- 排泄增加，K^+ 排泄减少；当体内醛固酮增多时，能减弱或抵消该药的作用

   B. Na^+ 和 Cl^- 排泄增加，K^+ 排泄减少；当切除肾上腺或体内醛固酮有变化时，不影响利尿作用

   C. 显著排泄 Na^+、Cl^-、K^+，作用于髓袢升支粗段

   D. 作用于远曲小管，使 Na^+、Cl^-、K^+ 排泄增加

   E. 利尿作用弱，起效慢而维持久

二、思考题

从呋塞米、氢氯噻嗪的作用部位、作用机制解释其利尿特点。

（周玖瑶）

Chapter 23　Drugs for diabetes

学习目标

　　1. **掌握**　胰岛素的临床应用和不良反应；磺酰脲类和二甲双胍的药理作用及机制、临床应用和不良反应。

　　2. **熟悉**　瑞格列奈、罗格列酮、阿卡波糖的主要药理作用和临床应用。

　　3. **了解**　其他口服降糖药的药理作用和临床应用。

1.　Diabetes mellitus

　　The incidence of diabetes mellitus (糖尿病) is growing rapidly both in China and worldwide. Diabetes is a heterogeneous group of syndromes characterized by an elevation of blood glucose caused by a relative or absolute deficiency of insulin. If left untreated, patients will undergo retinopathy (视网膜病变), nephropathy (肾脏病变), neuropathy (神经病变) and cardiovascular complications, which account for mortality of diabetes. Therefore, administration of insulin and oral hypoglycemic agents for diabetes are essential. Except for medications, diet and lifestyle modifications and exercises also play significant roles.

　　The American Diabetes Association (ADA) recognizes four types of diabetes: type 1 diabetes (T1DM), type 2 diabetes (T2DM), gestational diabetes, and diabetes due to other causes. The major characteristics of T1DM and T2DM are summarized in Table 23-1.

Table 23-1　Comparison of T1DM and T2DM

	(T1DM)	(T2DM)
Age of onset	Usually during children or puberty	Commonly over 35 years old
Prevalence	5%-10%	90%-95%
Pathogenesis	B cells are destroyed by immune-mediated processes, viruses or chemical toxins	Insulin resistance, be influenced by genetic factors, aging, obesity, unhealthy lifestyle
Insulin secretion	Absolute deficiency of insulin	Gradually decrease with progressing of diabetes
Clinical features	Classical symptoms (polydipsia, polyphagia, polyuria, weight loss)	The metabolic changes be milder than T1DM
Medications	Must rely on exogenous insulin	Oral hypoglycemic agents, insulin when necessary

189

2. Insulin and its analogs

Insulin consists of two peptide chains that are connected by disulfide bonds. It is synthesized as a precursor (proinsulin) that undergoes proteolytic cleavage (蛋白水解) to form insulin and C-peptide.

Initially, the insulin used in clinics were extracted from pancreas of porcine or bovine. Human insulin is produced by recombinant DNA technology. Nowadays, insulin analogs such as lispro, aspart, glulisine, glargine and detemir are widely used. They origin from modifications of amino acid sequences of human insulin to get different pharmacokinetic properties.

【Secretion】Both insulin and C-peptide are secreted by B cells of the pancreas. Measurement of circulating C-peptide provides a better index of insulin levels. Secretion of insulin is most commonly triggered by high blood glucose, also by certain amino acids, other hormones, and autonomic mediators. In general, glucose is taken up by glucose transporter into B cells, and then phosphorylated by glucokinase. The products enter mitochondrial respiratory chain and generate ATP, which blocks K^+ channel. The decreased outflow of K^+ leads to membrane depolarization and influx of Ca^{2+}. Finally, excess intracellular Ca^{2+} stimulates pulsatiles insulin exocytosis (Figure 23-1).

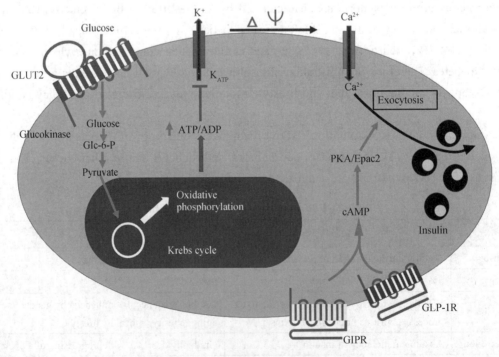

Figure 23-1   Process of insulin secretion

【Pharmacodynamics】

(1) Insulin promotes synthesis, while inhibits decomposition of fat, thus reducing the generation of free fatty acids and ketones (酮体). Insulin also facilitates the transport of fatty acids to increase its utilization.

(2) Insulin lowers blood glucose level by promoting the synthesis and storage of glycogen (糖原), accelerating the oxidation and fermentation of glucose, and inhibiting glycogen decomposition and gluconeogenesis (糖异生).

(3) Insulin inhibits the decomposition of proteins, and promotes the synthesis of proteins via increasing the transport of amino acids.

(4) Insulin also accelerates the heart rate, and strengthens myocardial contractility.

(5) Insulin promotes the entry of potassium into cells and reduces the blood potassium concentration.

【Clinical indications】

(1) **Type 1 diabetes**   Insulin is still the most important drug for the treatment of type 1 diabetes mellitus.

(2) **The newly diagnosed type 2 diabetes**   Insulin should be used at the beginning, with or without oral agents, for those with significant high level of blood glucose and HbA1c, or with obvious symptoms.

(3) **Type 2 diabetes**   If the patients do not respond well to diet control or oral agents, insulin injection is needed.

(4) **Diabetes mellitus with various acute or serious complications**   such as ketoacidosis (酮症酸中毒) and non-ketotic hyperosmotic coma (非酮症高渗性昏迷).

(5) **Diabetes mellitus with various comorbidities**   such as severe infections, consumptive diseases, high fever, pregnancy, trauma (外伤) and operation.

【Insulin preparations】 Several types of insulin preparations are available. They show different absorption and pharmacokinetic profiles. Figure 23-2 summarizes the onset of action, timing of peak level, and duration of action for the commonly used preparations. Long-term treatment of insulin relies predominantly on subcutaneous injection. In special settings, insulin should be administered intravenously. The major features of commonly used insulin preparations can be found in Table 23-2.

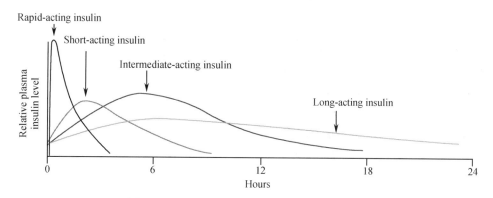

Figure 23-2   Properties of insulin formulations

Table 23-2　The widely used insulin preparations

Forms		Structure	Administration
Rapid-acting insulin	Lispro, aspart, glulisine	Have minor modifications of structure according to human insulin, leading to more rapid absorption and lower risk of hypoglycemia than regular insulin after SC injection	Be administered to mimic the prandial (餐时) release of insulin, offering flexible treatment regimens. Usually not used alone but with a long-acting insulin to ensure postprandial glucose control. Be administered subcutaneously, or intravenously in emergency, also in external insulin pump (胰岛素泵).
Short-acting insulin	Regular insulin	Soluble crystalline zinc insulin, associating as hexamers (六聚体) in aqueous solution at a neutral pH	Be injected subcutaneously 30-45 minutes before a meal. In emergencies IV injection is practicable
Intermediate-acting insulin	Neutral protamine hagedorn (NPH)	A suspension of crystalline zinc insulin combined at neutral pH with the positively charged polypeptide protamine (鱼精蛋白), forming a less-soluble complex, leading to delayed absorption and intermediate duration of action	Be used for basal control with SC injection (never IV) in all forms of diabetes except diabetic ketoacidosis and emergency hyperglycemia (高血糖). Usually given along with rapid-acting insulin for mealtime control
Long-acting insulin	Glargine, detemir	The lower isoelectric point (等电点) of glargine leads to precipitation at the injection site and extension of action. The addition of a fatty-acid side chain to detemir enhances association to albumin, thus slows dissociation from albumin. Both have slow onset and flat, prolonged hypoglycemic effect with no peak	Must be given subcutaneously and never be mixed in the same syringe (注射器) with other insulins

【 Adverse reactions 】

(1) **Hypoglycemia (低血糖)**　It is the most serious and common adverse reactions of excess dose of insulin. Early symptoms include hunger, sweating, tachycardia (心动过速), anxiety, tremor (震颤) and so on. Severe signs consist coma, shock, brain injury, and even death. In order to prevent the serious consequences of hypoglycemia, patients should be taught to be familiar with the reactions. The mild individuals can drink sugar water or take food, while those serious ones should be injected with 50% glucose immediately.

(2) **Allergic reactions (过敏反应)**　Allergic reactions may be induced by the structural difference between animal insulin and human insulin, or the low purity of the preparations. These can be avoided with high purity preparations or human insulin. The reactions may be alleviated with H_1 receptor blockers, or glucocorticoids in severe cases.

(3) **Insulin resistance (胰岛素抵抗)**　The acute insulin resistance is mainly caused by infection, trauma, operation and other stress states. In these occasions, large number of free fatty acids and ketones in the blood inhibit the uptake and utilization of glucose, leading to decreased action of insulin. It is essential to deal with the incentives, adjust the acid-base balance and increase the dose of insulin.

The chronic insulin resistance refers to patients who need more than 200U insulin every day with no complications. For these patients, insulin sensitizers may be better choice.

(4) Weight gain   As an anabolic hormone, insulin may be associated with modest weight gain in the treatment of both type 1 and type 2 diabetes.

3. Oral agents

Sulfonylureas (磺酰脲类)

The primary sulfonylureas used today include glyburide (格列本脲), glipizide (格列吡嗪), glimepiride (格列美脲), gliquidone (格列喹酮), gliclazide (格列齐特), and so on.

【Pharmacokinetics】 All sulfonylureas are effectively absorbed from the GI tract. The plasma binding is 90%-99%. The agents are metabolized by the liver and excreted in the urine. Their half-lives are short (3-5 hours), and their hypoglycemic effects are evident for 12-24 hours.

【Pharmacodynamics】

(1) Lower blood glucose level   These agents lower blood glucose level in normal individuals and those with remaining islet function, but not in patients of T1DM and resection of pancreas. The action is dependent on functioning B cells. The detailed mechanism include: ①stimulation of insulin release by binding with its receptor in B cells and blocking the receptor-coupled ATP-sensitive K^+ channels, leading to depolarization and Ca^{2+} influx (Figure 23-3). ②Decrease of glycogen levels. ③Increase in peripheral insulin sensitivity.

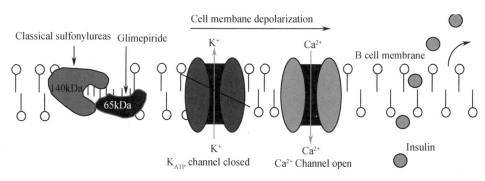

Figure 23-3   Major mechanisms of action of sulfonylureas

(2) Effect on water excretion   Glyburide and chlorpropamide (氯磺丙脲) show antidiuretic effect through promotion the secretion of ADH.

(3) Effect on coagulation   Some of the sulfonylureas can weaken platelet adhesion and stimulate the synthesis of plasminogen.

【Clinical indications】

(1) It is used for patients of T2DM with remaining islet function that do not respond well to diet control alone.

(2) Chlorpropamide can be used for diabetes insipidus patients to decrease the urine volume.

【Adverse reactions】Common adverse reactions include skin allergy, gastrointestinal discomfort, lethargy (嗜睡), jaundice (黄疸) and liver damage. Leukopenia, thrombocytopenia and hemolytic anemia are occasionally reported. Therefore, it is necessary to check the hepatic function and hemogram (血象) regularly.

Hypoglycemia is serious adverse reaction due to overdose of drugs. They should be used with caution in elderly patients and those with hepatic or renal insufficiency due to delayed excretion and accumulation of drugs.

Biguanides (双胍类)

Metformin (二甲双胍) is the only currently available biguanide. It can significantly decrease blood glucose levels in diabetic patients, with little effect on normoglycemic states. The main mechanism include: ①reduction of hepatic glucose output by inhibiting hepatic gluconeogenesis. ②Decrease of intestinal absorption of sugars and increase of peripheral glucose uptake and utilization. ③Reduce of hyperlipidemia.

Metformin is recommended as the drug of choice for newly diagnosed T2DM, especially for the obese ones and those do not respond well to diet control. It can be used alone or in combination with other oral agents or insulin.

The drug is well absorbed orally, does not bind to plasma proteins, and is excreted unchanged in the urine.

The adverse reactions are largely gastrointestinal, such as loss of appetite (食欲缺乏), nausea, abdominal discomfort, and diarrhea. Lactic acidemia (乳酸酸中毒) and ketosis (酮血症) are serious effects.

Glinides (格列奈类)

This class of agents includes repaglinide (瑞格列奈) and nateglinide (那格列奈).

【Pharmacokinetics】These agents are well absorbed after oral administration 1 to 30 minutes before meals. The glinides are metabolized to inactive products by CYP3A4 in the liver, 92% of which may be excreted through intestine.

【Pharmacodynamics】The glinides bind to a distinct site to the sulfonylurea receptor on the B cells, block the ATP-sensitive K^+ channels, and finally culminate the release of insulin. They have rapid onset and short duration of action as compared to the sulfonylureas. They are particularly effective in the early release of insulin after a meal.

【Clinical indications】The glinides can be used for patients of T2DM, including elderly and diabetic nephropathy.

【Adverse reactions】There is a lower incidence of hypoglycemia in glinides than sulfonylureas. Severe hypoglycemia has been reported in patients taking repaglinide in combination with lipid-lowering drug gemfibrozil, so the concurrent use should be avoided.

Thiazolidinediones (TZDs, 噻唑烷酮类)

As insulin resistance is one of the major pathophysiological changes of diabetes, insulin sensitizers have been widely used. The members of this class include pioglitazone (吡格列酮), rosiglitazone (罗格列酮), englitazone (恩格列酮), and so on.

【Pharmacokinetics】Both pioglitazone and rosiglitazone are absorbed within 2-3 hours after oral administration. They are largely bound to serum albumin and metabolized by CYP450 isozymes. Piglitazone and its metabolites are excreted mainly in the feces, while rosiglitazone mainly in the urine.

【Pharmacodynamics】

(1) Improve insulin resistance and reduce hyperglycemia　TZDs can alleviate insulin resistance in skeletal muscle, adipose tissue and liver, especially in combination with metformin or sulfonylureas. Thus TZDs can significantly reduce fasting and postprandial blood glucose, HbA1c and free fatty acid levels.

TZDs are known to target the nuclear hormone receptor peroxisome proliferator-activated receptor-γ (PPARγ), a group of nuclear receptors which are involved in regulation of adipocyte production, secretion of fatty acids, and glucose metabolism.

(2) Improve dyslipidemia　TZDs can significantly reduce triglycerides, increase the level of total cholesterol and HDL-C in patients of T2DM.

(3) Improve functions of B cells　TZDs can increase the area and density of pancreas, and decrease apoptosis of B cells. Rosiglitazone lowers free fatty acid level, which may be toxic to pancreas.

【Clinical indications】TZDs are mainly used for patients of T2DM or insulin resistance. They can be prescribed as monotherapy or in combination with other oral agents or insulin.

【Adverse reactions】The common adverse reactions of TZDs include drowsiness, muscle and bone pain, headache, gastrointestinal symptoms, with low incidence of hypoglycemia. However, some serious adverse reactions have limited the use of these agents. Troglitazone (曲格列酮) was withdrawn due to a number of deaths from hepatotoxicity. Rosiglitazone was also withdrawn in the USA and European Union because of potential increased risk of cardiovascular events. Other countries have made strict warnings and restrictions on its use.

α-glucosidase inhibitors (α-糖苷酶抑制剂)

The drugs in this class are acarbose (阿卡波糖) and voglibose (伏格列波糖). They reversibly inhibit the activity of α-glucosidase in the intestinal brush border. This enzyme is responsible for the hydrolysis of oligosaccharides to glucose and other sugars. Inhibition of this enzyme slows the digestion of carbohydrates from the GI tract, reduces intestinal absorption of glucose and lowers postprandial plasma glucose level.

α-glucosidase inhibitors are taken at the beginning of meals. They are indicated as adjuncts to diet and exercise in T2DM patients as monotherapy, or in combination with insulin and (or) other oral hypoglycemic agents.

Acarbose is poorly absorbed. It is metabolized primarily by intestinal bacteria. The major adverse reactions related to α-glucosidase inhibitors are malabsorption (吸收不良), flatulence (胀气), diarrhea (腹泻), and abdominal bloating (腹胀). Mild to moderate elevations of hepatic transaminases have been reported with acarbose. They should be avoided in patients with colonic ulceration, inflammatory bowel disease, or intestinal obstruction.

Dipeptidyl peptidase-Ⅳ (DPP-Ⅳ) inhibitors

Sitagliptin (西格列汀) and alogliptin (阿格列汀) are orally active DPP-Ⅳ inhibitors used in clinics. DPP-Ⅳ is responsible for the inactivation of incretin hormones such as glucagon-like peptide-1(GLP-1). GLP-1 stimulates insulin secretion, inhibits glucagon release, protects B cells, delays gastric emptying, and reduces food intake. Therefore, prolonging the activity of GLP-1 results in increased insulin release in response to meals and a reduction in inappropriate secretion of glucagon.

DPP-Ⅳ inhibitors may be used for the treatment of T2DM as monotherapy or in combination with other oral agents or insulin. They are well absorbed after oral administration. The majority of sitagliptin is excreted unchanged in the urine.

In general, DPP-Ⅳ inhibitors are well tolerated, with the most common adverse reactions being nasopharyngitis (鼻咽炎) and headache. Rates of hypoglycemia are comparable to those with placebo.

重 点 小 结

药物	药理作用	临床应用	不良反应
胰岛素	促进肝脏、脂肪、肌肉等靶组织的糖原和脂肪储存	①T1DM。②新诊断的 T2DM。③T2DM经饮食或口服降糖药未能控制者。④糖尿病发生严重或急性并发症者。⑤糖尿病伴有应激状态。⑥细胞内缺钾	低血糖、过敏反应、胰岛素抵抗、体重增加
磺酰脲类：格列美脲	刺激胰岛 B 细胞释放胰岛素，降低血糖	胰岛功能尚存的 T2DM 且仅靠饮食控制无效者	低血糖、肝功能异常
格列奈类：瑞格列奈	促进胰岛素生理性分泌曲线的恢复	T2DM，包括老年和糖尿病肾病患者	较低的低血糖发生率
双胍类：二甲双胍	促进脂肪组织摄取葡萄糖，减少肠道对糖的吸收	新诊断的 T2DM 患者，尤其肥胖者	胃肠道反应、乳酸酸中毒、酮血症少见

目 标 检 测

题库

一、选择题

（一）单项选择题

1. 下列哪一种糖尿病不需首选胰岛素治疗（　　　）
   A. 合并严重感染的中度糖尿病　　　B. 需行手术治疗的糖尿病　　　C. 轻度及中度糖尿病
   D. 1 型糖尿病　　　E. 妊娠期糖尿病

2. 对于使用胰岛素进行治疗的患者应告知其警惕（　　　）
   A. 低血糖的发生　　　B. 酮症酸中毒的发生　　　C. 过敏反应
   D. 消化道反应　　　E. 肝肾功能损害

医药大学堂
WWW.YIYAODXT.COM

3. 体态肥胖的成年 2 型糖尿病患者初治首选（ 　　 ）
　　A. 饮食控制 　　　　　　　　　B. 多休息 　　　　　　　　　C. 口服双胍类降糖药
　　D. 口服磺脲类降糖药 　　　　　E. 注射胰岛素

4. 磺脲类降糖药主要用于下列哪种情况（ 　　 ）
　　A. 饮食控制无效的 2 型糖尿病 　　　B. 1 型糖尿病
　　C. 糖尿病酮症酸中毒 　　　　　　　D. 1 型糖尿病伴眼底病变
　　E. 肥胖且饮食控制无效的糖尿病

5. 罗格列酮降糖的基本作用机制是（ 　　 ）
　　A. 阻滞 ATP 敏感的钾通道
　　B. 减少葡萄糖在小肠的吸收及糖原异生
　　C. 竞争性激活过氧化物酶 – 增殖体受体
　　D. 抑制胰高血糖素的释放
　　E. 抑制胰岛素降解

6. 下列可用于治疗尿崩症的降糖药是（ 　　 ）
　　A. 氯磺丙脲 　　B. 瑞格列奈 　　C. 甲苯磺丁脲 　　D. 二甲双胍 　　E. 苯乙双胍

7. 下列有关瑞格列奈的叙述，错误的是（ 　　 ）
　　A. 可以模仿胰岛素的生理性分泌 　　　B. 是一种促胰岛素分泌剂
　　C. 半衰期短，适于降餐后血糖 　　　　D. 对功能受损的胰岛细胞有保护作用
　　E. 禁用于糖尿病肾病患者

（二）多项选择题

8. 胰岛素对脂代谢的影响有（ 　　 ）
　　A. 促进脂肪合成并抑制其分解 　　　B. 减少游离脂肪酸和酮体
　　C. 增加脂肪酸的转运，使其利用增加 　　D. 可致酮症酸中毒
　　E. 减少脂类的吸收

9. 对双胍类药物叙述不正确的是（ 　　 ）
　　A. 可以减少食物中糖的吸收 　　　B. 促进组织摄取葡萄糖
　　C. 主要用于重度糖尿病 　　　　　D. 可促进肌肉组织中糖的有氧氧化
　　E. 可引起严重的高乳酸血症

二、思考题

常用的促胰岛素分泌剂有哪些？试比较其异同点。

（王芙蓉）

Chapter 24　Thyroid and antithyroid drugs

 学习目标

　　1.**掌握**　甲状腺激素的药理作用；硫脲类抗甲状腺药的药理作用及机制、临床应用和不良反应。

　　2.**熟悉**　抗甲状腺药的分类及代表药物；其他抗甲状腺药如碘剂、放射性碘、β受体阻断药治疗甲状腺功能亢进的作用特点。

　　3.**了解**　甲状腺激素的生物合成、分泌过程。

　　The thyroid is a small gland located in neck. It's responsible for helping to regulate many physiological processes, such as metabolism, energy generation and mood. Thyroid hormones (甲状腺激素) are two hormones produced and released by the thyroid gland, namely triiodothyronine (T_3, 三碘甲状腺原氨酸) and thyroxine (T_4, 甲状腺素). Hypothyroidism (甲状腺功能减退症) is caused by the decrease of synthesis and secretion of thyroid hormones and needs thyroid hormones replacement therapy. While hyperthyroidism (overactive thyroid, 甲状腺功能亢进症) occurs when the thyroid gland produces too much of the thyroid hormones and needs antithyroid drugs (抗甲状腺药) treatment timely.

1. Thyroid hormones

　　Thyroid hormones are tyrosine-based hormones and active substance, which ensure regulation of the metabolism, growth and development of the body. T_4 contains 4 molecules of iodide and T_3 contains 3 molecules of iodide. The iodine in T_3 and T_4 is an active ingredient from food, water and drug, which can be quickly absorbed and enter the blood circulation. Thyroid drugs include thyroid tablets (甲状腺片) of animal origin and synthetic levothyroxine sodium tablets (左甲状腺素钠片), the former are mainly composed of T_4 and T_3, while the latter are synthetic T_4. Thyroid drugs are used to supplement the low thyroid hormones levels in people with hypothyroidism whose thyroid gland do not produce enough thyroid hormones to meet the needs of the body.

　　The effects of T_4 last longer than T_3, while T_3 is approximately 10 times more active than T_4 in the body, and T_4 can be converted to T_3 in peripheral tissues. Therefore, although the thyroid produces two hormones, T_3 and T_4, synthetic T_4 is most commonly prescribed to treat hypothyroidism.

WWW.YIYAODXT.COM

1.1 Biosynthesis, storage, secretion and regulation of thyroid hormones

In humans, thyroid hormones T_3 and T_4 are synthesized in the follicular cells of thyroid gland (甲状腺滤泡细胞) in a process that crucially involves the thyroglobulin (甲状腺球蛋白). Thyroglobulin is a precursor to thyroid hormones, its tyrosine residues are combined with iodine and the protein is subsequently cleaved. The process is as follows (Figure 24-1).

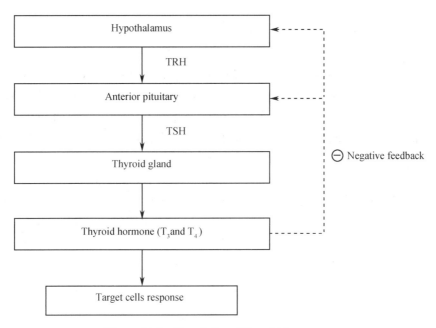

Figure 24-1   Regulation of thyroid hormones

(1) **Intake of iodine**   Iodine ions (I^-) enter the thyroid follicular cells from blood by the iodine pump.

(2) **Biosynthesis and storage of thyroid hormones**   The first is the activation of iodine. I^- is oxidized by thyroid peroxides (甲状腺过氧化物酶) to an intermediate of active iodine (I^0) or iodine oxide (I^+). The second is the iodination of tyrosine residues on thyroglobulin. The third is the coupling reaction. Attachment of an iodine molecule to a tyrosine residue produces monoiodotyrosine (MIT); attachment of two iodine molecules produces diiodotyrosine (DIT). In the presence of peroxides, T_4 is formed when two molecules of DIT are coupled, and T_3 is formed when one MIT and DIT are coupled. Subsequently, the generated T_4 and T_3 molecules are combined with thyroglobulin and are stored in the colloid of thyroid gland cells.

(3) **Release and secretion of the thyroid hormones**   The colloid is subsequently cleaved by proteases to release thyroglobulin from its T_3 and T_4 attachments, and then the active T_4 and T_3 are released into the bloodstream. Thyroid hormone receptors in cell membrane, mitochondria and nucleus, which are distributed in the cells of pituitary, heart, liver, kidney, skeletal muscle, lung, intestine and other organs and tissues. Thyroid hormones play important roles in regulating gene expression mediated by T_3 receptors in the nucleus and promoting synthesis of some related mRNA and proteins. Generally, the ratio of T_4 to T_3 within thyroglobulin is approximately 5 : 1, so most of the hormone released is T_4, and most

of the T_3 is derived from the metabolism of T_4 in peripheral tissues.

(4) Regulation of the thyroid hormones levels in the blood The synthesis and secretion of thyroid hormones are regulated by the hypothalamus-pituitary-thyroid axis (下丘脑-垂体-甲状腺轴). Thyrotropin-releasing hormone (TRH, 促甲状腺激素释放激素) secreted by hypothalamus can promote the secretion of thyroid-stimulating hormone (TSH, 促甲状腺激素) by pituitary. TSH can promote the proliferation of thyroid cells and the synthesis and release of T_3 and T_4, and increase the concentration of T_3 and T_4 in blood. However, when the concentration of T_3 and T_4 in blood increases, it will produce a negative feedback regulation on the synthesis and release of TRH in hypothalamus and TSH in pituitary.

1.2 Pharmacokinetics

T_3 and T_4 can be easily absorbed by oral administration, and the bioavailability is 50%-75% and 90%-95% respectively. The plasma protein binding rates of both T_3 and T_4 are more than 99%. However, the affinity of T_3 to the protein is lower than that of T_4, and its free amount is 10 times more than that of T_4. In addition, 30% of T_4 can be converted to T_3 by deiodination reaction (脱碘反应) in peripheral tissues. Therefore, the effect of T_3 is faster and stronger, and the duration time is shorter than that of T_4; while the effect of T_4 is slower and weaker, and the duration time is longer than T_3.

The plasma half-life of T_3 is 1-2 days, and the onset time is 6 hours after administration. The plasma half-life of T_4 is 6-7 days, and the curative effect will reach a peak in 7-10 days. Thyroid hormones are metabolized mainly by the deiodination reaction in the mitochondria of liver cells and kidney cells, and the glucuronic acid and sulfuric acid conjugated metabolites are excreted through the kidney. Thyroid hormones can cross the placenta and pass through breast milk, so pregnant and lactating women should use them with caution.

1.3 Pharmacodynamics

Thyroid hormones exert their physiologic actions through control of DNA transcription and protein synthesis. T_3 and T_4 diffuse into the cell nucleus and bind to thyroid receptor proteins attached to DNA. This hormone nuclear receptor complex activates gene transcription and synthesis of messenger RNA and cytoplasmic proteins.

(1) Maintaining growth and development Thyroid hormones are critical for optimal growth, development, function, and maintenance of all body tissues especially for bone and nervous system. These actions depend on protein synthesis and the potentiating of the secretion and action of growth hormone. Hypothyroidism in infants and young children will lead to short stature, short limbs and mental retardation, known as dwarfism (侏儒症) or cretinism (克汀病). Hypothyroidism in adults may lead to myxedema (黏液性水肿), decreased excitability of the central nervous system, memory loss and so on. Rarely, severe hypothyroidism may lead to myxedema coma, characterized by bradycardia, hypothermia, hypotension, and decreased level of consciousness.

(2) Regulation of metabolism Thyroid hormones promote substance oxidation, increase oxygen consumption, as well as basal metabolic rate and heat production. People with hyperthyroidism are afraid of heat, sweating, hyperorexia, emaciation, palpitation and so on. People with hypothyroidism always possess low basal metabolic rate and some symptoms such as hypohidrosis and intolerance to cold.

(3) Increase of the sensitivity of the sympathetic-adrenal system　In patients with hyperthyroidism, the increased response to catecholamine may cause some neurological and cardiovascular symptoms, such as emotional agitation, tremor, insomnia, fast heart rate and cardiac output, high blood pressure and so on.

1.4　Clinical indications

(1) Hypothyroidism　For cretinism in newborns, infants and young children, the sooner they are treated with thyroid hormones, the better outcome they will get. These patients need to be supplemented with oral thyroid tablets (main ingredients are T_4 and T_3) throughout their lifetime. If the treatment is too late, mental retardation and dwarfism will continue and need lifelong medication. For patients with myxedema, they need a low dose of oral thyroid tablets and then gradually increase the amount to an adequate therapeutic dose. For those who are in the term of myxedema coma, T_3 must be injected immediately and then with oral administration after awakening.

(2) Simple goiter (单纯性甲状腺肿)　Simple goiter is an enlargement of the thyroid gland. It is usually not a tumor or cancer and needs to be treated according to the etiology. Those caused by iodine deficiency need to be supplemented with iodine agents. Those for some unknown reasons may be given an appropriate amount of thyroid hormones replacement therapy, which can inhibit the excessive secretion of TSH from the pituitary and relieve the compensatory effects of TSH on producing hyperplasia and hypertrophy of thyroid gland.

(3) Other uses　In T_3 inhibition test for thyroid function, those whose iodine uptake percentage-decrease value are lower than 50% before medication can be diagnosed as a simple goiter; while the percentage-decrease value more than 50% can be diagnosed as hyperthyroidism. T_4 is also used to inhibit the proliferation of residual thyroid cancerous tissue and reduce the recurrence after thyroid cancer surgery.

1.5　Adverse reactions

Excessive thyroid hormones may lead to palpitation (心悸), fear of heat, sweating, hand tremor, insomnia and so on. In some serious cases, there are symptoms such as diarrhea, fast heart rate and irregular heartbeat, and even angina pectoris and myocardial infarction. Once the above symptoms occur, it should stop the drug immediately and use β receptor antagonist for symptomatic treatment, and then begin to continue treatment at a low dose of T_4 a week later.

2. Antithyroid drugs

Antithyroid drugs can interfere with the synthesis and release of thyroid hormones and treat hyperthyroidism. Antithyroid drugs include thioamides (硫脲类), iodine and iodide (碘和碘化物), radioactive iodine (放射性碘) and β receptor blockers.

Thioamides (硫脲类)

Common drugs used to treat hyperthyroid conditions are propylthiouracil (丙硫氧嘧啶), carbimazole (卡比马唑) and its active metabolite methimazole (甲巯咪唑).

【Pharmacokinetics】Thioamides can be quickly absorbed orally, the protein binding rates are about 75%, and can be widely distributed *in vivo* and easy to enter milk and pass through the placenta. Thioamides are mainly metabolized in the liver with an elimination half-life of 2 hours, and partially conjugated to glucuronic acid and excreted through the kidney. The half-life of methimazole is 6-13 hours. Carbimazole is a derivative of methimazole, and it does not work until it is converted to methimazole *in vivo*.

【Pharmacodynamics】

(1) Inhibition of the synthesis of thyroid hormones   Methimazole and propylthiouracil inhibit thyroid peroxidase (甲状腺过氧化物酶), and prevent oxidation of iodine, iodization and coupling of tyrosine in thyroid gland, so as to reduce the synthesis of thyroid hormones. However, they have no effect on the synthesized thyroid hormones. The symptoms of hyperthyroidism can be controlled after 2-3 weeks of treatment, and need 1-3 months of medication for the basal metabolic rate to return to normal.

(2) Inhibition of the conversion of T_4 to T_3 in peripheral tissues   Thioamides can quickly control the T_3 level in serum. Therefore, they are the preferred drugs in severe hyperthyroidism or thyroid crisis.

(3) Inhibition of immunity   At present, it is believed that the pathogenesis of hyperthyroidism is related to the abnormal autoimmune function, that is, the abnormal production of thyroid stimulating immunoglobulin (TSI). Thioamides can slightly inhibit the production of immunoglobulin. Therefore, they also have a certain therapeutic effect on the etiology of hyperthyroidism.

【Clinical indications】

(1) Treatments for hyperthyroidism (甲亢的治疗)   Thioamides are suitable for patients with mild illness, and those not suitable for surgery or use of radioactive iodine, such as children, adolescents and postoperative patients. If the dose of the drugs is appropriate, the symptoms of hyperthyroidism can be controlled within 1-2 months. Until the basal metabolic rate is close to normal level, the drug may be reduced to the maintenance dose, and the course of treatment takes 1-2 years.

(2) Preoperative preparation of hyperthyroidism (甲亢的术前准备)   Preoperative use of thioamides in patients with hyperthyroidism can make thyroid function close to normal, reduce surgical anesthesia and postoperative complications, and prevent the occurrence of thyroid crisis.

(3) Treatment of thyroid crisis (甲状腺危象的治疗)   Infection, trauma, surgery, emotional agitation and other inducing factors, can cause a prompt and massive release of thyroid hormones into the blood, which will lead to high fever, collapse, heart failure, pulmonary edema, electrolyte disorders and so on, some serious cases may lead to death, known as thyroid crisis. In addition, large doses of iodine and other treatment methods, and high-dose thioamides may be used as adjuvant therapy to block the synthesis of thyroid hormones.

【Adverse reactions】About 3%-12% of patients may experience adverse reactions. The occurrence risk of propylthiouracil and methimazole is less than that of carbimazole. The allergic reactions such as itching and drug eruptions are common in patients. The most severe adverse reaction is agranulocytosis, which usually occurs 2-3 months after treatment, and peripheral hemogram (外周血象) should be examined regularly during treatment.

If there is a sore throat or fever in patients, the drug should be stopped immediately. At the same time, attention should be paid to the difference between the low white blood cell counts caused by hyperthyroidism itself. A low white blood cell count indicates the presence of one or more serious health problems, such as hyperthyroidism, leukemia, aplastic anemia (再生障碍性贫血), or an infectious disease. In addition, long-term use of thioamides may decrease the level of blood thyroid hormones, which in turns stimulates hyperplasia of the glandular epithelium and enlargement of thyroid follicles due to the compensatory feedback increase of TSH. The drugs can pass easily through the placenta and into breast milk. Therefore, thioamides should be used cautiously in pregnant women, and should be prohibited in breast-feeding women and patients with nodular goiter complicated with hyperthyroidism and thyroid cancer.

Iodine (碘) and iodides (碘化物)

Potassium iodide (碘化钾) and compound iodine solution (复方碘溶液) are commonly used to treat certain thyroid conditions such as hypothyroidism and hyperthyroidism, and can also be used to prevent thyroid damage after a nuclear radiation emergency.

【Pharmacodynamics】Different doses of iodine and iodide have different effects on thyroid function. Low dose of iodine is involved in the synthesis of thyroid hormones, and used for the prevention of simple goiter. However, a large of dose of iodine produces antithyroid effects mainly by inhibiting proteolysis of thyroglobulin, makes T_3 and T_4 unable to dissociate from thyroglobulin and reduces the synthesis and release of TSH. High doses of iodine seem to have fast and strong effects on the thyroid gland.

The drugs often initiate pharmacological effects in 1-2 days, and reach the maximum effect in 10-15 days. Long-term use of iodine or iodide will inhibit the uptake of iodine of thyroid cells, decrease the concentration of intracellular iodide, and then may lose its antithyroid effect. So iodide cannot be used alone in the treatment of hyperthyroidism.

【Clinical indications】

(1) Prevention and treatment of iodine deficiency disorders　Supplementation of low dose of iodine can prevent and treat simple goiter and dementia caused by iodine deficiency.

(2) Preoperative preparation in hyperthyroidism　Generally, a large dose of iodine given two weeks before surgery can degenerate thyroid tissue, decrease the blood vessels and toughen the gland, which will help to reduce the bleeding after thyroid surgery.

(3) Treatment of thyroid crisis　Iodide added into 10% glucose solution by intravenous drip, or oral compound iodine solution can be used intermittently to treat thyroid crisis within two weeks, and thioamides should be used together.

【Adverse reactions】

(1) Allergic reaction　It can occur immediately or a few hours later, and the main manifestations are angioneurotic edema (血管神经性水肿), upper respiratory tract edema and severe laryngeal edema.

(2) Chronic iodine poisoning (慢性碘中毒)　The main manifestations are a metallic taste in the mouth, burning sensation in the throat, eye irritation and increased saliva secretion.

(3) Iodine-induced thyroid dysfunction (碘诱发的甲状腺功能紊乱)　Long-term use of iodide may induce hyperthyroidism. In addition, iodine can pass through the placenta and enter the breast milk and cause goiter in newborns and infants, so pregnant women and lactating women should use it with caution.

Radioactive iodine (放射性碘)

The radioactive iodine used in the clinic is ^{131}I, and its half-life is about 8 days. More than 99% of the drug ^{131}I can be eliminated within 56 days.

【Pharmacodynamics】 The thyroid gland has a strong ability to absorb iodine. ^{131}I can be absorbed and concentrated by the thyroid gland quickly and produce γ and β rays within the thyroid tissue. The β rays from ^{131}I (account for 99% of all rays) have a range of nearly 2 mm in the tissue, and the radiation damages are limited in the thyroid gland but rarely damages the surrounding tissues. The γ rays from ^{131}I can be determined *in vitro* and often used to examine the iodine uptake function of the thyroid gland.

【Clinical indications】

(1) **Treatment of hyperthyroidism**   It is used for those who are not suitable for surgery or recurrent patients after surgery, and those who are ineffective or allergic to thioamides. Generally, the drug will take effect after 1 month, and the thyroid function may return to normal after 4 months.

(2) **Thyroid function test**   Low dose of iodine is used to detect thyroid function.In patients with hyperthyroidism, the iodine uptake rate is high and the peak time of iodine uptake moves forward; on the contrary, the iodine uptake rate is low and the peak time of iodine uptake will delay.

【Adverse reactions】 The most common adverse reactions of radioactive iodine may seem ironic, and it may cause hypothyroidism, so the dose should be strictly controlled. The radioactive iodine often kills an excessive amount of thyroid cells, leaving the thyroid unable to produce enough hormones. Once hypothyroidism occurs, thyroid hormones T_3 or T_4 should be supplemented. ^{131}I may have carcinogenic effect in children, and is not suitable for patients under 20 years' old, pregnant women, lactating women and those with impaired renal function. In addition, patients with thyroid crisis, infiltrative exophthalmos (浸润性突眼) and iodine uptake dysfunction of thyroid are prohibited.

β receptor blockers

【Pharmacodynamics】 Propranolol and other β receptor blockers are adjuvant drugs for treatment of hyperthyroidism and thyroid crisis, and can also be used for preoperative thyroid preparation. In hyperthyroidism, the sensitivity of the body to catecholamine increases, leading to symptoms such as nervousness, impatience, tremor, fast heart rate, increased cardiac output and so on. The β receptor blockers not only inhibit the above sympathetic activation symptoms by blocking the receptors, but also reduce the secretion of thyroid hormones and inhibit the conversion of T_4 to T_3 in peripheral tissues.

【Clinical indications】 β receptor blockers are suitable for patients with hyperthyroidism who are not suitable for antithyroid drugs and ^{131}I treatment. Intravenous injection of β receptor blockers, especially the drugs with no intrinsic parasympathetic activity can help patients get through the critical period in case of thyroid crisis. The curative effects of β receptor blockers become quicker and more significant when in combination with thioamides. They can also be used before thyroid surgery, which can make the gland unable to enlarge and easy to be treated with surgery.

【Adverse reactions】 Attention should be paid to prevent the adverse reactions on tracheal smooth muscle and cardiovascular system, etc.

重 点 小 结

类别	药物	药理作用	临床应用	不良反应
甲状腺激素	三碘甲状腺原氨酸(T_3)和甲状腺素(T_4)	维持生长发育，促进代谢：促进物质氧化，增加耗氧量，提高基础代谢率；提高交感－肾上腺系统的敏感性	甲状腺功能低下，如克汀病；黏液性水肿；单纯性甲状腺肿；T_3抑制试验	过量甲状腺激素可引起甲亢症状，严重者可致腹泻、脉搏快而不规律、心绞痛和心肌梗死
抗甲状腺药	硫脲类	抑制甲状腺过氧化物酶，减少甲状腺激素合成；抑制外周组织T_4转化为T_3，控制T_3水平；抑制免疫	甲亢的治疗，甲亢术前准备，甲状腺危象的治疗	过敏反应，如瘙痒、药疹等；严重不良反应为粒细胞缺乏症，应定期检查血象
	碘和碘化物	小剂量碘参与甲状腺激素合成；大剂量碘抑制蛋白水解酶并能负反馈抑制TSH分泌，减少甲状腺激素的合成、释放	小剂量预防碘缺乏病；大剂量用于甲亢术前准备和甲状腺危象治疗	过敏反应，慢性碘中毒，可诱发甲状腺功能紊乱
	放射性碘(^{131}I)	^{131}I释放的β射线在组织内射程约2mm，能破坏甲状腺细胞，产生抗甲状腺作用；释放的γ射线用于甲状腺功能检查	甲亢的治疗；甲状腺功能检查	甲状腺功能减退；其放射性损伤对儿童可能有致癌作用
	β受体阻断药	阻断β受体，拮抗儿茶酚胺的作用，改善甲亢症状；还能抑制外周组织T_4脱碘变为T_3	配合硫脲类辅助治疗甲亢	心脏抑制，诱发支气管哮喘

目 标 检 测

题库

一、选择题

（一）单项选择题

1. 甲状腺激素主要用于（　　　）
   　　A. 甲亢危象　　　　　　　　　　B. 重症甲亢
   　　C. 甲状腺功能低下的替代治疗　　D. 糖尿病
   　　E. 甲状腺术前准备

2. 治疗克汀病的药物是（　　　）
   　　A. 甲硫氧嘧啶　　　　B. 甲巯咪唑　　　　C. 大剂量碘剂
   　　D. 甲状腺素片　　　　E. 放射性碘

3. 丙硫氧嘧啶治疗甲亢的主要作用机制是（　　　）
   　　A. 抑制甲状腺分泌　　　　　　　B. 抑制甲状腺摄碘
   　　C. 抑制甲状腺激素的生物合成　　D. 抑制甲状腺激素释放
   　　E. 破坏甲状腺组织

4. 不宜用作甲亢常规治疗的药物是（　　　　）

   A. 碘化物　　　　　　　　　B. 甲硫氧嘧啶　　　　　　C. 丙硫氧嘧啶

   D. 甲巯咪唑　　　　　　　　E. 卡比马唑

5. 具有治疗黏液性水肿作用的药物是（　　　　）

   A. 卡比马唑　　　　　　　　B. 甲巯咪唑　　　　　　　C. 丙硫氧嘧啶

   D. 甲状腺素片　　　　　　　E. 大剂量碘

（二）多项选择题

6. 硫脲类的主要不良反应包括（　　　　）

   A. 皮疹　　　　　　　　　　B. 粒细胞缺乏　　　　　　C. 甲状腺功能减退

   D. 高血压　　　　　　　　　E. 瘙痒

7. 关于 T_3 和 T_4 的描述，下列说法正确的是（　　　　）

   A. T_4 即甲状腺素

   B. T_3 即三碘甲状腺原氨酸

   C. T_4 比 T_3 作用慢，维持时间长

   D. T_4 可在外周组织脱碘转化为 T_3

   E. T_4 和 T_3 均通过亲和靶细胞上的甲状腺激素受体影响相关基因转录和蛋白表达发挥作用

二、思考题

从药理作用和临床应用角度比较各类抗甲状腺药的特点。

（陶小军）

Chapter 25 Adrenocortical hormones

 学习目标

1. **掌握** 糖皮质激素类药物的药理作用、临床应用和不良反应。
2. **熟悉** 糖皮质激素类药物的作用机制。
3. **了解** 促肾上腺皮质素及皮质激素抑制药的药理作用和临床应用。

1. Overview

The adrenal gland consists of the cortex and the medulla. The latter secretes epinephrine, while the former synthesizes and secretes adrenocortical hormones. The adrenal cortex is divided into three zones. The outer zona glomerulosa (球状带) synthesizes mineralocorticoids (盐皮质激素), which are responsible for water and salt metabolism. The middle zona fasciculate (束状带) secretes gulcocoricoids (糖皮质激素), which are involved with normal metabolism and resistance to stress. The inner reticularis (网状带) produces adrenal androgens. Secretion of adrenocorticosteroids is regulated by hypothalamic corticotropin-releasing hormone (CRH), and the following pituitary adrenocorticotropic hormone (ACTH). Adrenocorticosteroids serve as feedback inhibitors of CRH and ACTH secretion (Figure 25-1).

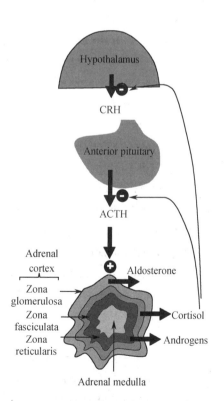

Figure 25-1 Regulation of corticosteroid secretion

2. Glucocorticoids

Glucocorticoids possess various actions, which are dependent on the dosage. In physiological states, the body secrets a small amount of glucocorticoids, which are essential for the carbohydrate, protein and lipid metabolism, and fluid and electrolyte balance. More glucocorticoids are secreted in stressful state to help the body to adapt to the strong stimulus. At high dose, glucocorticoids exert lots of pharmacological actions, except for the effects on metabolism, which are related to adverse reactions.

【Pharmacokinetics】Synthetic glucocorticoids preparations are well absorbed when administered orally, intravenously, intramuscularly, or topically. After absorption, greater with than 90% of cortisol in plasma is reversibly bound to protein under normal circumstances, either with corticosteroid-binding globulin (CBG), or with albumin. Only the fraction of corticosteroid that is unbound and active can be transfered into cells.

Corticosteroids are metabolized by the liver, and the metabolites are excreted by the kidney. The half-life of steroids may increase dramatically in patients with hepatic or renal dysfunction.

【Physiological functions】

(1) **Glucose metabolism** Glucocorticoids elevate blood glucose levels through promoting gluconeogenesis (糖异生) in the liver and skeletal muscle, decreasing utilization of glucose in the periphery, and slowing the decomposition of glucose. Due to the effects on glucose metabolism, glucocorticoids can worsen glycemic control in patients with overt diabetes and can precipitate the onset of hyperglycemia in susceptible patients.

(2) **Protein metabolism** They stimulate protein catabolism, thus providing the building block needed for glucose synthesis. The breakdown of protein in thymus, skeletal muscle, bone and other tissues increase excretion of nitrogen from urine, leading to negative nitrogen balance. High dose of glucocorticoids still inhibits anabolism of protein. Therefore, chronic administration of glucocorticoids is associated with muscle wasting, osteoporosis, skin thinning, and impaired wound healing.

(3) **Lipid metabolism** The lipolytic effect of glucocorticoids lead to an increase in free fatty acids levels. In pharmacological setting, corticosteroids result in dramatic redistribution of body fat, which is increased fat in the face (moon facies), back and neck (buffalo hump), and supraclavicular area, coupled with a loss of fat in the extremities.

(4) **Fluid and electrolyte balance** Aldosterone is by far the most potent endogenous corticosteroid with respect to fluid and electrolyte balance. Glucocorticoids also show weak effects on resorption of sodium and excretion of potassium by activating mineralcorticoids receptors. Other effects include antagonism of ADH (抗利尿激素), increase of glomerular filtration rate, decrease of absorption of calcium from intestine, inhibition of resorption of calcium from tubules, etc.

【General mechanisms of glucocorticoids】The lipid-soluble glucocorticoids diffuse across the cell membrane and bind to specific intracellular cytoplasmic glucocorticoid receptors (GR) in target tissues (Figure 25-2). The inactive GR is complexed with other proteins, including heat-shock protein

(HSP) 70 and HSP90. Steroid binding results in GR activation, dimerization (二聚体化) and translocation to the nucleus, where the hormone-receptor complex attaches to glucocorticosteroid response element (GRE) or negative GRE (nGRE), specific DNA sequences within the regulatory regions of affected genes. By binding with GRE or nGRE, the steroid-receptor complex acts as a transcription factor to initiate or inhibit transcription of a gene, thereby changing the levels and array of corresponding proteins. The genes that are responsive to glucocorticoids include lipocortin, COX-2, inducible nitric oxide synthase, inflammatory cytokines, adhesion molecules, and so on.

As a consequence of the time required to modulate gene expression and protein synthesis, most effects of corticosteroids are not immediate but become apparent after several hours, even several days. In addition, corticosteroids may exert some of their immediate effects by nongenomic mechanisms.

【Pharmacodynamics】

(1) **Anti-inflammatory actions** Glucocorticoids can dramatically reduce the inflammatory response induced by mechanical, physical, chemical, immunological and infectious factors. In the early stage of acute inflammation, glucocorticoids improve red, swelling, hot, pain and other symptoms by decreasing permeability of capillaries, reducing congestion and exudation, inhibiting leukocyte infiltration (浸润) and phagocytosis (吞噬反应), and abating the release of various inflammatory factors. In

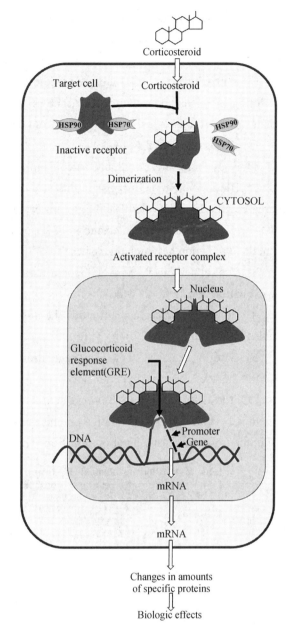

Figure 25-2　Possible mechanisms for glucocorticoids

the late stage of inflammation, glucocorticoids can inhibit the proliferation of capillaries and fibroblasts (成纤维细胞), and suppress formation of collagen and granulation, prevent adhesion and scar formation and alleviate sequelae. However, inflammatory reactions contribute to defense and repair of the body. So the anti-inflammatory actions of glucocorticoids may lead to diffusion of infection and delayed healing of wound.

(2) **Immunosuppressive and anti-allergic effects** (免疫抑制和抗过敏作用)　Glucocorticoids inhibit multiple steps of immunological reactions, including cellular and humoral immunity. The detailed mechanisms are complex and unclear, among which the suppression of peripheral lymphocytes and macrophages is known to play a role. In clinics, glucocorticoids are of great values in treating diseases that result from undesirable immune reactions. These diseases range from conditions that predominantly result from humoral immunity, such as urticaria (荨麻疹), to those that are mediated by cellular immune

mechanisms, such as transplantation rejection.

In addition, glucocorticoids interfere with mast cell degranulation (肥大细胞脱颗粒), lead to decreased release of histamine, serotonin and bradykinin. Thus the symptoms of allergic reactions are relieved.

(3) Anti-shock actions Glucocorticoids can be used in many types of serious shocks due to the inhibition of release of inflammatory factors, decrease of formation of myocardial depressant factor, enhancement of tolerance to endotoxins, and so on.

(4) Effects on other systems

1) Body temperature Glucocorticoids may lower body temperature quickly and strongly.

2) Blood system Glucocorticoids stimulate the hematopoietic function of bone marrow, thus increasing the blood levels of hemoglobin, erythrocytes, platelets, and polymorphonuclear leukocytes. The steroids cause decrease in eosinophils, basophils, monocytes and lymphocytes by redistributing them from the circulation to lymphoid tissues.

3) Central nervous system Glucocorticoids also excite central nervous system (CNS) and decrease the excitation threshold of CNS.

4) Bone Chronic glucocorticoids therapy can cause bone loss, myopathy and osteoporosis, even leading to bone fracture.

5) Cardiovascular system The regulation on fluid and electrolytes metabolism and lipolysis can lead to atherosclerosis and hypertension.

【Clinical indications】 Several semisynthetic derivatives of the glucocorticoids have been developed according to their relative potencies in sodium retention, effects on glucose metabolism, anti-inflammatory potency and duration of action. These are summarized in Table 25-1.

Table 25-1 Pharmacological effects and duration of action of representative corticosteroids

Agents		Potencies			Equivalent dose (mg)[a]	Half-life (min)	Duration of action (h)
		Sodium retention	Glucose metabolism	Anti-inflammation			
Short acting (8-12 hours)	Hydrocortisone (氢化可的松)	1.00	1.00	1.00	20.00	90	8-12
	Cortisone (可的松)	0.80	0.80	0.80	25.00	30	8-12
Intermediate acting (12-36 hours)	Prednisone (泼尼松)	0.80	4.00	3.50	5.00	60	12-36
	Prednisolone (泼尼松龙)	0.80	4.00	4.00	5.00	200	12-36
	Methylprednisolone (甲基泼尼松龙)	0.50	5.00	5.00	4.00	180	12-36
	Triamcinolone (曲安奈德)	0	5.00	5.00	4.00	>200	12-36
Long acting (36-72 hours)	Betamethasone (倍他米松)	0	20.00-30.00	25.00-35.00	0.60	100-300	36-54
	Dexamethasone (地塞米松)	0	20.00-30.00	30.00	0.75	100-300	36-54

Activities are all relative to that of hydrocortisone which is considered to be 1; a means the dose relationships apply only to oral or intravenous administration, as glucocorticoid potencies may differ greatly following intramuscular or intraarticular administration

(1) Severe infectious and inflammatory diseases　Although the use of glucocorticoids as anti-inflammatory agents does not address the underlying cause of the disease, the suppression of inflammation is of enormous clinical utility and has made these drugs among the most frequently prescribed agents.

　1) Severe and acute infections　The use of immunosuppressive glucocorticoids in infectious diseases may seem paradoxical. Therefore, glucocorticoids are only used for severe and acute infections, such as toxic bacillary dysentery (中毒性细菌性痢疾), toxic pneumonia (中毒性肺炎), fulminant epidemic meningitis (暴发性流行性脑膜炎), septicemia (败血症), etc. In these setting, sufficient and efficient antibacterial agents must be used in combination with glucocorticoids, the latter relieve inflammatory reactions, enhance the tolerance to toxins, thus lower the mortality. For infections induced by virus, the use of glucocorticoids is also limited, except for SARS and other serious ones.

　2) Chronic inflammation　Inflammations in important organs can lead to adhesion and scar, then severe dysfunction and scar contracture. Administration of glucocorticoids at the early stage is helpful for the prevention of sequelae in tuberculous meningitis (结核性脑膜炎), pericarditis (心包炎), encephalitis (脑炎), traumatic arthritis (损伤性关节炎), orchitis (睾丸炎), iritis (虹膜炎), keratitis (角膜炎), retinitis (视网膜炎), severe burn (烧伤), and so on.

(2) Immuno-related diseases

　1) Autoimmune diseases　Glucocorticoids are widely used for a variety of autoimmune diseases, such as severe rheumatic fever (严重风湿热), rheumatic myocarditis (风湿性心肌炎), rheumatoid arthritis (类风湿关节炎), systemic lupus erythematosus (系统性红斑狼疮), nephrotic syndrome (肾病综合征), and so on. In these situations, glucocorticoids are often used in combination with other regimens, which offer better long-term control than steroids alone.

　2) Allergies　The onset of action of glucocorticoids in allergic diseases is delayed, and patients with severe allergic reactions such as anaphylaxis require immediate therapy with epinephrine. Glucocorticoids are beneficial in the treatment of allergic diseases with limited duration, such as allergic rhinitis, serum sickness, urticaria, contact dermatitis, drug, serum and transfusion allergic reactions, and angioneurotic edema. For bronchial asthma, steroids are applied topically to the respiratory tract through inhalation in order to minimize systemic effects.

　3) Organ transplantation (器官移植)　Glucocorticoids can be used 1-2 days before organ transplantation to prevent graft rejection. High dose of steroids are used in combination with other immunosuppressive agents at the time of transplant surgery. Most patients are kept on a maintenance regimen that includes lower doses of glucocorticoids.

(3) Shock　For septic shock, high dose of glucocorticoids can be used early, in conjunction with efficient and sufficient antibacterial agents. The use of steroids should be terminated once microcirculation is improved and symptoms of shock are relieved. For anaphylactic shock (过敏性休克), glucocorticoids can be used in severe cases or those do not respond well to epinephrine. For other types of shock, steroids can be given besides regimens aimed at primary diseases.

(4) Hematopathy (血液病)　Glucocorticoids show efficacy for acute lymphocytic leukemia (急性淋巴细胞性白血病) in children. They are also available for aplastic anemia (再生障碍性贫血), granulocytopenia (粒细胞减少症), thrombocytopenia (血小板减少症), and allergic purpura (过敏性紫癜). Combined therapy is essential to decrease recurrence.

(5) Topical use (局部应用)　For eczema, anal pruritus, contact dermatitis, psoriasis, hydrocortisone and prednisolone are often applicated in the formation of ointment, cream or lotion. For strain of skeletal muscles, ligaments or joints, hydrocortisone or prednisone acetate can be injected intramuscularly, or into joint cavity to relieve the inflammatory symptoms. For the treatment of ocular or respiratory diseases, eyedrops or inhalants may be more suitable.

(6) Replacement therapy (替代疗法)   Low dose of glucocorticoids can be supplemented throughout the lifetime for patients with decreased or diminished secretion of steroids, such as primary adrenal insufficiency (原发性肾上腺皮质功能减退), Addison's diseases, hypofunction of anterior pituitary or hypothalamus, acute adrenal insufficiency, adrenalectomy (肾上腺切除术后), bilateral adrenal hemorrhage, neoplastic infiltration of the adrenal glands (肾上腺肿瘤), and so on.

【Adverse reactions】Generally, glucocorticoids are associated with various adverse reactions, which come from either prolonged use or abrupt cessation. As the duration of glucocorticoid therapy increases beyond 1 week, adverse reactions increase in a time-dependent and dose-dependent manner. Given the number and severity of potential side reactions, the decision to address glucocorticoids regimen always requires a careful consideration of the relative risks and benefits in each patient. After therapy is initiated, the minimal dose needed to achieve a given therapeutic effect must be determined by trial and error, and must be reevaluated periodically. Patients must be monitored carefully.

(1) Continued use of supraphysiological doses of glucocorticoid

1) Iatrogenic adrenal hyperfunction (医源性肾上腺皮质功能亢进)   Long and high dose of steroids administration may led to carbohydrate and lipid metabolism disorders, fluid and electrolyte abnormalities. The major manifestation include hyperglycemia, hypertension, atherosclerosis, centripetal distribution of body fat (脂肪向心性分布), puffy face (满月脸), buffalo back (水牛背), thin skin, increased body hair growth, edema (水肿), hypokalemia (低血钾), etc. These can be managed with insulin, hypoglycemic agents or antihypertensives. Diets with low proportion of glucose and salt, enough protein and calcium may be helpful.

2) Increased risk of infection (诱发感染)   Due to multiple effects to inhibit the immune system and the inflammatory response, glucocorticoid use is associated with an increased susceptibility to infection and a risk for reactivation of latent infections, especially in those with low immunity. In the presence of known infections, glucocorticoids should be administered only if absolutely necessary and concomitantly with appropriate and effective antimicrobial or antifungal therapy.

3) Possible risk of peptic ulcers   Because of the properties to stimulate secretion of gastric acid and pepsin, glucocorticoid may induce peptic ulcers, even leading to hemorrhage and perforation. It should be cautious for peptic ulcer formation in patients receiving corticosteroids therapy, especially if administered concomitantly with nonsteroidal anti-inflammatory drugs.

4) Osteoporosis (骨质疏松) and osteonecrosis (骨坏死)   Osteoporosis, a frequent serious complication of glucocorticoid therapy, occurs in patients of all ages, especially in children, elderly, and postmenopausal women. Patients may feel pain, and some will develop osteoporotic fractures. Glucocorticoids decrease bone density by multiple mechanisms, including inhibition of gastrointestinal absorption of Ca^{2+}, suppression of protein synthesis and promotion of protein decomposition, and inhibition of bone formation due to suppressive effects on osteoblasts and stimulation of resorption by osteoclasts. Calcium supplementation by diet and vitamin D intake of 800 IU/d are recommended to decrease the risk of osteroporosis. Osteonecrosis is also reported with glucocorticoid therapy. The femoral head is affected most frequently, with joint pain and stiffness as the earliest symptoms. Most affected patients ultimately require joint replacement. Although the risk increases with the duration and dose of glucocorticoid therapy, osteonecrosis also can occur when high doses of glucocorticoids are given for

short periods of time.

5) Cataracts (青光眼)　Increased frequency of cataract occurs with long-term and high dose of glucocorticoids therapy, with children particularly at risk. The cataracts may progress despite reduction or cessation of therapy. Patients on steroids regimen should receive examination of ocular pressure, fundus oculi and visual field to detect glucocorticoid-induced cataracts.

6) Muscular atrophy (肌肉萎缩), impaired wound healing (伤口愈合延缓), decreased growth in children (儿童生长发育迟缓)　These are related with the increase of protein catabolism, and decrease of protein synthesis. The inhibition of formation of granulation tissues accounts for impaired wound healing. Growth retardation in children can result from administration of relatively small doses of glucocorticoids, which can be restored by growth hormone.

7) Emotional disturbances (精神障碍)　These include nervousness, insomnia, changes in mood or psyche, and overt psychosis. Therefore, steroids should be contraindicated or used cautiously in patients with previous psychiatric illness or epilepsy.

(2) Withdrawal reactions (停药反应)

1) Iatrogenic adrenal insufficiency (医源性肾上腺皮质功能不全)　This is the most severe complication of steroid cessation. With HPA axis being suppressed by prolonged therapy, overly rapid withdrawal of corticosteroids causes acute adrenal insufficiency which can even be lethal. Many patients recover from glucocorticoid-induced HPA suppression within several weeks to months; in some individuals the time can be a year or longer. Therefore, to lower the risk of iatrogenic acute adrenal insufficiency, protocols for discontinuing corticosteroid therapy in patients receiving long-term treatment with corticosteroids have been proposed. The dose must be tapered according to the individual, possible through trial and error. Generally, it takes several months to two years to terminate the use of corticosteroids gradually. During this period, supplementation of sufficient steroids is essential in case of infection, operation, trauma and other stressful settings. Continual use of ACTH for 7 days after cessation of corticosteroids is also helpful.

2) Exacerbation of the diseases or flare-up of the underlying disease　Abrupt withdrawal of corticosteroids may also lead to aggravation of primary diseases. Then high dose of steroids is needed for the retreatment until most of the symptoms are alleviated. So the gradual withdrawal is crucial.

【Contraindications】Glucocorticoids should be contraindicated in patients with active peptic ulcer (活动性消化性溃疡), bone fracture, corneal ulcer (角膜溃疡), hypercorticism (肾上腺皮质功能亢进), severe hypertension, diabetes, severe psychosis or epilepsy, and infections induced by varicella, measles, fungal that cannot be treated with antibacterial agents.

3. Mineralocorticoids

The common mineralocorticoids include aldosterone (醛固酮) and desoxycorticosterone (去氧皮质酮). The major function for mineralocorticoids is to maintain the fluid and electrocyte balance, especially sodium and potassium.

【Pharmacodynamics】Mineralocorticoids act on the distal tubules and collecting ducts of the kidney to enhance reabsorption of sodium, bicarbonate, and water from the tubular fluid. Conversely, mineralocorticoids decrease reabsorption of potassium, which, with H^+, is then lost in the urine. Enhancement of sodium reabsorption and potassium excretion by aldosterone also occurs in gastrointestinal mucosa, skeletal muscle, sweat and salivary glands.

The detailed mechanism is that aldosterone binds with the specific receptor in the epithelial cells of distal convoluted tubules, translocates into nucleus, and promotes the transcription of the target mRNA. Then the expression of aldosterone induced protein increase, which enhances the activity of sodium channel in epithelial cells, leading to increased number and frequency for the opening of sodium channel and increased resorption of sodium.

Elevated aldosterone levels may cause alkalosis and hypokalemia, whereas retention of sodium and water leads to an increase in blood volume and blood pressure, and edema. Hyperaldosteronism is treated with spironolactone (螺内酯). On the contrary, deficiency of mineralocorticoid is especially predisposed to Na^+ loss and volume depletion through excessive sweating in hot environments, leading to hypotension and vascular collapse.

【Clinical Indications】Mineralocorticoid is administered for chronic adrenal insufficiency in combination with hydrocortisone. In this situation, supplementation of 6-10g salt each day is essential.

4. Corticotropin

Corticotropin (adrenocorticotropin, ACTH) is synthesized and secreted by the anterior pituitary, and regulated by CRH released from hippocampus. The major function of ACTH is to maintain the normal structure and function of adrenal gland. Lack of ACTH leads to decreased or diminished secretion of corticosteroids, even atrophy of adrenal cortex. The ACTH of synthetic origin can only be administered intravenously. The adrenal cortex initiates secretion 2 hours after injection. ACTH can be used to detect the responsiveness of adrenal gland to pituitary, and to promote the functional recovery of adrenal cortex in termination of corticosteroids.

5. Inhibitors of biosynthesie or function of adrenocortcoids

Hypercortisolism is most frequently caused by pituitary adenomas that overproduce ACTH (Cushing's disease) or by adrenocortical tumors or bilateral hyperplasias that overproduce cortisol (Cushing's syndrome). Although surgery is the treatment of choice, it is not always effective, and adjuvant therapy with inhibitors of steroidogenesis becomes necessary. In these settings, ketoconazole, metyrapone, etomidate, and mitotane are clinically useful. Sometimes they can even replace the partial adrenalectomy. All of these agents possess the common risk of precipitating acute adrenal insufficiency; thus, they must be used in appropriate doses, and the status of the patient's HPA axis must be carefully monitored. Agents that act as glucocorticoid receptor antagonists (antiglucocorticoids) show similar pharmacological effects. Mineralocorticoid antagonists are discussed in the other chapter.

Mitotane (米托坦)

Mitotane selectively impairs cells in the zona fasciculate and reticularis of adrenal cortex, including normal cells and those from adenomas. The atrophy and necrosis of these cells result in decreased secretion of glucocorticoids, but not mineralcorticoids. It is used to treat inoperable adrenocortical carcinoma, recurrent tumor after surgery and postoperative tumor as an adjunctive approach. GI disturbances, inhibition of CNS and ataxia are the major toxicities.

Metyrapone (美替拉酮)

Metyrapone is a relatively selective inhibitor of 11β-hydroxylase, which converts 11-deoxycortisol to cortisol, and 11-deoxyhydrocortisone to hydrocortisone in the glucocorticoid biosynthesis. Thus the level of plasma cortisol and hydrocortisone are decreased. Metyrapone has been used to treat the hypercorticism resulting from either adrenal neoplasms or tumors producing ACTH ectopically. Chronic administration of metyrapone can cause hirsutism, hypertension, nausea, headache, sedation, and rash.

Ketoconazole (酮康唑)

Ketoconazole, an antifungal agent, strongly inhibits adrenal and gonadal steroidogenesis, primarily because of its inhibition of the activity of 17α-hydroxylase. Ketoconazole is the best tolerated and most effective inhibitor of steroid hormone biosynthesis in patients with hypercortisolism. Cushing's syndrome and prostatic carcinoma are the major indications of ketoconazole. Side effects include hepatic dysfunction, which ranges from asymptomatic elevations of transaminase levels to severe hepatic injury.

Antiglucocorticoids

Mifepristone (米非司酮), a progesterone receptor antagonist, also inhibits the GR at higher dose, blocking feedback regulation of the HPA axis and secondarily increasing endogenous ACTH and cortisol levels. This agent has been studied as a potential therapeutic agent in a small number of patients with hypercortisolism (皮质醇增多症). It is considered investigational and is restricted to patients with inoperable causes of cortisol excess that have not responded to other agents.

重 点 小 结

药物	药理作用	临床应用	不良反应
糖皮质激素类药物	①调控物质代谢。②抗炎。③免疫抑制。④抗过敏。⑤抗休克。⑥刺激骨髓造血。⑦降低体温。⑧提高中枢兴奋性。	①替代疗法。②严重感染或炎症，防止炎症后遗症，局部应用。③自身免疫性疾病、器官移植排斥反应。④过敏反应。⑤多种类型休克。⑥血液病。⑦发热	①医源性肾上腺皮质功能亢进。②诱发或加重感染。③诱发癫痫或精神病发作。④骨质疏松。⑤心血管系统并发症。⑥消化系统并发症。⑦医源性肾上腺皮质功能不全、反跳现象

题库

目 标 检 测

一、选择题

（一）单项选择题

1. 糖皮质激素适用于下列哪种疾病的治疗（　　）
   A. 原因不明的高热 　　　　B. 风湿性心肌炎 　　　　C. 支气管哮喘
   D. 角膜溃疡 　　　　　　　E. 骨折

2. 肾上腺皮质激素诱发和加重感染的主要原因是（　　）
   A. 抑制 ACTH 的释放
   B. 促使多种病原微生物繁殖
   C. 用量不足，无法控制症状
   D. 患者对激素不敏感而未出现相应的疗效
   E. 抑制炎症反应和免疫反应，降低机体的防御功能

3. 糖皮质激素可引起除下列哪一种外的病症（　　）
   A. 精神病 　　　　　　　　B. 风湿病 　　　　　　　C. 高血糖
   D. 骨质疏松 　　　　　　　E. 低血钾

4. 糖皮质激素的停药反应是（　　）
   A. 严重精神障碍 　　　　　B. 消化道溃疡 　　　　　C. 骨质疏松
   D. 医源性肾上腺皮质功能不全 　E. 糖尿病

5. 长期应用糖皮质激素可引起（　　）
   A. 高血钙 　　　　　　　　B. 低血钾 　　　　　　　C. 高血钾
   D. 高血磷 　　　　　　　　E. 钙、磷排泄减少

6. 糖皮质激素用于严重感染的目的在于（　　）
   A. 加强抗菌药的抗菌作用
   B. 提高机体抗病毒能力
   C. 抗炎、抗毒、抗过敏、抗休克
   D. 加强心肌收缩力，改善微循环
   E. 提高机体免疫力

7. 糖皮质激素用于慢性炎症的目的在于（　　）
   A. 具有强大的抗炎作用，促进炎症消散
   B. 抑制肉芽组织生长，防止粘连和疤痕
   C. 促进炎症区血管收缩，降低其通透性
   D. 稳定溶酶体膜，减少蛋白水解酶的释放
   E. 抑制花生四烯酸释放，使炎症介质 PG 合成减少

（二）多项选择题

8. 糖皮质激素类药物促进蛋白分解，可引起（　　）
   A. 胃、十二指肠溃疡 　　　B. 肌肉萎缩 　　　　　　C. 伤口愈合迟缓
   D. 骨质疏松 　　　　　　　E. 水肿

医药大学堂
WWW.YIYAODXT.COM

9. 长期使用糖皮质激素突然停药可引起（　　　）

　　A. 肾上腺皮质萎缩或功能不全　　　B. 应激状态下易发生肾上腺危象

　　C. 原病恶化　　　　　　　　　　　D. 原病复发

　　E. 感染扩散

二、思考题

长期使用糖皮质激素进行治疗的患者在饮食上应当注意什么？

（王芙蓉）

Chapter 26　Estrogens and androgens

学习目标

1. **掌握** 雌激素类和雄激素类药物的药理作用、临床应用及不良反应。
2. **熟悉** 孕激素类药物的药理作用、作用特点及临床应用。
3. **了解** 同化激素的作用；氯米芬、他莫昔芬的药理作用及临床应用。

Sex hormones, also known as sex steroids, are critical regulators produced in the body, mainly affecting the growth or function of the reproductive organs or sexual features. Natural sex steroids made by the gonads include the estrogens (雌激素), progestogens (孕激素), and androgens (雄激素) in females and males, summarized in Figure 26-1. They can activate their corresponding receptors. The two main classes of sex steroids are androgens and estrogens.

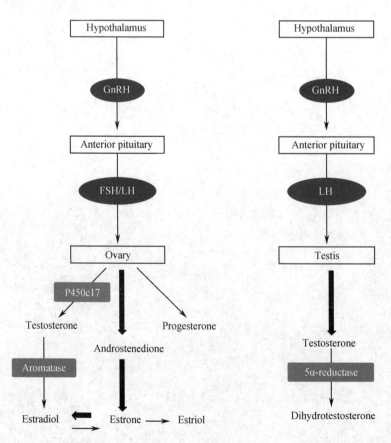

Figure 26-1　The representative sex hormones in females (left) and males (right)

1. Estrogens

Estrogens interact with estrogen receptor. Estrogenic activity is shared by a great number of chemical substances. The major estrogen secreted by the ovary in women is estradiol. It belongs to natural estrogens. Most estriol (雌三醇) and estrone (雌酮) are natural estrogens from oxidized estradiol in liver or in peripheral tissues from androstenedione and other androgens, and some estrone is produced in the ovary. Natural estrogens are inactive orally and are metabolized rapidly in liver. Synthetic estrogens include steroidal and nonsteroidal compounds, such as quinestrol (炔雌醚), ethinylestradiol (炔雌醇), and diethylstilbestrol (己烯雌酚). The most important effect of these alterations has been to improve their oral effectiveness.

【Pharmacokinetics】Natural estrogens are inactive by the oral route because of rapid metabolism in liver. Estradiol is the most potent natural estrogen. Significant amounts of estrogens and their active metabolites are excreted in the bile and reabsorbed from the intestine. Orally administered estrogens will have a high ratio of hepatic to peripheral effects. The hepatic effects of estrogen can be minimized by routes that avoid first-pass liver exposure. Synthetic estrogens, especially ethinylestradiol, are metabolized very slowly and active through oral administration.

【Pharmacodynamics】

(1) **Female reproductive system**　In females, estrogens are important for normal reproductive development. Estrogens induce the growth of uterus (子宫), fallopian tubes (输卵管), vagina (阴道) and mammary glands. Precisely, estrogens stimulate the development of the endometrium (子宫内膜) and the muscles in uterus. In the fallopian tubes, estrogens stimulate the development of a thick muscular wall. Additionally, estrogens stimulate the vaginal epithelium to get thickened, stratified and cornified. In the breasts, estrogens are responsible for controlling lactation (泌乳) and other changes during adolescence (青春期) and pregnancy. Estrogens are responsible for the appearance of secondary sexual characteristics and additional estrogen administration suppresses pituitary-gonadal secretion.

(2) **Metabolic effects**　Estrogens have many metabolic effects. Estrogens can cause mild salt and water retention (水钠潴留). Estrogens are instrumental in bone formation, promoting positive calcium balance with vitamin D, calcium and other hormones, and help to preserve bone strength and prevent bone loss. Also, estrogens decrease low-density lipoprotein (LDL) cholesterol and increase high-density lipoprotein (HDL) cholesterol. Estrogens impair glucose tolerance. Estrogens increase circulating clotting factors (凝血因子) II, VII, IX, and X, resulting in enhancing the coagulability of blood.

(3) **Other effects**　Estrogens could induce the synthesis of progesterone receptors. Administration of estrogens stimulates central components of the stress system, such as corticotropin-releasing hormone, promoting a sense of well-being to estrogen-deficient women. Estrogens also modulate sympathetic nervous system control of smooth muscle function.

【Clinical indications】

(1) **Hormone replacement therapy**　Estrogens can be used for the treatment of symptoms of menopause (绝经期). Females at menopause stage suffer from a number of physical, psychological and

emotional consequences. Estrogens may help relieve symptoms, such as hot flashes, mood swings and sleep disorders. The combination of androgens and estrogens is highly effective in perimenopausal syndrome (围绝经期综合征) and osteoporosis (骨质疏松症).

(2) Hypogonadism Estrogens can be used in the treatment of estrogen-deficient young females. Hypogonadism is characterized by diminished function of the gonads and delayed growth of secondary sex characteristics. Estrogens can stimulate the development of secondary sexual characteristics. Treatment attempts to mimic the physiology of puberty (青春期). It is initiated with small doses of estrogen and is slowly increased to adult doses and then maintained until the age of menopause.

(3) Other uses Additional estrogens can reduce lactation when an infant is no longer breast-feeding. Estrogens can be used for hemostasis and regulating bleeding cycle in dysfunctional uterine bleeding. Estrogens combined with progestogens can prevent ovulation (排卵). High-dose estrogens are effective for the treatment of advanced breast cancer (晚期乳腺癌). Estrogens can counteract the effects of androgens in the body, thereby decreasing acnes. Also, estrogens is the most commonly used for the management of advanced prostatic carcinoma.

【Adverse reactions】Estrogen therapy may result in a number of common symptoms, such as nausea (恶心), bloating and vomiting. Estrogen therapy is a major cause of postmenopausal uterine bleeding. Long-term estrogen therapy can increase the risk of endometrial carcinoma. Moreover, a small increase in the incidence of breast cancer may occur with prolonged therapy. Estrogen therapy may also cause hypertension.

2. Antiestrogens

These drugs have estrogen antagonist effects.

Clomifene (氯米芬)

Clomifene is a nonsteroidal triphenylethylene derivative, acting as a selective estrogen receptor modulator. Clomifene exerts the antiestrogenic effect in the uterus. It is mainly used for infertility (不育) through inducing ovulation. Clomifene blocks estrogen receptors, resulting in the increase of gonadotropins stimulating ovulation. Clomifene may cause reversible ovarian enlargement as one of the common adverse reactions.

Tamoxifen (他莫昔芬)

Tamoxifen is a nonsteroidal selective estrogen receptor modulator in the triphenylethylene family. Tamoxifen acts as a potent estrogen antagonist in breast and is mainly used for the treatment of estrogen receptor-positive breast cancer in postmenopausal women. Interestingly, tamoxifen exerts agonist on bone, preventing osteoporosis in postmenopausal women. It can also be used for the prevention of breast cancer. Common adverse reactions include hot flushes and vomiting.

3. Progestogens

Progestogens are a class of steroid hormones interacting with the progesterone receptor. Progesterone is a naturally steroid involved in the menstrual cycle, pregnancy, and embryogenesis of humans and other species. It also serves as a precursor to the estrogens, androgens, and adrenocortical steroids. A variety of progestational compounds have been synthesized, and all of them differ from progesterone in one or more respects. Synthetic progestogens include megestrol (甲地孕酮), norethisterone (炔诺酮) and norgestrel (炔诺孕酮). Progestins are synthetic forms of progesterone, causing progesterone-like effects.

【Pharmacokinetics】Progesterone is rapidly absorbed following administration by any route. Especially, progesterone is inactive orally, because it is almost completely metabolized in liver. It is most effective injected intramuscularly or administered sublingually. It is excreted in the urine. Most of the synthetic progestins are orally active and metabolized slowly. They are extensively metabolized to inactive products that are excreted mainly in the urine.

【Pharmacodynamics】Progesterone induces secretory changes in the endometrium, prepares the uterus for nidation (着床) and maintains pregnancy. Progesterone stops muscular contractions in the fallopian tubes once the egg has been transported. Progesterone can also stimulate acini proliferation in the mammary glands. Progesterone can compete with aldosterone for the mineralocorticoid receptor, leading to an increased secretion of aldosterone by the adrenal cortex. Progesterone decreases the plasma levels of many amino acids, leading to increased urinary nitrogen excretion. Progesterone can also cause a slight rise in body temperature during the luteal phase.

【Clinical indications】

(1) **Dysfunctional uterine bleeding**　A progestin in relatively large doses stops bleeding.

(2) **Endometriosis (子宫内膜异位症)**　Continuous administration of progestin induces an anovulatory state, treating the chronic pelvic pain and preventing bleeding in the ectopic sites.

(3) **Birth control**　Progestin can be used with estrogens to prevent pregnancy through the inhibition of ovulation. Chronic use of combination agents depresses ovarian function.

(4) **Habitual abortion (习惯性流产)**　Progestin therapy may be applied in patients with progesterone deficiency.

(5) **Endometrial cancer**　Progestins can prevent the endometrium from building up too much and becoming cancerous.

【Adverse reactions】Adverse reactions include breast engorgement (肿胀), headache, and mood swings. Continuous administration can cause irregular bleeding. Large dosage given in early pregnancy can cause masculinization (男性化).

4. Androgens

Testosterone is a potent androgen secreted by the testis. In men, approximately 8mg of testosterone is produced daily. The testis also secretes small amounts of another potent androgen, dihydrotestosterone (双氢睾酮), and other weak androgens, namely, androstenedione (雄烯二酮) and dehydroepiandrosterone (普拉睾酮). Methyltestosterone (甲睾酮) and testosterone propionate (丙酸睾酮) are derivatives of testosterone. Some synthetic androgens with higher anabolic (同化) activity and lower androgenic activity are called as anabolic steroids (同化激素). These drugs include nandrolone phenylpropionate (苯丙酸诺龙), stanozolol (司坦唑醇) and methandienone (美雄酮). Androgens enter cells and bind to cytosolic androgen receptors.

【Pharmacokinetics】In many target tissues, testosterone is converted to dihydrotestosterone by 5α-reductase. Small quantities of estradiol can be produced from testosterone by P450 aromatase. Testosterone is inactive orally because of rapid metabolism in liver. It is excreted in urine. Methyltestosterone has a longer duration of action.

【Pharmacodynamics】Testosterone is necessary for normal development of the male fetus and is responsible for the appearance of secondary sexual characteristics. These include growth of facial and body hair, deepening of the voice, development of the prostate and seminal vesicles, and prominent musculature. Testosterone promotes anabolic actions, stimulating rapid bone and skeletal muscles growth. Testosterone accelerates erythropoiesis (红细胞生成). In women, the administration of androgens sometimes reduces the excretion of nitrogen into the urine, indicating an increase in protein synthesis or a decrease in protein breakdown within the body.

【Clinical indications】

(1) **Testicular failure (睾丸功能不全)**　The primary clinical use of the androgens is for replacement therapy (替代疗法) in hypogonadism of male patients, improving secondary sex characteristics.

(2) **Aplastic anemias (再生障碍性贫血)**　Androgens, including methyltestosterone and testosterone propionate, can stimulate red blood cell production to treat certain anemias.

(3) **Dysfunctional uterine bleeding**　Androgens can affect the effect of estrogens, resulting in the bleeding stop.

(4) **Advanced breast cancer**　Androgens can interfere with the effect of estrogens, resulting in improving symptoms of some patients.

(5) **Osteoporosis**　Anabolic steroids have proportionately greater anabolic effects, promoting rapid growth of bone.

(6) **Use as protein anabolic agents**　Androgens and anabolic steroids have been used in conjunction with dietary measures and exercises in an attempt to reverse protein loss after trauma, surgery, or prolonged immobilization and in patients with debilitating diseases.

(7) **Use as growth stimulators**　Androgens can be used to stimulate growth in boys with delayed puberty.

【Adverse reactions】Androgens should not be used in infants. Replacement therapy in men may cause acne, sleep apnea, and erythrocytosis (红细胞增多症). Virilization in women and increased libido in men are predictable effects. Long term usage may cause hepatic damage.

重 点 小 结

类别	药物	药理作用	临床应用	不良反应
雌激素类	雌二醇、雌酮、雌三醇、炔雌醚、炔雌醇、己烯雌酚	激动雌激素受体：促女性性器官发育成熟，维持第二性征；形成月经周期；调节排卵、乳腺发育、乳汁分泌	围绝经期综合征、骨质疏松、性腺功能低下、功能性子宫出血、回乳、乳腺癌、避孕等	恶心、呕吐、子宫出血、提高子宫内膜癌发生率、高血压等
抗雌激素类	氯米芬、他莫昔芬	竞争性拮抗雌激素受体：抑制或减弱雌激素作用	不孕、晚期乳腺癌、抗骨质疏松等	卵巢肥大等
孕激素类	黄体酮、甲地孕酮、炔诺酮、炔诺孕酮	激动孕激素受体：助孕、安胎、促进乳腺发育等	功能性子宫出血、子宫内膜异位症、习惯性流产、避孕、抗子宫内膜癌等	乳房肿胀、头痛、女性胎儿男性化等
雄激素类和同化激素类	睾酮、甲睾酮、丙酸睾酮、苯丙酸诺龙、司坦唑醇、美雄酮	激动雄激素受体：促男性性器官发育成熟，维持第二性征；促进蛋白质合成；刺激骨髓造血功能	替代疗法、功能性子宫出血、晚期乳腺癌、再生障碍性贫血等	女性男性化、男性女性化等

目 标 检 测

题库

一、单项选择题

1. 由卵巢成熟滤泡分泌的雌激素是（　　　）
    A. 甲地孕酮 　　　　　　B. 炔诺酮 　　　　　　C. 炔雌醇
    D. 雌二醇 　　　　　　　E. 丙酸睾酮

2. 以下属于抗雌激素类药的是（　　　）
    A. 氯米芬 　　　　　　　B. 前列腺素 　　　　　C. 苯乙酸睾酮
    D. 己烯雌酚 　　　　　　E. 苯丙酸诺龙

3. 孕激素类药常用于（　　　）
    A. 晚期乳腺癌 　　　　　B. 习惯性流产 　　　　C. 回乳
    D. 睾丸功能发育不全 　　E. 乳房胀痛

4. 治疗再生障碍性贫血宜选用（　　　）
    A. 黄体酮 　　　　　　　B. 丙酸睾酮 　　　　　C. 炔诺孕酮
    D. 他莫昔芬 　　　　　　E. 雌三醇

二、多项选择题

5. 同化激素包括（　　　）

　　A. 苯丙酸诺龙　　　　　　　B. 美雄酮　　　　　　　　C. 司坦唑醇

　　D. 炔诺酮　　　　　　　　　E. 睾酮

（彭　芙）

Chapter 27　Drugs affecting the respiratory system

PPT

The common symptoms of respiratory diseases include wheezing, coughing, expectoration (咳痰) and respiratory failure. Antiasthmatic drugs (平喘药), antitussives (镇咳药) and expectorants (祛痰药) can relieve the corresponding symptoms and effectively prevent the complications occurring.

1. Antiasthmatic drugs

Bronchial asthma (支气管哮喘) is a chronic inflammatory disease of the airways characterized by recurrent wheezing and shortness of breath and a variable degree of airway obstruction. The pathological changes of asthma include chronic bronchitis mainly dominated by eosinophil infiltration, reversible airway obstruction, airway hyperreactivity (气道高反应性) and bronchial remodeling. The pathophysiology of asthma involves inflammation, allergy, disorders in neuroregulation, heredity, drugs, environment, psychological factors, etc.

Antiasthmatic drugs refer to a class of drugs that can alleviate or prevent asthma attacks, which include bronchodilators (支气管扩张药), anti-inflammatory drugs for asthma (抗炎平喘药), and anti-allergic drugs for asthma (抗过敏平喘药).

1.1　Bronchodilators

Bronchodilators relax the bronchi, reduce respiratory resistance and relieve asthma. The drugs include β adrenoceptor agonists, methylxanthines and muscarinic receptor antagonists.

1.1.1　β adrenoceptor agonists

The β receptor agonists include selective and non-selective β_2 receptor agonists, which are important

医药大学堂
WWW.YIYAODXT.COM

in the treatment of asthma. The non-selective β receptor agonists have strong cardiovascular adverse reactions, such as isoproterenol (异丙肾上腺素) and epinephrine, which are now rarely used for asthma. However the selective β_2 agonists such as salbutamol (沙丁胺醇), have less adverse reactions and are the first choice for asthma control.

Other β_2 agonists such as terbutaline (特布他林), which are often used orally or inhaled, and subcutaneous injection can be used to control the acute attack of asthma. A small amount of clenbuterol (克伦特罗) can produce significant antiasthmatic effect, and the adverse reactions are mild. Formoterol (福莫特罗) and salmeterol (沙美特罗) are long-acting selective β_2 agonists with strong and long-lasting effects, and the effects can last for 12 hours after a single dose.

【Pharmacodynamics】The β receptor agonists relax bronchial muscle and enlarge airway caliber by the activation of β receptors in bronchial smooth muscle cells, stimulate adenylate cyclase (腺苷酸环化酶) and increase the formation of intracellular cyclic adenosine monophosphate (cAMP), which activate cAMP-dependent protease and reduce intracellular Ca^{2+} concentration. The β_2 agonists have very high selectivity for β_2 receptors in respiratory smooth muscle, and their effects on β_2 receptors in bronchial smooth muscle are much greater than the β_1 receptors in heart, so the cardiac excitability of β_2 agonists is lower than β receptor agonists.

【Clinical indications】Selective β_2 receptor agonists such as salbutamol are used to control frequent or chronic asthma symptoms. After inhaling salbutamol, it can directly act on bronchial smooth muscle and quickly control the symptoms of asthma.

【Adverse reactions】There are few adverse reactions in general treatment, and sinus tachycardia and muscle tremor may be seen occasionally.

1.1.2　Methylxanthines

Methylxanthines are the second type of bronchodilators that have direct relaxation effect on airway smooth muscle. The commonly used methylxanthines are aminophylline (氨茶碱), cholinophylline (胆茶碱) and diprophylline (二羟丙茶碱).

【Pharmacokinetics】The gastrointestinal absorption of methylxanthines is rapid and complete, with the mean peak time of 3 hours, and the therapeutic blood concentration of 10-20μg/ml. The half-life of methylxanthines is about 6 hours for adults and 3.7 hours for children. About 90% of methylxanthines are metabolized in the liver by demethylation and oxidation reaction, and 10% of the drugs are excreted from urine in their original form.

【Pharmacodynamics】

(1) Relaxation of bronchial smooth muscle phosphodiesterase (扩张支气管平滑肌)　Aminophyllines increase the production of cAMP by inhibition of phosphodiesterase (磷酸二酯酶), the enzyme that can catalyze the decomposition of cAMP in bronchial smooth muscle cells and relax the smooth muscle. By promoting endogenous release of epinephrine, aminophyllines also act on β_2 receptors and relax the bronchial smooth muscle, and inhibit the bronchial contraction induced by endogenous adenosine by blocking adenosine receptors.

(2) Anti-inflammatory effect　Long-term uses of low-dose aminophyllines inhibit airway responsiveness and inflammation.

(3) Enhancement the contractile force of respiratory muscles　Aminophyllines increase the contraction of septum muscle and prevent respiratory muscle fatigue caused by respiratory tract obstruction.

【Clinical indications】

(1) Bronchial asthma　Aminophyllines are mainly used in the maintenance treatment of chronic asthma to prevent acute attack. Aminophyllines are often used for intravenous injection in patients whose asthma cannot be controlled by β₂ receptor agonists alone.

(2) Chronic obstructive pulmonary disease   Aminophyllines can significantly relieve the symptoms in patients with shortness of breath.

(3) Central sleep apnea syndrome (CSA,中枢性呼吸睡眠暂停综合征)   CSA is a sleep-related disorder in which the breathing repeatedly stops and starts during sleep, typically for 10 to 30 seconds either intermittently or in cycles, and is usually associated with the reduction in blood oxygen saturation. Aminophyllines belong to a group of drugs known as bronchodilators, which relax the muscles in the bronchial tubes of the lungs and are beneficial to treat CSA.

【Adverse reactions】 The safe dose ranges of aminophyllines are narrow and there are many adverse reactions. The common adverse reactions of aminophyllines are nausea, vomiting, loss of appetite and other gastrointestinal reactions, as well as restlessness, insomnia, irritability and other central symptoms. Rapid intravenous injection of aminophyllines may cause tachycardia (心动过速), arrhythmia, a sudden drop in blood pressure, delirium, convulsions, coma, and even respiratory depression and cardiac arrest (心脏骤停). Therefore, intravenous injection of aminophyllines should be fully diluted and injected slowly. In addition, strict control of the dose is still a basic measure to avoid the toxic reactions.

1.1.3   Inhaled anticholinergic drugs(吸入性抗胆碱药)

There are three M receptors in respiratory tract, M₁, M₂ and M₃ receptors. Atropine is a non-selective M receptor blocker, which not only acts on all M receptor subtypes in the airway, but also blocks the M receptors in the whole body. Therefore, atropine has many side effects and cannot be used in the treatment of asthma.

However, non-selective M receptor blockers, ipratropium bromide (异丙托溴铵) and oxitropium bromide (氧托溴铵) inhalation have selective dilation effect on the bronchial smooth muscles, and can be used in those who are resistant to β₂ receptor agonists, especially in the elderly. In addition, tiotropium bromide (噻托溴铵), a long-acting selective M₁ and M₃ receptor blocker, has strong antiasthmatic effects with few adverse reactions. The half-life of tiotropium bromide is about 5 days and the therapeutic effects can last for 24 hours.

1.2   Anti-inflammatory antiasthmatic drugs

The anti-inflammatory antiasthmatic drugs represented by glucocorticoids (糖皮质激素) can inhibit the production of airway inflammatory mediators and the inflammatory response, and have become first-line drugs for their effects of long-term prevention and treatment of asthma attack. Glucocorticoids are strong anti-inflammatory drugs with many adverse systemic reactions, while inhaled corticosteroids can play strong local anti-inflammatory effects with few adverse reactions. The inhaled corticosteroids include beclomethasone (倍氯米松), triamcinolone acetonide (曲安奈德), budesonide (布地奈德), fluticasone propionate (丙酸氟替卡松), etc.

【Pharmacokinetics】 For an example, after inhalation of beclomethasone, only 10%-20% of beclomethasone enter the lungs, and 80%-90% of the drug are deposited in oropharyngeal region (口咽部). After being swallowed, most of the drug is metabolized in the liver, the bioavailability is less than 20%, and the half-life is about 15 hours. About 70% of the metabolites are excreted through the bile and 10%-25% through the kidneys.

【Pharmacodynamics】Glucocorticoids are a class of steroid hormones that bind to the glucocorticoid receptors almost every vertebrate animal cell. Glucocorticoids can effectively decrease the transcription of inflammation-related genes and inhibit inflammatory molecules and inflammatory cells involved in inflammatory response of asthma.

(1) Inhibition of a variety of inflammatory and immune cells. The cells involved in the pathogenesis of asthma include neutrophils, eosinophils, pulmonary macrophages, mast cells, T lymphocytes and B lymphocytes, etc. In addition, glucocorticoids inhibit the interaction between inflammatory cells and endothelial cells and reduce the microvascular permeability of the inflammatory cells.

(2) Inhibition of the production of inflammatory cytokines (TNF-α, IL-1, IL-6), adhesion molecules (E-selectin and intercellular adhesion molecules) and inflammatory mediators (leukotrienes, prostaglandins, thromboxane A_2, platelet activating factor) involved in the pathogenesis of asthma. In addition, glucocorticoids reduce the release of lysosomal hydrolase by lysosomal membrane stabilization.

(3) Inhibition of airway hyperresponsiveness induced by inhaled antigens, cold air and exercise-induced bronchoconstriction in asthma patients.

(4) Enhancement of the sensitivity on bronchial and vascular smooth muscle to catecholamine which is helpful to relieve bronchospasm and mucosal swelling.

【Clinical indications】Glucocorticoid inhalers (糖皮质激素吸入剂) are used in patients with chronic asthma whose bronchospasm cannot be effectively controlled by bronchodilators, which can reduce and alleviate the attack of the disease, but cannot stop the acute symptoms of asthma. After aerosol inhalation, the dose of oral corticosteroids can be reduced or gradually replaced by inhaler corticosteroids.

【Adverse reactions】A small number of patients seem to have oral fungal infection, hoarseness and other local reactions.

1.3　Anti-allergic antiasthmatic drugs

These drugs mainly inhibit the release of inflammatory mediators and bronchospasm induced by non-specific stimuli. Anti-allergic antiasthmatic drugs include inflammatory cell membrane stabilizers (炎症细胞膜稳定药) and regulators of leukotrienes (白三烯调节药). Some of the drugs are also histamine receptor antagonists.

Sodium cromoglycate (色甘酸钠)

【Pharmacodynamics】As an inflammatory cell membrane stabilizer, sodium cromoglycate can specifically inhibit activation of mast cells and the release of inflammatory mediators such as substance P, bradykinin, histamine and 5-hydroxytryptamine (5-HT) induced by antigen, as well as rapid and delayed-type hypersensitivity. Therefore, sodium cromoglycate is used to prevent the symptoms of asthma. When it is used regularly, it will lessen the number and severity of asthma attacks by reducing inflammation in the lungs. It can also inhibit bronchospasm induced by sulfur dioxide, cold air, and exercise and so on.

Other anti-inflammatory, anti-allergic and antiasthmatic drugs, such as tranilast (曲尼司特), which have similar mechanism to sodium cromoglycate. Ketotifen (酮替芬), not only inhibits the release of inflammatory mediators, but also blocks histamine H_1 receptor, so it has some preventive effects on various types of asthma. Nedocromil sodium (奈多罗米钠) is a drug considered as mast cell stabilizer which acts to prevent wheezing, shortness of breath, and other breathing problems caused by asthma for its strong anti-inflammatory effect and mild adverse reactions.

【Clinical indications】Anti-allergic antiasthmatic drugs are mainly used as preventive drugs for asthma, but they cannot stop the acute attack. In addition, these drugs work slowly, and may take up to several days or even weeks to reach their maximum effect.

【Adverse reactions】A few patients may have symptoms of throat and tracheal irritation after use of the inhalation.

1.4　Regulators of leukotrienes

Leukotrienes are metabolites of arachidonic acid via 5-lipoxygenase (5-脂加氧酶), which are closely related to bronchial inflammation in asthma.Cysteinyl leukotriene receptor-1 antagonists (半胱氨酰白三烯受体−拮抗药) and 5-lipoxygenase inhibitors are called regulators of leukotrienes and used for the treatment of chronic asthma. The commonly used cysteinyl leukotriene receptor-1 antagonists are zafirlukast, montelukast (孟鲁司特), and pranlukast (普仑司特). Zileuton (齐留通) is an orally active inhibitor of 5-lipoxygenase, and thus inhibits formation of leukotrienes, and used for the maintenance treatment of asthma.

Zafirlukast(扎鲁司特)

【Pharmacodynamics】As a cysteinyl leukotriene receptor-1 antagonist, zafirlukast inhibits the inflammatory effects of leukotriene C_4, D_4 and E_4, and inhibits airway inflammation-induced bronchospasm and antigen-induced bronchoconstriction.

【Clinical indications】Regulators of leukotrienes are used for prevention and treatment of chronic asthma, or as an alternative to glucocorticoids and β_2 receptor agonists, but they are not suitable to control acute asthma.

【Adverse reactions】Zafirlukast is well tolerated and may induce mild headache, gastrointestinal reaction and elevated liver transaminase levels, which can disappear after drug withdrawal.

2. Antitussives

Drugs that act in the central or peripheral nervous system to inhibit cough reflexes are antitussives. Cough is a protective reflex of the upper respiratory tract. Beneficial cough promotes the excretion of sputum and foreign matter in the respiratory tract and keeps the respiratory tract unobstructed. Therefore, antitussives are not suitable to the symptom of much more sputum and thick sputum, so as to avoid bronchial obstruction caused by sputum retention. However, antitussives are commended when severe and frequent coughs seriously affect life, rest, and may cause other problems with breathing. According to the pharmacodynamics, there are two types of antitussives, central antitussives and peripheral antitussives.

2.1 Central antitussives（中枢性镇咳药）

Central antitussives can be divided into two categories: addictive and non-addictive drugs. The former is morphine alkaloids and its derivatives with strong antitussive effects and addiction, which acts inside the central nervous system to suppress the responsiveness of one or more sensory afferent response components of the central reflex pathway for cough, while the latter is not addictive drugs and frequently used to treat cough.

2.1.1 Addictive antitussives（成瘾性镇咳药）

Many antitussives, including codeine and pholcodine (福尔可定), are derived from opioids and may be addictive.

Codeine（可待因）

【Pharmacokinetics】The oral bioavailability of codeine is 40%-70%, the peak time is about 1 hour, about 15% is converted to morphine by demethylation reaction and combined with glucuronic acid in liver, the metabolites are excreted by the kidneys into urine, and the serum half-life of codeine is 3-4 hours.

【Pharmacodynamics】Codeine is an opioid and an agonist of the μ-opioid receptor. It acts on the central nervous system to play analgesic effect and antitussive effect. Codeine selectively inhibits cough center of medulla oblongata, and its effect is strong and rapid. The antitussive effect is 1/10 of morphine, and its analgesic effect is also much lower than morphine.

【Clinical indications】Codeine is suitable for severe dry cough (干咳) caused by various causes, especially for those with pleurisy and dry cough with chest pain, but it is not commended for those with thick or large amounts of sputum.

【Adverse reactions】Addiction is the main adverse reaction of codeine; therefore it should not be used for a long time. Other adverse reactions are nausea, vomiting, lightheadedness, constipation, drowsiness, vertigo and inhibition of the respiratory center in large doses.

2.1.2 Non-addictive antitussive drugs（非成瘾性镇咳药）

Non-addictive antitussive drugs also inhibit cough center in the central nervous system but with no analgesic and addictive effects. The commonly used non-addictive antitussive drugs are as follows.

Dextromethorphan（右美沙芬）

Dextromethorphan is methyl ether of dextrorotatory isomer of levorphanol, a codeine analog. Its antitussive effect is similar to that of codeine, but has no analgesic effect. Dextromethorphan is mainly used for dry cough, which is induced by colds, bronchitis, pharyngitis, and other upper respiratory tract infections. There are few adverse reactions such as itching, nausea, drowsiness and dizziness, etc. It takes effects 15-30 minutes after oral administration, and the effects can last for 3-6 hours.

Pentoxyverine（喷托维林）

Pentoxyverine is an antitussive drug containing amino group, its antitussive effect is 1/3 of codeine. It has a direct inhibitory effect on the cough center of medulla oblongata, and has a mild atropine-like effect and local anesthetic effects; its anticholinergic properties can theoretically relax the pulmonary alveoli, reduce phlegm production, and relieve bronchial smooth muscle spasm and decrease airway resistance, so it also has peripheral antitussive effect. Pentoxyverine is mainly used for dry cough and paroxysmal cough during respiratory tract inflammation, but it is prohibited in patients with excessive phlegm. The adverse reactions are mild, such as dizziness, dry mouth, constipation, allergic reactions of the skin like itching, rashes and hives are rare.

2.2 Peripheral antitussives (外周性镇咳药)

Peripheral antitussives act outside the central nervous system to inhibit cough by suppressing the responsiveness of one or more vagal sensory receptors that produce cough reflex, and are used to replace the addictive antitussive drugs such as codeine or morphine.

Benproperine (苯丙哌林)

Benproperine mainly blocks the stretch receptor of lung-pleura and inhibits pulmonary-vagal reflex, so as to relieve bronchospasm. After oral administration, the efficacy of benproperine may maintain for about 7 hours and can be exerted within 15-60 minutes. Its antitussive effect is 2-4 times stronger than that of codeine and can be used for cough caused by a variety of causes. Its common adverse reactions are fatigue, dizziness, transient oral and throat numbness, etc.

Other peripheral antitussive drugs include benzonatate (苯佐那酯), narcotine (那可丁), dioxopromethazine (二氧丙嗪) and so on.

3. Expectorants

Expectorants aim to make coughing up mucus easier, but they cannot actually stop coughing. They always make sputum thinner, reduce viscosity and cough easily. Expectorants reduce the thickness or viscosity of bronchial secretions thus increasing mucus flow that can be removed more easily through coughing. Expectorants also reduce the stimulation of respiratory mucosa, and indirectly play antitussive and antiasthmatic effect and are beneficial to the control of secondary infection. Expectorants include irritating expectorants (刺激性祛痰药) and mucolytics (黏痰溶解药). The common adverse reactions are nausea and gastrointestinal discomfort.

3.1 Irritating expectorants

Irritating expectorants stimulate the gastric mucosa (e.g., ammonium chloride, 氯化铵) or bronchial mucosa (guaifenesin，愈创木甘油醚), promote the dilution and secretion of sputum and make it easy to cough. Nausea and gastrointestinal discomfort after oral administration are their common adverse reactions.

3.2 Mucolytics

Mucolytics decrease the viscosity or thickness of sputum or secretions from the respiratory tract and make it easy to cough. The drugs are suitable for dyspnea caused by thick sputum and difficulty in expectoration. Both acetylcysteine (乙酰半胱氨酸) and carbocisteine (羧甲司坦) are mucolytics that reduce the viscosity of sputum to relieve the symptoms of chronic obstructive pulmonary disorders. They can break the disulfide bond in mucus sputum, thus reduce the viscosity of sputum and make it easy to be excreted. Their adverse reactions are similar to that of irritating expectorants.

重 点 小 结

类别	药物	药理作用	临床应用	不良反应
平喘药	支气管扩张药	β_2受体激动药：选择性扩张支气管平滑肌，控制哮喘发作	急性哮喘，慢性哮喘	窦性心动过速，肌肉震颤
		茶碱类平喘药：抑制磷酸二酯酶，扩张支气管平滑肌，抗炎，增强呼吸肌收缩力	急性哮喘，慢性哮喘	安全范围窄，不良反应较多，如心动过速、不安、失眠等
		吸入性抗胆碱平喘药：选择性阻断支气管M_1受体，扩张支气管平滑肌	β_2受体激动药疗效不佳时的替代用药	口干等
	抗炎平喘药	糖皮质激素类：抑制多种免疫细胞、炎症细胞以及炎性趋化因子、黏附分子、炎症介质等的产生，降低气道高反应性，增强支气管及血管平滑肌对儿茶酚胺的敏感性	慢性哮喘，预防哮喘，单用不能缓解急性发作	口腔真菌感染、声音嘶哑等局部反应
	抗过敏平喘药	炎症细胞膜稳定药：稳定肥大细胞膜，减少5-羟色胺、缓激肽、组胺、P物质等炎症介质释放，降低气道高反应性	预防哮喘	咽喉和支气管刺激
		白三烯调节药：拮抗半胱氨酰白三烯受体1，拮抗白三烯类的炎症反应，降低气道高反应性	轻度至中度慢性哮喘，预防哮喘，单用不能缓解急性发作	头痛、胃肠道反应、血清转氨酶升高等
镇咳药	中枢性镇咳药	成瘾性镇咳药：抑制延髓咳嗽中枢，镇咳作用快而强	严重干咳，不宜用于痰多或痰液黏稠者	成瘾性，呼吸抑制，偶有恶心、呕吐、便秘等
		非成瘾性镇咳药：抑制延髓咳嗽中枢，抑制外周咳嗽神经反射	干咳、阵咳，不宜用于痰多或痰液黏稠者	无成瘾性，偶有头晕、口干等
	外周性镇咳药	抑制外周咳嗽神经反射，解除支气管平滑肌痉挛	干咳	疲乏、眩晕、嗜睡等
	祛痰药	刺激性祛痰药：口服后，刺激胃黏膜或支气管，促进支气管腺体分泌，使痰液稀释，易于咳出	痰液不易咳出者	恶心、呕吐以及胃肠刺激
		黏痰溶解药：使黏痰中的酸性黏蛋白或黏痰中的二硫键断裂，降低痰液黏稠度，易于咳出	痰液不易咳出者	恶心、胃肠刺激

目 标 检 测

一、选择题

（一）单项选择题

1. 下列属于通过抑制磷酸二酯酶活性发挥平喘作用的药物是（　　）
   A. 沙丁胺醇　　　　　　B. 异丙托溴铵　　　　　　C. 硝苯地平
   D. 胆茶碱　　　　　　　E. 麻黄碱
2. 通过激动 β_2 受体发挥平喘作用的药物是（　　）
   A. 硝苯地平　　　　　　B. 异丙托溴铵　　　　　　C. 沙丁胺醇
   D. 氨茶碱　　　　　　　E. 色甘酸钠
3. 通过抑制肥大细胞过敏介质释放发挥平喘作用的药物是（　　）
   A. 可待因　　　　　　　B. 色甘酸钠　　　　　　　C. 肾上腺素
   D. 氨茶碱　　　　　　　E. 特布他林
4. 可待因临床适用于治疗（　　）
   A. 剧烈无痰干咳　　　　B. 多痰性咳嗽　　　　　　C. 长期慢性咳嗽
   D. 哮喘　　　　　　　　E. 心绞痛
5. 属于糖皮质激素类的平喘药是（　　）
   A. 沙丁胺醇　　　　　　B. 丙酸倍氯米松　　　　　C. 胆茶碱
   D. 肾上腺素　　　　　　E. 孟鲁司特

（二）多项选择题

6. 下列属于黏痰溶解药的是（　　）
   A. 溴己新　　　　　　　B. 碘化钾　　　　　　　　C. 乙酰半胱氨酸
   D. 愈创木甘油醚　　　　E. 氯化铵
7. 仅用于哮喘预防和慢性哮喘治疗而对急性哮喘发作无效的药物是（　　）
   A. 沙丁胺醇　　　　　　B. 丙酸倍氯米松　　　　　C. 氨茶碱
   D. 色甘酸钠　　　　　　E. 扎鲁司特

二、思考题

急性哮喘和慢性哮喘分别如何选择治疗药物？

（陶小军）

Chapter 28　Drugs acting on the gastrointestinal system

学习目标

1．掌握　抗消化性溃疡药的分类、作用特点和临床应用。
2．熟悉　镇吐药的作用机制和临床应用。
3．了解　促胃肠动力药、泻药、止泻药、利胆药的主要作用与临床应用。

1．Drugs for peptic ulcers

Peptic ulcer disease (PUD) is characterized by discontinuation in the inner lining of the gastrointestinal tract because of gastric acid secretion or pepsin. It extends into the muscularis propria layer of the gastric epithelium. It usually occurs in the stomach and proximal duodenum, involving the lower esophagus, distal duodenum or jejunum. In all these conditions, mucosal erosions or ulceration arise when the caustic effects of aggressive factors (e.g., acid, pepsin, and bile) exceed the defensive factors of gastrointestinal mucosa (e.g., mucus and bicarbonate secretion, prostaglandins, blood flow, and the processes of restitution and regeneration after cellular injury). Moreover, non-steroidal anti-inflammatory drugs and *Helicobacter pylori* infection are the two major factors disrupting the mucosal resistance to injury. Drugs used for the treatment of PUD may be divided into four major categories.

1.1　Antacids

Antacids (抗酸药) are weak bases that react with excessive gastric hydrochloric acid to form a salt and water. An ideal antacid should have a long-lasting effect and be non-absorbable, and should not produce gas or case the adverse reactions of diarrhea and constipation. The commonly used antacids include magnesium hydroxide (氢氧化镁), magnesium trisilicate (三硅酸镁), magnesium oxide (氧化镁), aluminum hydroxide (氢氧化铝), calcium carbonate, sodium bicarbonate, etc.

医药大学堂
WWW.YIYAODXT.COM

1.2   Drugs against gastric acid secretion

Gastric acid is mainly secreted by gastric parietal cells (胃壁细胞), which express histamine H_2 receptors, choline M_1 receptors and gastrin (胃泌素) receptors. Gastric acid secretion can be regulated by many endogenous substances including neurotransmitter acetylcholine, gastrin, histamine, and prostaglandins (前列腺素). Activation of H_2, M_1, or gastrin receptors triggers a series of biochemical reactions, which in turn activate H^+-K^+-ATPase (also known as proton pump) on the tubular membrane of gastric parietal cells. The proton pump, by consuming ATP, pumps out H^+ from the gastric parietal cells to the gastric cavity, and meanwhile transfers K^+ to the gastric parietal cells for H^+-K^+ exchange, leading to formation of gastric acid (Figure 28-1). Therefore, H_2 receptor blockers, M receptor blockers, gastrin receptor blockers, and H^+-K^+-ATPase inhibitors can all inhibit gastric acid secretion.

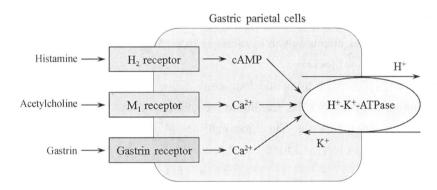

Figure 28-1   Mechanisms of gastric acid secretion

1.2.1 H_2 receptor blockers

These drugs selectively block the H_2 receptors in gastric parietal cells, and thus inhibit gastric acid secretion. Their actions are stronger and longer-lasting than M receptor blockers with less adverse reactions. Using them for PUD usually has a relatively short course of treatment. Additionally, combination of antacids and H_2 receptor blockers is more effective than using H_2 receptor blockers alone. The commonly used H_2 receptor blockers include cimetidine (西咪替丁), ranitidine (雷尼替丁), famotidine (法莫替丁), nizatidine (尼扎替丁), etc.

1.2.2 H^+-K^+-ATPase inhibitors(proton pump inhibitors)

Proton pump inhibitors (质子泵抑制剂) can specifically bind to H^+-K^+-ATPase and irreversibly suppress its activity, thereby exerting a strong and long-lasting reducing effect on gastric acid secretion. They can also reduce pepsin secretion and have antibacterial activity against *Helicobacter pylori*. The first generation of proton pump inhibitors is omeprazole; the second generation is lansoprazole (兰索拉唑); and the third generation is rabeprazole (雷贝拉唑).

Omeprazole (奥美拉唑)

【Pharmacokinetics】This drug has a short serum half-life of about 1 hour. However, the duration of gastric acid inhibition lasts up to 24 hours due to the irreversible inactivation of the proton pump. Omeprazole undergoes rapid first-pass and systemic hepatic metabolism and has negligible renal clearance.

【Pharmacodynamics】 After oral administration, this drug is concentrated in the highly acidic environment of secretory tubules of gastric parietal cells, and is converted into sulfinamide (亚磺酰胺) compounds. The disulfide bonds of these sulfonamide compounds irreversibly combine with the thiol group of H^+-K^+-ATPase to form an enzyme-sulfinamide complex, which inhibits the proton pump function and blocks the final common pathway of acid secretion.

【Clinical indications】 Omeprazole can be used for gastric and duodenal ulcers, postoperative ulcers, reflux esophagitis (反流性食管炎), stress ulcers, acute gastric mucosal hemorrhage, and gastrinoma (胃泌素瘤).

【Adverse reactions】 Headache, dizziness, dry mouth, nausea, bloating, and insomnia are common adverse reactions. Occasionally, rash and peripheral neuritis may occur.

1.2.3　M receptor blockers

Pirenzepine (哌仑西平) can reduce gastric acid secretion by blocking the M_1 choline receptor on gastric parietal cells. This drug was used to treat PUD many years ago. Now it is rarely used for PUD clinically because of its weak effects and anticholinergic side effects.

1.2.4　Gastrin receptor blockers

Proglumamine (丙谷胺) with a chemical structure similar to gastrin can competitively block the gastrin receptor on gastric parietal cells, leading to reduction in gastric acid and pepsin secretion and to protection of gastric mucosa. However, the clinical efficacy of proglumamine is weaker than H_2 receptor blockers, and thus it has been less used for the treatment of PUD.

1.3　Mucosal protective agents

Prostaglandins (mainly PGI_2 and PGE_2) can activate their receptors on the basal side of gastric mucosal epithelial cells, promote the secretion of mucus and bicarbonate ions, increase the blood flow of gastric mucosa, and enhance the resistance of mucosal cells to injury factors. These actions are beneficial for the healing of ulcer wound. Misoprostol (米索前列醇) is a methyl analog of PGE_1, and can decrease the basal secretion of gastric acid and inhibit the secretion induced of gastric acid by histamine, gastrin or food uptake.

1.4　Drugs against *Helicobacter pylori*

Helicobacter pylori is a kind of Gram-negative anaerobic (厌氧的) bacterium. Infection of this bacterium in the stomach has been sufficiently validated as the main cause of chronic gastritis. It can produce harmful substances, break down mucus, and cause tissue inflammation. Elimination of *Helicobacter pylori* can significantly reduce the recurrence rate of duodenal ulcer. *Helicobacter pylori* is sensitive to a variety of antibacterial agents *in vitro*, but single use of one antibacterial agent is less effective *in vivo*. Currently, a triple or quadruple therapy for 10-14 days is usually recommended to achieve favorable therapeutic efficacy in the clinic, that is, combination use of proton pump inhibitors with two or three antibacterial drugs such as clarithromycin (克拉霉素), amoxicillin (阿莫西林), metronidazole/tinidazole, tetracycline, furazolidone, and gentamicin.

2.　Drugs for regulating digestive function

2.1　Antiemetic drugs (镇吐药)

Vomiting is a complex reflection process. The medulla oblongata vomiting center (延髓呕吐中枢) and the chemoreceptor trigger zone (催吐化学感受区) are responsible for the vomiting reflex. Serotonin 5-HT_3, dopamine D_2, and M receptors are abundant in the chemoreceptor trigger zone. The nucleus of the solitary tract (孤束核) is also rich in 5-HT_3, D_2, M, and H_1 receptors. These receptors and their ligand transmitters control the vomiting reflex. Antiemetic drugs are mainly divided into four categories.

　　(1) H_1 receptor blockers　Diphenhydramine (苯海拉明) is used to prevent and treat motion vomiting and inner ear vertigo (内耳眩晕病). It is commonly used in conjunction with other antiemetic drugs for treatment of emesis due to chemotherapy.

　　(2) M receptor blocks　Scopolamine (东莨菪碱) is used to relieve nausea and vomiting. It is one of the best agents for the prevention of motion sickness.

　　(3) 5-HT_3 receptor blockers　Alosetron (阿洛司琼), ondansetron (昂丹司琼) and granisetron (格拉司琼) have good effects on vomiting caused by radiotherapy and chemotherapy.

　　(4) Dopamine D_2 receptor blockers　Chlorpromazine (氯丙嗪) and domperidone (多潘立酮) are used for nausea and vomiting caused by chemotherapy.

2.2　Prokinetic Drugs (促胃肠动力药)

Prokinetic drugs can enhance and coordinate gastrointestinal rhythmic movements. They are mainly used for gastrointestinal symptoms caused by poor gastrointestinal function. Prokinetic drugs are mainly divided into three categories.

　　(1) Pseudocholine drugs　Bethanechol chloride (氯贝胆碱) can not only enhance gastrointestinal motility, but also increase the secretion of saliva, gastric juice, and pancreatic juice.

　　(2) Dopamine D_2 receptor blockers　Within the gastrointestinal tract, dopamine receptor antagonism may potentiate cholinergic smooth muscle stimulation. Metoclopramide (甲氧氯普胺) and domperidone (多潘立酮) can stimulate esophageal peristalsis, increase lower esophageal sphincter pressure, and enhance gastric emptying.

　　(3) 5-HT_4 receptor agonists　Cisapride (西沙必利) can increase the tension of esophageal sphincter and gastrointestinal contractility, and improve the coordination of stomach and duodenal motility.

2.3　Laxatives (泻药)

Laxatives are drugs that stimulate bowel movements, soften stools, and lubricate the bowel to promote defecation. Clinically, they are mainly used to treat functional constipation. According to their pharmacodynamic properties, laxatives are mainly divided into three categories.

(1) Stimulant laxatives　These drugs include bisacodyl (吡沙可啶) and anthraquinones (蒽醌类). Their mechanisms of action include direct stimulation of the enteric nervous system and colonic electrolyte and fluid secretion.

(2) Osmotic laxatives　These drugs include magnesium sulfate (硫酸镁) and lactulose (乳果糖). High doses of osmotically active agents produce prompt bowel evacuation within 1-3 hours. The rapid movement of water into the distal small bowel and colon leads to a high volume of liquid stool followed by rapid relief of constipation.

(3) Lubricant laxatives　These drugs include liquid paraffin (液状石蜡) and glycerin.

2.4　Antidiarrheal drugs (止泻药)

Diarrhea is a common symptom of a variety of diseases, and appropriate antidiarrheal drugs may be given to relieve the above symptoms. The commonly used antidiarrheal drugs include loperamide (洛哌丁胺), opioids (阿片类), diphenoxylate (地芬诺酯), etc.

2.5　Choleretic drugs (利胆药)

Ursodeoxycholic acid (熊去氧胆酸) can inhibit cholesterol absorption and promote the dissolution of gallstones (胆结石). It is used clinically for the treatment of cholesterol gallstones, cholecystitis (胆囊炎), and cholangitis (胆管炎).

重 点 小 结

药物分类			代表药物
抗消化性溃疡药	抗酸药		氢氧化镁、氢氧化铝
	抑制胃酸分泌药	H₂ 受体阻断药	西咪替丁、雷尼替丁
		H⁺-K⁺-ATP 酶抑制药	奥美拉唑、兰索拉唑
		M 受体阻断药	哌仑西平
		胃泌素受体阻断药	丙谷胺
	胃黏膜保护药		米索前列醇
	抗幽门螺杆菌药		阿莫西林、克拉霉素
消化功能调节药	镇吐药	H₁ 受体阻断药	苯海拉明、茶苯海明
		M 受体阻断药	东莨菪碱、苯海索
		5-HT₃ 受体阻断药	阿洛司琼、昂丹司琼
		D₂ 受体阻断药	氯丙嗪、硫乙拉嗪
	促胃肠动力药	拟胆碱药	氯贝胆碱
		D₂ 受体阻断药	多潘立酮
		5-HT₄ 受体激动药	西沙必利
	泻药	刺激性泻药	吡沙可啶
		渗透性泻药	硫酸镁
		润滑性泻药	液状石蜡
	止泻药		洛哌丁胺、阿片制剂
	利胆药		熊去氧胆酸

目 标 检 测

一、选择题

（一）单项选择题

1. 不属于抗消化性溃疡药的是（　　　）
　　A. 乳酶生　　　　B. 氢氧化镁　　　　C. 丙谷胺　　　　D. 奥美拉唑　　　　E. 雷尼替丁

2. 西咪替丁抑制胃酸分泌的机制是（　　　）
　　A. 阻断 M 受体　　　　　　　B. 保护胃黏膜　　　　　　　C. 阻断 H_1 受体
　　D. 促进 PGE_2 合成　　　　　E. 阻断 H_2 受体

3. 哌仑西平为（　　　）
　　A. H_1 受体阻断药　　　　　B. H_2 受体阻断药　　　　　C. M_1 受体阻断药
　　D. α 受体阻断药　　　　　　E. β 受体阻断药

4. 硫酸镁导泻的机制是（　　　）
　　A. 对抗 Ca^{2+} 的作用
　　B. 激活 Na^+-K^+-ATP 酶
　　C. 扩张外周血管
　　D. 在肠腔内形成高渗而减少水分吸收
　　E. 分泌缩胆囊素，促进肠液分泌和蠕动

（二）多项选择题

5. 奥美拉唑的药理作用有（　　　）
　　A. 减少胃壁细胞分泌 H^+
　　B. 抑制 H^+-K^+-ATP 酶
　　C. 减少胃黏液分泌
　　D. 促进 HCO_3^- 分泌
　　E. 黏附于胃上皮细胞和溃疡基底膜，形成保护膜

二、思考题

简述常用抗消化性溃疡药的分类、作用机制及代表药。

（张　峰）

PPT

Chapter 29 Drugs acting on the uterine smooth muscles

学习目标

1. **掌握**　缩宫素的药理作用、临床应用。
2. **熟悉**　缩宫素的不良反应。
3. **了解**　前列腺素和麦角生物碱的药理作用。

Uterine stimulants (oxytocics) are medications given to cause a woman's uterus to contract, or to increase the frequency and intensity of the contractions. These drugs are applied to induce/start or augment/speed labor, facilitate uterine contractions following a miscarriage, induce abortion, or reduce hemorrhage following childbirth or abortion. Improper use can cause severe consequences associated with uterine rupture (子宫破裂) and asphyxia (窒息).

Oxytocin (缩宫素)

Oxytocin and vasopressin (加压素) are the only known hormones released by the human posterior pituitary gland (垂体后叶) to act at a distance.

【Pharmacokinetics】When orally given, oxytocin is easily destroyed by digestive enzymes in the digestive tract and becomes ineffective. So it is administered intravenously for initiation and augmentation of labor. It can be injected intramuscularly for control of uterine hemorrhage (子宫出血). It can pass through the placenta, and most of them are eliminated by the liver and kidneys.

【Pharmacodynamics】

(1) Stimulating uterine smooth muscle　Oxytocin can directly stimulate muscular contraction and frequency of uterine smooth muscle (子宫平滑肌). The contraction response depends on the uterine threshold of excitability. When properly administered, it can stimulate uterine contractions similar to those seen in normal labor (自然分娩). Oxytocin exerts a selective action on the uterine smooth muscle, particularly toward the end of pregnancy, during labor and immediately following delivery. Oxytocin can increase both the force and the frequency of uterine contractions in small doses (2-5U). Whereas, oxytocin in high doses (5-10U) can produce sustained contraction. Oxytocin also stimulates the release of prostaglandins and leukotrienes that augment uterine contraction.

(2) Other actions　Oxytocin causes contraction of myoepithelial cells surrounding mammary alveoli (乳腺腺泡), which leads to lactation. It can reduce the excretion of urine slightly due to its similarity to vasopressin.

医药大学堂
WWW.YIYAODXT.COM

240

【Clinical indications 】

(1) Initiation and augmentation of labor   Oxytocin is used to induce labor in such conditions, worsening preeclampsia (先兆子痫), intrauterine infection, uncontrolled maternal diabetes, or ruptured membranes after 34 weeks. It is also used to augment protracted labor.

(2) Uterine hemorrhage   Oxytocin can be used in the immediate postpartum period (产后期) to stop vaginal bleeding due to uterine atony (子宫张力缺乏).

【Adverse reactions 】 Oxytocin in relatively safe when used at recommended doses, and adverse reactions are uncommon. The potential adverse reactions include subarachnoid hemorrhage (蛛网膜下腔出血), increased heart rate, decreased blood pressure, cardiac arrhythmia (心律失常) and premature ventricular contraction (室性期前收缩), impaired uterine blood flow (子宫血流), and pelvic hematoma (盆腔血肿), etc. Excessive dosage or long term administration may result in high frequency or even continuous tetanic contraction (强直性收缩) of the uterus, uterine rupture, postpartum hemorrhage (产后出血), and water intoxication (水中毒), sometimes fatal.

Prostaglandins (前列腺素)

The prostaglandins (PG) are a group of physiologically active lipid compounds called eicosanoids having diverse hormone-like effects, and show a wide effect on cardiovascular, respiratory, digestive and reproductive systems. The brand used for stimulating uterine smooth muscle include dinoprostone (地诺前列酮, PGE_2, 前列腺素 E_2), dinoprost (地诺前列素, $PGF_{2\alpha}$, 前列腺素 $F_{2\alpha}$), sulprostone (硫前列酮), carboprost (卡前列素, 15- 甲 基 前 列 腺 素 $F_{2\alpha}$) and etc. Prostaglandins are important mediators of uterine activity. They have stimulated effects on the uterus in all stages of pregnancy, and the uterus is particularly sensitive before delivery. The effect on the early and middle pregnancy is stronger than that of oxytocin. The uterine contractions caused by prostaglandins are similar to physiological pains. While enhancing the rhythmic contraction of uterine smooth muscles, it can still contract the cervix. Therefore, in addition to full-term induction of labor, it can also cause high frequency and large-scale contraction in the uterus in early or mid-term pregnancy, resulting in an abortion effect. Common adverse reactions mainly include gastrointestinal excitation such as nausea, vomiting, and abdominal pain. It is not suitable for patients with bronchial asthma and glaucoma.

Ergot alkaloids (麦角生物碱)

Ergot alkaloids are compounds derived from the parasitic fungus *Claviceps purpurea*. The alkaloids are often divided into amine alkaloids [e.g., ergonovine(麦角新碱) and methylergonovine (甲基麦角新碱), methysergide (美西麦角), lergotrile (麦角腈)] and amino acid alkaloids[e.g., ergotamine (麦角胺)]. They have a wide range of physiological effects. They also exert a selective action on the uterine smooth muscle, and the contraction strength depends on the physiological state of the uterine. The pregnant uterus is sensitive to ergot alkaloids compared to the non-pregnant uterus. Unlike oxytocin, ergot-associated contractions are tonic rather than rhythmic, these agents cannot be used during labor. Tonic contraction of the uterus during labor can result in fetal hypoxia and even death. Therefore, Ergot alkaloids are not suitable for initiation and augmentation of labor. Among them, ergometrine has the fastest and strongest effect. The amino acid ergot alkaloids, especially ergotamine, can directly contract arterial and venous blood vessels, and in high doses even do harm to vascular endothelial cells, and long-term use can cause dry limb gangrene. The amino acid ergot alkaloids can also block alpha adrenergic receptors, which reverse the pressure-increasing effect of adrenaline. Current medical uses of ergot alkaloids include ergometrine to induce uterine contractions, ergotamine for migraine headaches. The ergot alkaloids are highly toxic and can result in nausea, vomiting, decreased circulation, rapid and weak pulse, and coma.

重 点 小 结

药物	药理作用	临床应用	不良反应
缩宫素	兴奋子宫平滑肌，促进排乳，抗利尿	催产和引产，产后止血	过量可引起子宫高频率甚至持续性强直收缩，可致胎儿窒息或子宫破裂等
麦角生物碱	兴奋子宫，收缩血管，阻断 α 受体	子宫出血，偏头痛，子宫复原	恶心、呕吐及血压升高；偶见过敏反应，严重者出现呼吸困难、血压下降。麦角流浸膏中含有麦角毒和毒角胺，长期使用可损害血管内皮细胞

题库

目 标 检 测

单项选择题

下列关于缩宫素药理作用的叙述，错误的是（　　　）

A. 抑制子宫平滑肌　　　　　B. 促进排乳　　　　　C. 促进前列腺素释放

D. 抗利尿　　　　　E. 兴奋子宫平滑肌

（董世芬）

医药大学堂
WWW.YIYAODXT.COM

Chapter 30 Antihistamines

 学习目标

　　1.**掌握** 抗组胺药的概念、分类；苯海拉明、氯雷他定、法莫替丁的药理作用及机制、临床应用和不良反应。

　　2.**熟悉** 氯苯那敏、西替利嗪、雷尼替丁的药理作用和临床应用。

　　3.**了解** 组胺的生理功能。

1. Overview

　　Histamine (组胺) is an amine formed by the decarboxylation (脱羧反应) of the amino acid histidine (组胺酸). It is found at high concentration in mast cells (肥大细胞) and basophils (嗜碱性粒细胞). In mast cells, histamine is stored in granules (颗粒). Various types of stimuli (刺激), such as trauma (组织损伤), higher temperature, certain toxins from organisms, can trigger its release. By combining with histamine receptors (H_1, H_2, H_3 and H_4), histamine mediates a wide range of cellular responses, including allergic and inflammatory reactions, gastric acid secretion, and neurotransmission in the brain (Figure 30-1).

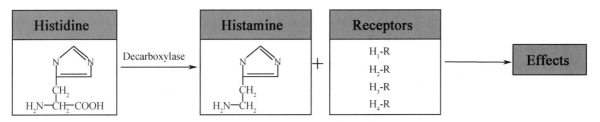

Figure 30-1　Summary of histamine

　　The agents that inhibit the action of histamine are called antihistamines (抗组胺药) or histamine receptor blockers (组胺受体阻断药). They have opposite physiological effects to the histamine, reduce the release of histamine and block the receptor-mediated response of histamine. Both H_1 receptor blockers and H_2 receptor blockers are used widely clinically.

243

2. H₁ antihistamines

The H₁ receptor blockers can be divided into first-generation and second-generation drugs. The second-generation drugs are fewer lipids soluble and do not penetrate the blood-brain barrier. The first-generation H₁ receptor blockers include diphenhydramine (苯海拉明), promethazine (异丙嗪) and chlorpheniramine (氯苯那敏). The second-generation drugs include cetirizine (西替利嗪), loratadine (氯雷他定) and astemizole (阿司咪唑).

【Pharmacodynamics】

(1) **The antagonism of H₁ receptor**   Since inhibiting most of the effects of histamine on smooth muscles and strongly prevent capillary permeability (毛细血管通透性) and formation of edema (水肿) and wheal, they suppress the flare component of the triple response (三重反应) and itching.

(2) **Anticholinergic effects**   Many of the first-generation H₁ receptor antagonists tend to inhibit responses to acetylcholine that are mediated by muscarinic receptors.

(3) **Central inhibition**   The older first-generation H₁ receptor antagonists can inhibit the central nervous system. The common manifestations include diminished alertness, slowed reaction times, and somnolence (嗜睡).

(4) **Local anesthetic effect**   Some H₁ receptor antagonists have local anesthetic activity. However, this effect requires much high concentrations.

【Clinical indications】

(1) **Allergic and inflammatory conditions**   Oral H₁ receptor blockers are useful in controlling allergic rhinitis (过敏性鼻炎), allergic conjunctivitis (结膜炎) and urticaria (荨麻疹).

(2) **Motion sickness and nausea**   Certain H₁ receptor blockers are the most effective agents for prevention of motion sickness.

(3) **Insomnia**   Many first-generation antihistamines are used in the treatment of insomnia.

【Adverse reactions】

(1) **Inhibition of central nervous system**   The most common side effect of the first generation of H₁ antagonists is sedation. Other untoward central actions include dizziness (眩晕), tinnitus (耳鸣), lassitude (乏力), blurred vision (视物模糊), etc.

(2) **Symptoms of anti-cholinergic receptors**   The most frequent side effects of some first-generation H₁ antagonists include nausea, vomiting, constipation or diarrhea, urinary retention (尿潴留) or frequency (尿频), etc.

(3) **Others**   Several antihistamines had teratogenic effects (致畸作用) in animal studies.

3. H₂ antihistamines

At present, four agents, cimetidine (西咪替丁), ranitidine (雷尼替丁), famotidine (法莫替丁), and nizatidine (尼扎替丁), are commonly used in clinic.

【Pharmacodynamics】The H_2 antihistamines block H_2 receptors in the stomach, thereby completely inhibit basal (基础的), food-stimulated and nocturnal (夜间的) gastric acid secretion, induced by histamine or gastrin (胃泌素). However, they only partially inhibit gastric acid secretion induced by acetylcholine (乙酰胆碱).

【Clinical indications】

(1) Peptic ulcer (消化性溃疡)　H_2 antihistamines are effective in the healing of duodenal and gastric ulcers, and are widely used in combination with antimicrobial drugs.

(2) Zollinger-Ellison syndrome (卓–艾综合征)　With H_2 receptor antagonists, the hypersecretion of gastric acid can be kept at safe level in patients with Zollinger-Ellison syndrome.

(3) Gastroesophageal reflux disease (胃食管反流性疾病)　Even at low doses, H_2 receptor antagonists is effective for prevention and treatment of gastroesophageal reflux disease.

【Adverse reactions】The H_2 receptor antagonists generally are well tolerated, with a low incidence of adverse reactions. Side effects usually are minor and include diarrhea, headache, drowsiness, fatigue, muscular pain, and constipation. Taking high-dose cimetidine for a long-term can lead to female galactorrhea (溢乳) and impotence (阳痿) in male. Moreover, caution should be done when they are used during pregnancy. Both cimetidine and ranitidine inhibit hepatic CYPs, while, ranitidine has a lower affinity.

重 点 小 结

类别	药物	药理作用	临床应用	不良反应
H_1 受体阻断药	第一代：苯海拉明、氯苯那敏	阻断 H_1 受体，抗组胺、抗胆碱、镇静、催眠	以皮肤黏膜症状为主的变态反应性疾病，晕动病和呕吐、失眠	头晕、嗜睡、乏力，抗胆碱样副作用
	第二代：氯雷他定、西替利嗪	阻断过敏介质的释放	以皮肤黏膜症状为主的变态反应性疾病，过敏性哮喘	较少，过量可致心律失常
H_2 受体阻断药	雷尼替丁、法莫替丁	阻断 H_2 受体，抑制胃酸分泌	消化性溃疡、胃食管反流性疾病，其他胃酸分泌过多的疾病	较少

目 标 检 测

一、选择题

（一）单项选择题

1. 下列哪个药物具有明显的镇静催眠作用（　　　）

　　A. 氯苯那敏　　　B. 氯雷他定　　　C. 西替利嗪　　　D. 氮卓斯汀　　　E. 非索非那定

2. 下列哪个药物属于第二代 H_1 受体阻断药（　　　）

　　A. 异丙嗪　　　B. 苯海拉明　　　C. 氯苯那敏　　　D. 曲吡那敏　　　E. 西替利嗪

3. 法莫替丁抗消化性溃疡的主要药理作用是（　　　）

    A. 抗幽门螺杆菌　　　　　　　　B. 保护胃黏膜　　　　　　　　C. 抑制胃酸分泌

    D. 中和胃酸　　　　　　　　　　E. 抑制胃肠蠕动

（二）多项选择题

4. 下列哪些 H_1 受体阻断药可引起嗜睡、视物模糊等不良反应（　　　）

    A. 异丙嗪　　　B. 苯海拉明　　　C. 氯苯那敏　　　D. 氯雷他定　　　E. 西替利嗪

二、思考题

从苯海拉明、氯雷他定对 H_1 受体的选择性解释其药理作用与特点。

（王志琪）

Chapter 31　Drugs for anemia

学习目标

1. **掌握**　口服铁剂、叶酸、维生素 B_{12} 的临床应用。
2. **熟悉**　常用口服铁剂及其不良反应。
3. **了解**　红细胞生成素的临床应用。

Anemia means that the number of red blood cells or the content of hemoglobin (血红蛋白) in the circulating blood is lower than the normal level. Anemia is caused by poor hematopoiesis (造血), excessive destruction of red blood cells, or loss of blood. Common clinical anemias include iron deficiency anemia (IDA, 缺铁性贫血), megaloblastic anemia (巨幼红细胞性贫血), and aplastic anemia (再生障碍性贫血). IDA can be treated with iron preparations. Megaloblastic anemia can be treated with folic acid and vitamin B_{12}. Aplastic anemia is caused by reduced bone marrow hematopoiesis. Drug treatment is currently not ideal for aplastic anemia and will not be discussed in this chapter.

1. Iron preparations

Iron is an important raw material for heme synthesis in the mature stage of red blood cells. The iron required by the human body can be obtained from food, that is, exogenous iron. Iron in food is high-valent iron or organic iron. Stomach acid, fructose, cysteine, and vitamin C in food can reduce it to divalent iron and promote its absorption. Insufficient intake of iron or chronic blood loss causes body iron deficiency, which affects the synthesis of hemoglobin and causes IDA. Oral iron preparation (铁剂) is the first choice in the treatment of IDA. Clinically used oral iron preparations include ferrous sulfate (硫酸亚铁), ferrous fumarate (富马酸亚铁), ferrous gluconate (葡萄糖酸亚铁), ferrous succinate (琥珀酸亚铁), 10% ferric ammonium citrate (枸橼酸铁铵), and iron dextran (右旋糖酐铁). Common adverse reactions of oral iron preparations are gastrointestinal irritation symptoms, such as nausea, vomiting, upper abdominal pain, and diarrhea. Taking oral iron preparations after meals can reduce these adverse reactions. In addition, oral iron can also cause constipation.

2. Folic acid

Folic acid (叶酸) is a water-soluble B-group vitamin. Under the catalytic action of dihydrofolate reductase (二氢叶酸还原酶), folic acid forms active tetrahydrofolate (四氢叶酸), which acts as a transporter of one-carbon groups such as methyl ($-CH_3$) and formyl (-CHO) and thereby participating in the synthesis of purines (嘌呤) and pyrimidines (嘧啶). Animal cells cannot synthesize folic acid by themselves and must obtain folic acid from food. Inadequate folic acid intake or increased folic acid requirements, alcoholism (酒精中毒) and alcoholic cirrhosis (酒精性肝硬化), drugs, genetic factors, and intestinal diseases can cause folic acid deficiency. The deficiency of folic acid leads to the metabolic disorder of one-carbon groups and thereby affecting the synthesis of nucleotides. Thymine (胸腺嘧啶) nucleotide synthesis is most affected, resulting in reduced DNA synthesis in the nucleus and reduced cell division and proliferation. However, due to the less effect on RNA and protein synthesis, the cell's DNA/RNA ratio is decreased, and the cells become larger, the cytoplasm is enriched, and the chromatin is loosely dispersed in the nucleus. Red blood cells are the most affected cells, causing megaloblastic anemia. Clinically, folic acid is often combined with vitamin B_{12} for the treatment of megaloblastic anemia caused by various reasons, especially for nutritional megaloblastic anemia (营养性巨幼红细胞性贫血), gestational and infantile megaloblastic anemia. But folic acid is not effective for the megaloblastic anemia caused by dihydrofolate reductase inhibitors including methotrexate (甲氨蝶呤) and pyrimethamine (乙胺嘧啶). In this case, calcium leucovorin (亚叶酸钙) should be used. For megaloblastic anemia caused by malignant anemia (恶性贫血) and vitamin B_{12} deficiency, the application of folic acid cannot reduce the symptoms of the nervous system, but it can improve the haemogram (血象), so it can also be used as an auxiliary medicine.

3. Vitamin B_{12}

Vitamin B_{12} is necessary for cell division and maintenance of the myelin sheath (髓鞘) integrity of neural tissue. Vitamin B_{12} deficiency can lead to a deficiency of folic acid, and induce the synthesis of abnormal fatty acids, which affects the synthesis of normal sphingomyelin (神经鞘磷脂) and finally causes neurological symptoms. Clinically, vitamin B_{12} is mainly used for the treatment of malignant anemia and megaloblastic anemia. Vitamin B_{12} can also be used as an adjuvant treatment for neurological diseases such as neuritis (神经炎) and neuroatrophy (神经萎缩) and liver diseases.

4. Erythropoietin

Erythropoietin (EPO, 促红细胞生成素) is produced by the interstitial cells around the renal proximal convoluted tubules. EPO can combine with EPO receptor on the surface of erythroid stem cells (红细胞系干细胞) and then stimulate the formation of the cells, promote the maturation of erythrocytes, release reticulocytes from bone marrow, and increase erythrocytes and hemoglobin. Recombinant human erythropoietin (rhEPO) is currently used in clinical practice. It is mainly used for renal anemia and perioperative red blood cell mobilization. It can cause hypertension due to the rapid rise of red blood cells and the increase of blood viscosity. It also induce the increase of blood concentration of alanine aminotransferase (ALT, 谷丙转氨酶) and aspartate aminotransferase (AST, 谷草转氨酶), nausea and vomiting.

重 点 小 结

药物	药理作用	临床应用
铁剂	作为原料参与血红素合成	缺铁性贫血
叶酸	参与嘌呤、嘧啶等合成	巨幼红细胞性贫血
维生素 B_{12}	参与细胞分裂，维持神经组织髓鞘完整性	恶性贫血及巨幼红细胞性贫血
促红细胞生成素	促进红细胞和血红蛋白生成	肾功能不全所致贫血及外科围手术期的红细胞动员

目 标 检 测

题库

单项选择题

1. 硫酸亚铁可用于治疗（　　　　）
　　A. 恶性贫血　　　　　　　　　B. 缺铁性贫血　　　　　　　C. 再生障碍性贫血
　　D. 巨幼红细胞性贫血　　　　　E. 肾功能不全所致贫血
2. 叶酸治疗巨幼红细胞性贫血的机制是叶酸（　　　　）
　　A. 为红细胞的组成成分
　　B. 为合成血红蛋白的主要原料
　　C. 使血红素增加
　　D. 参与 DNA 的合成，促进红细胞发育成熟
　　E. 促进红细胞分裂

3. 治疗甲氨蝶呤诱发的巨幼红细胞性贫血主要用（　　）

    A. 维生素 B_{12} B. 叶酸   C. 硫酸亚铁

    D. 亚叶酸钙   E. 促红细胞生成素

4. 治疗恶性贫血主要用（　　）

    A. 维生素 B_{12} B. 叶酸   C. 硫酸亚铁

    D. 亚叶酸钙   E. 促红细胞生成素

（马秉亮）

Chapter 32　General considerations of antimicrobial agents

 学习目标

1. **掌握** 抗生素药理相关基本术语；抗菌药物的作用机制；细菌耐药性的产生机制。
2. **熟悉** 抗菌药物合理应用的基本原则；抗菌药物的联合应用。
3. **了解** 机体、药物、病原微生物三者的关系；细菌耐药性的传播方式。

Chemotherapy is defined as the chemical treatment of a given disease caused by pathogens (e.g., microorganisms, parasites, and cancer cells) and is widely used in the treatment of cancer. Thus, a chemotherapeutic agent is refined to any chemical agent used for a given disease caused by pathogens. Antimicrobial drugs are chemotherapeutic agents with the ability to suppress the infecting microorganisms. They are the greatest contribution of the 20th century to therapeutics. An ideal antimicrobial drug has specific characteristics, such as good effect, selectively toxicity, and reasonably priced. Understanding the relationship of Host-drug-pathogen in chemotherapy can help us to select the best drugs for diseases(Figure 32-1).

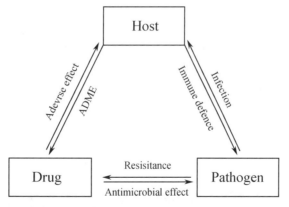

Figure 32-1　The relationship of host-drug-pathogen in chemotherapy

Drugs kill or inhibit pathogens and may develop adverse reactions. Pathogens can be resistant to drugs and infect hosts. Hosts can be against pathogens through the immune system. Hosts can absorb, distribute, metabolize and excrete drugs

1. Terminology

(1) Antimicrobial agents (抗菌药物) These are chemical substances that can kill or inhibit the growth of microorganisms.

(2) Antibiotics (抗生素) These are substances that are derived from certain microorganisms and can kill or inhibit the growth of other microorganisms.

(3) Bactericidal drugs (杀菌药) These drugs such as penicillins (青霉素类), cephalosporins (头孢菌素类)and aminoglycosides (氨基糖苷类), refer to antimicrobial agents that can kill their target bacteria. Particularly, these drugs are essential for the successful treatment of infections in immunocompromised patients.

(4) Bacteriostatic drugs (抑菌药) These drugs such as tetracycline (四环素) and chloramphenicol (氯霉素), refer to antimicrobial agents that cause a reversible arrest of growth of bacteria. These drugs are generally limiting the growth spread of infections with immune defenses.

(5) Spectrum of activity (抗菌谱) It refers to the variety and range of targeted microorganisms of antimicrobial agents. Antimicrobial agents acting only on a limited group of microorganisms are defined as narrow-spectrum antimicrobial agents (e.g., penicillin G, isoniazid). Broad-spectrum antimicrobial agents, such as tetracycline and chloramphenicol, act on a wide diversity of microorganisms. Broad-spectrum antimicrobial use may lead to the development of a superinfection (二重感染).

(6) Anti-microorganism activity It refers to the ability of antimicrobial agents to kill or suppress the growth of microorganisms.

(7) Minimum inhibitory concentration (MIC，最低抑菌浓度) It is the lowest concentration of antibiotic that inhibits bacterial growth.

(8) Minimum bactericidal concentration (MBC，最低杀菌浓度) It is the lowest concentration of antimicrobial agent that kills 99.9% of bacteria.

(9) The post-antibiotic effect (PAE，抗生素后效应) It is continual inhibition of bacterial growth after exposure to an antimicrobial agent in a short time. After short-time treatment, even the drug concentration falls below MIC or reaches zero, there is still a persistent suppression of microbial growth.

(10) The first expose effect (首次接触效应) It refers to the strong antibacterial effect of an antimicrobial agent for the first-time exposure to bacteria, and continual drug treatment or retreatment in a short time cannot exert the same effect. Then, the obvious antibacterial effect needs a time interval (e.g., hours) to appear again.

2. Mechanisms of action

Most antimicrobial drugs currently in clinical use have unique modes of actions, selectively killing or inhibiting the growth of microbial targets. Mechanisms of action of common antimicrobial agents are summarized in Figure 32-2.

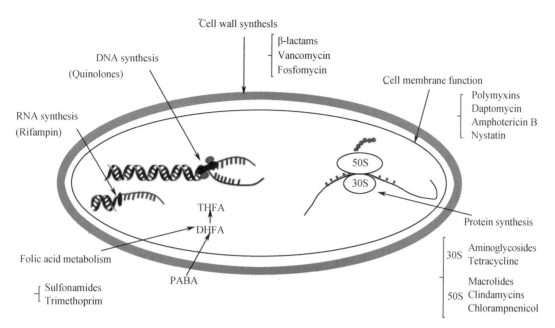

Figure 32-2 Actions of antimicrobial agents at different sites
They could kill or inhibit microorganisms through the inhibition of cell wall synthesis, protein synthesis, nucleic acid synthesis, folic acid metabolism or cell membrane function

2.1 Inhibitors of cell wall biosynthesis

Several different classes of antibacterial drugs inhibit synthesis of bacterial walls. These drugs are bactericidal and mainly suppress peptidoglycan biosynthesis. Gram-positive bacteria have a relatively thick cell wall, composed of peptidoglycan (肽聚糖), while the peptidoglycan layer in Gram-negative bacteria is thin. Peptidoglycan synthesis is divided into three steps. It starts in the cytoplasm, with synthesized N-acetylglucosamine (NAG，N–乙酰葡糖胺) and N-acetylmuramic acid (NAM，N–乙酰胞壁酸). Membrane-embedded undecaprenyl phosphate synthesis occurs in the cytoplasmic side. Transglycosylation (转糖) produces glycan strands, and transpeptidation (转肽) links the peptides to form a 3D network, finally resulting in the formation of peptidoglycan layer. Penicillin-binding proteins (PBP，青霉素结合蛋白) catalyze formation of cross-links between peptidoglycan chains. β-lactams (β-内酰胺类) mainly bind to PBPs, inhibiting transpeptidation. Vancomycin (万古霉素) binds to the D-Ala-D-Ala terminal of the nascent peptidoglycan pentapeptide side chain, creating a structural blockage and suppressing transglycosylation. Vancomycin also structurally blocks transpeptidation. Fosfomycin (磷霉素) blocks the formation of UDP-N-acetylmuramic acid. Because human cells do not make peptidoglycan, this mode of action is an excellent example of selective toxicity.

2.2 Inhibitors of membrane function

A small group of antibacterial agents target the bacterial membrane as their mode of action. The polymyxins (多黏菌素类) are bactericidal drugs and interact with lipopolysaccharide of Gram-negative bacteria, finally disrupting cell membranes. Daptomycin (达托霉素) is a cyclic lipopeptide and inserts in the bacterial cell membrane, resulting in the leakage of K^+ from bacteria and killing the bacterial cells.

Ergosterol is one of the essential fungal cell membrane constituents. For most fungi, the predominant membrane sterol is ergosterol. The fungicidal actions of amphotericin B (两性霉素B) and nystatin (制霉菌素) rely on ergosterol in fungal cell membranes, resulting in the formation of artificial pores. The imidazoles (咪唑类) are broad-spectrum antifungal drugs and inhibit cytochrome lanosterol-α-demethylase, an enzyme that converts lanosterol (羊毛甾醇) to ergosterol, resulting in the perturbation of the fungal cell membrane. Unfortunately, the membrane-targeting mechanism is not a selective toxicity, and these drugs also target and damage the membrane of cells in the kidney and nervous system when administered systemically.

2.3 Inhibitors of protein biosynthesis

The cytoplasmic ribosomes in bacteria consists of a large (50S) and a small (30S) subunit. Aminoglycosides and tetracycline bind to the 30S subunit of bacterial ribosomes, inhibiting protein synthesis. Precisely, aminoglycosides are bactericidal and interfere with protein synthesis in at least 3 ways. ① Blocking formation of the initiation complex. ② Inducing misreading of the code on the mRNA template. ③ Arresting breakup of 70S ribosomes. Tetracycline is bacteriostatic and binds reversibly to acceptor (A) site of 30S subunit, preventing aminoacyl-tRNA attaching to the A site of ribosome-mRNA complex. Macrolides (大环内酯类), clindamycin (克林霉素) and chloramphenicol bind to the 50S subunit of bacterial ribosomes, resulting in the inhibition of protein synthesis. Precisely, macrolides and clindamycin share a common binding site on the 50S ribosome, inhibiting translocation (移位) and transpeptidation (转肽). Chloramphenicol binds reversibly to the 50S subunit of the bacterial ribosome and inhibits transpeptidation through peptidyl transferase (肽酰基转移酶).

2.4 Inhibitors of nucleic acid synthesis

Some antibacterial drugs inhibit nucleic acid synthesis. RNA polymerase is an extremely useful enzyme for transcription. Rifampin (利福平) blocks RNA polymerase activity, interrupting RNA synthesis. DNA gyrase (促旋酶) introduces negative supercoiling into bacterial DNA, and topoisomerase Ⅳ (拓扑异构酶) modulates the segregation of newly replicated chromosomes. Quinolones (喹诺酮类) are synthetic antimicrobial agents. Quinolones block DNA gyrase and topoisomerase Ⅳ activity, interfering with DNA synthesis. Quinolones mainly inhibit DNA gyrase in Gram-negative bacteria and inhibit topoisomerase Ⅳ in Gram-positive bacteria.

2.5 Inhibitors of metabolic pathways

Bacteria synthesize folic acid, which is essential for the synthesis of purine and thymidylate nucleic acids. Precisely, p-aminobenzoic acid (对氨基苯甲酸, PABA) is a constituent. Dihydropteroate synthase (二氢叶酸合成酶) and dihydrofolate reductase (二氢叶酸还原酶) catalyze important reactions for forming folic acid. Dihydropteroate synthase catalyzes the formation of dihydrofolic acid, while dihydrofolate reductase catalyzes the formation of tetrahydrofolic acid (四氢叶酸). Sulfonamides (磺胺类) are the oldest synthetic antimicrobial agents and structural analogues of PABA. Sulfonamides competitively suppress dihydropteroate synthetase and block the synthesis of dihydrofolic acid, leading to the inhibition of folate required for DNA synthesis. Trimethoprim (甲氧苄啶) is a synthetic antimicrobial agent and an inhibitor of dihydrofolate reductase. It blocks the synthesis of tetrahydrofolic acid, suppressing a later step in the folic acid metabolic pathway.

3. Resistance

Drug resistance refers to an adaptive response of microorganisms to the antimicrobial agent, which means microorganisms begin to tolerate an amount of drug used to halt their growth. Types of resistance include intrinsic resistance (固有耐药) and acquired resistance (获得性耐药) according to the origin. Intrinsic resistance refers to a natural resistance existing on chromosome. This is generally a group of species characteristics, such as Gram-negative bacilli to basic penicillins and anaerobic bacteria to aminoglycosides. Namely, an entire bacterial species may be resistant to a drug before its introduction. Acquired resistance refers to the development of resistance through mutation and selection after drug treatment for a period of time, such as the acquisition of β-lactamases (β-内酰胺酶) in bacteria resistant to most β-lactams (β-内酰胺类抗生素). Namely, bacteria that were once sensitive to a drug become resistant. Cross-resistance (交叉耐药) refers to that, when certain microorganisms acquire resistance to one drug, they can acquire resistance to other drugs without exposure. For an example, resistance to erythromycin (红霉素) means resistance to lincomycin (林可霉素). Interestingly, multidrug-resistant (MDR, 多药耐药) microbes, with one or more resistance mechanisms, are resistant to multiple antimicrobials. For example, having an efflux pump that can export multiple antimicrobial drugs is a common way for microbes to be resistant to multiple drugs by using a single resistance mechanism. Gram-negative bacteria that produce extended-spectrum β-lactamases show resistance to all penicillins, cephalosporins and monobactams (单环类). The mechanism of resistance, acquisition of a new low-affinity PBP, provides methicillin-resistant *Staphylococcus aureus* (MRSA) with resistance to most β-lactams.

Acquired resistance may be developed because of mutation or gene transfer. Mutation is a stable and heritable genetic change in microorganisms. For an example, DNA gyrase gene mutation in bacteria results in resistance to quinolones, and RNA polymerase gene mutation in bacteria leads to resistance to rifampin. Gene transfer refers to the resistance gene passed from one microorganism to the others. Resistance gene may enter microorganisms through transduction (转导), transformation (转化) or conjunction (接合). Transduction refers to the process that bacteriophage carrying resistance genes from one microorganism infects another, resulting in the movement of resistance genes from one microorganism to another. Transformation refers to the process that the sensitive organism can imbibe "naked" DNA carrying resistance genes in solution from a resistant microorganism, developing resistance. Conjunction refers to the direct passage of resistance gene through conferring DNA between living cells in contact by way of sex pilus (菌毛) or a bridge.

Microbes are constantly evolving through multiple ways to develop resistance to antimicrobial agents. There are several common mechanisms for drug resistance as summarized in Figure 32-3.

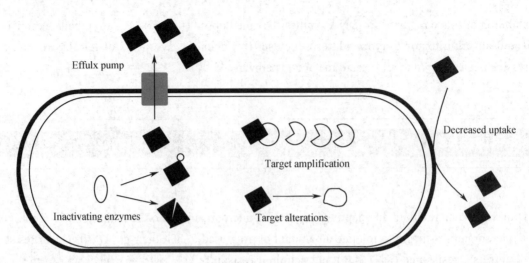

Figure 32-3   Multiple strategies of microbes developing resistance to common antimicrobial drugs

Microbes can become resistant through inactivating drugs, altering targets, reducing drug uptake and even changing metabolic pathways

3.1   Drug inactivation

Bacteria may produce enzymes to chemically modify an antimicrobial agent, thereby inactivating it. β-lactamases induce hydrolysis of the β-lactam ring, resulting in the loss of antibacterial activity of β-lactams. Acetyltransferases catalyze the transfer of adenylyl groups to aminoglycosides, impairing the antibacterial activity. These reactions destroy the effective chemical structure of antimicrobial agents.

3.2   Decreased accumulation

Bacteria may develop resistance through blocking the accumulation of an antimicrobial agent. A common mechanism of Gram-negative bacteria is to limit the uptake of antimicrobial agents, such as β-lactams and chloramphenicol, through altering the number or structure of porins in the outer membrane. Also, the outer membrane of Gram-negative bacteria can block the entrance of some antimicrobial agents with large molecular weights. Additionally, many bacteria produce efflux pumps to transport the antibacterial drugs out of membrane, decreasing the drug concentration.

3.3   Target modification

Because antimicrobial agents have very specific targets, the alteration of targets can confer resistance to related antibacterial drugs. For example, MRSA can produce PBP2a instead of PBP to participate into peptidoglycan synthesis, leading to the decreased binding of most β-lactams to their targets. Additionally, a chromosomal mutation producing a DNA gyrase or topoisomerase Ⅳ with reduced affinity for quinolones in bacteria can make bacteria resistant to quinolones. Resistance to trimethoprim can result from overproduction of dihydrofolate reductases. Then, the increase of targets would abate the effect of antimicrobial agents.

3.4   Others

Bacteria may develop resistance to trimethoprim or sulfonamides through the alteration of metabolic pathways. Some bacteria lack the enzymes required for folate synthesis from PABA, depending on exogenous sources of folate, so they are not susceptible to sulfonamides.

4. Principles in selecting an antimicrobial agent

Selection of the most appropriate antimicrobial agent must be rational, leading to successful chemotherapy. Improper selection of drug, dose, route or duration of treatment may fail to cure an infection. The choice relies on the particulars of the pathogen, the drug and the patient.

4.1   Precise diagnosis

Clinical diagnosis and microbial examination should be made promptly and precisely, directing the application of drugs. Each antimicrobial agent has a specific spectrum of activity. An antimicrobial agent should be selected according to the pathogen of infections. Obviously, antibacterial agents could not treat viral infections.

4.2   Drug factors

Specific properties of antimicrobial agents can affect clinical efficacy. A narrow-spectrum drug inhibiting the definitive pathogen is preferred to the antimicrobial agent with a broad spectrum. A bactericidal antimicrobial agent is preferred to bacteriostatic one for patients with impaired immune defense. A less toxic antimicrobial agent is preferred. An antimicrobial agent with high oral bioavailability is preferable for less severe infections. An antimicrobial agent with the ability to attain high concentration at the infection site is preferable.

4.3   Patient factors

Attention must be paid to the condition of the patient. Age may affect kinetics. For an example, inefficient excretion of chloramphenicol in the newborn can induce gray baby syndrome (灰婴综合征). Additionally, tetracycline deposits in the developing teeth and bone, especially for teens below the age of 6 years. Organ function should be assessed. For an example, antimicrobial agents excreted by kidney are not preferable for patients with impaired renal function, and antimicrobial agents metabolized by liver are not preferable for patients with impaired hepatic function. Genetic factors should be considered. For an example, chloramphenicol may produce hemolysis in G-6-PD deficient patient. Host immune system should be considered. For an example, bactericidal drugs are preferable in immunocompromised patients.

4.4 Prophylaxis (预防给药)

Prophylaxis should be restricted to cases where the pathogen can commonly lead to infection or produce devastating results. Prophylaxis against specific organisms is preferable. Prevention of infection in high risk situations is sometimes necessary. Improper prophylactic uses may result in drug resistance and successive infections.

4.5 Avoiding unreasonable use of drugs

If inadequate doses of nonsynergistic drugs are used, emergence of resistance may be promoted. Toxicity of one agent may be enhanced by another, such as gentamicin (庆大霉素) and cephalothin (头孢噻吩). Additionally, vancomycin and tobramycin (妥布霉素) produce exaggerated kidney failure. Combination of drugs with the increasing toxicity should be mostly avoided. Using improper broad-spectrum antimicrobial agents may increase chances of superinfections.

5. Combined use of antimicrobial agents

More than one antimicrobial agent is frequently used for complicated infections. The objectives of using antimicrobial combinations are to achieve effective synergism, to reduce severity of adverse reactions, to prevent emergence of resistance, and to broaden the spectrum.

5.1 Objectives of using antimicrobial combinations

Drug combinations are often used: ①for unknown pathogen infection. ②For multiple microbes infection. ③For infection by pathogens easy to develop resistance (e.g., tuberculosis, 结核病). ④For reducing toxicity of single drug treatment.

5.2 General conditions of using antimicrobial combinations

When antimicrobial agents are applied together, the anti-microorganism effect may be indifference (无关), addition (相加), synergism (协同) and antagonism (拮抗). A classic example of synergistic combinations is trimethoprim and sulfamethoxazole (磺胺甲噁唑). Individually, these two drugs provide only bacteriostatic inhibition of bacterial growth, but combined, the drugs are bactericidal. Generally, bacteriostatic agents are often additive in combination (e.g., combination of tetracyclines and erythromycin/chloramphenicol). Bactericidal drugs are sometime synergistic (e.g., penicillin G used with streptomycin/gentamicin). The inhibition of cell wall synthesis may enhance the penetration of aminoglycosides into the bacteria. Combination of a bactericidal with a bacteriostatic drug may be synergistic or antagonistic. Penicillin G used with tetracycline/chloramphenicol exerts an antagonistic effect. Penicillin G used with sulfonamide display a synergistic effect. Erythromycin and clindamycin/

chloramphenicol compete with the same target, and the combination of these drugs can demonstrate the antagonistic effect. Attention must be paid to the improper combination. Combination of drugs with an antagonistic effect should not be applied into clinical treatment.

重 点 小 结

药物	抗菌药物作用机制	细菌耐药性产生机制	代表性现象举例
β-内酰胺类、万古霉素、磷霉素	抑制细胞壁合成	产生灭活酶	β-内酰胺酶水解 β-内酰胺类抗生素
氨基糖苷类、大环内酯类、四环素、林可霉素类、氯霉素	抑制蛋白质合成	药物靶点改变	PBP 变为 PBP2a
喹诺酮类、利福平	抑制核酸合成	药物积累减少	主动外排功能增强
磺胺类、甲氧苄啶	影响叶酸代谢	改变代谢途径等	细菌摄取外源性叶酸

目 标 检 测

题库

一、选择题

（一）单项选择题

1. 评价一种化疗药物的临床价值，主要采用下列哪种指标（   ）
   A. 抗菌谱   B. 化疗指数   C. 最低抑菌浓度
   D. 最低杀菌浓度   E. 抗生素后效应

2. 抗菌活性是指（   ）
   A. 药物的抗菌范围   B. 血药浓度
   C. 药物的抑菌或杀菌能力 D. 抑制肿瘤的 LD_{50}
   E. 首次接触效应

3. 耐药性是指（   ）
   A. 连续用药机体对药物产生不敏感现象
   B. 连续用药细菌对药物的敏感性降低甚至消失
   C. 反复用药患者对药物产生精神性依赖
   D. 长期用药细菌对药物缺乏选择性
   E. 长期用药机体对药物产生生理性依赖

4. 属于抑制细菌细胞壁合成的杀菌药是（   ）
   A. 头孢菌素类   B. 氨基糖苷类
   C. 四环素类   D. 氯霉素类

5. 属于静止期杀菌药的是（   ）
   A. 青霉素类   B. 多黏菌素类   C. 磺胺类
   D. 大环内酯类   E. 头孢菌素类

（二）多项选择题

6. 抗菌药的作用机制包括（　　　）

　　A. 阻碍细菌细胞壁合成　　　　　B. 抑制 DNA 合成

　　C. 抑制细菌蛋白质合成　　　　　D. 使细胞壁通透性增加

　　E. 糖肽类　　　　　　　　　　　F. 阻碍叶酸形成

7. 抑制细菌蛋白质合成的抗菌药物包括（　　　）

　　A. 林可霉素类　　　　　　B. 氨基糖苷类　　　　　C. 四环素类

　　D. 氯霉素类　　　　　　　E. 磺胺类

二、思考题

试从抗菌作用特点及机制解释繁殖期杀菌药分别与静止期杀菌药、速效抑菌药联用后的效果。

（彭　芙）

Chapter 33 β-lactam antibiotics and other inhibitors of cell wall synthesis

PPT

学习目标

1. 掌握　青霉素 G 的药理作用及机制、临床应用及不良反应；半合成青霉素类药物的分类、作用特点及临床应用；各代头孢菌素的作用特点、临床应用及不良反应。

2. 熟悉　其他 β-内酰胺类抗生素的作用特点及临床应用；β-内酰胺酶抑制剂和 β-内酰胺类抗生素的复方制剂。

3. 了解　达托霉素、磷霉素的药理作用、临床应用及不良反应。

Several different classes of antibacterial agents block steps in the biosynthesis of peptidoglycan, such as β-lactams, glycopeptides (糖肽类), fosfomycin, cycloserine (环丝氨酸), and bacitracin (杆菌肽). Antibacterial agents that target cell wall biosynthesis are bactericidal in their action. Their mode of actions are summarized in Figure 33-1.

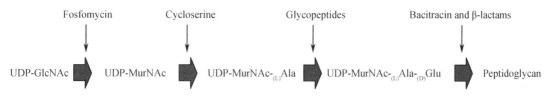

Figure 33-1　Drugs inhibit bacterial cell wall synthesis

1. β-lactam antibiotics

β-lactam antibiotics are anti-microorganism agents with β-lactam ring in their structure. β-lactam antibiotics, especially penicillins and cephalosporins, are considered as preferable choices to treat many infections, for the reason that these drugs are bactericidal with few adverse reactions. These drugs share features of chemistry, pharmacodynamics, pharmacology, and immunologic characteristics, including penicillins, cephalosporins, monobactams, carbapenems (碳青霉烯类), and cephamycins (头霉素类). β-lactamase inhibitors resemble β-lactam molecules, and are often used with other β-lactams. The administration of a bacteriostatic agent, such as tetracycline, may antagonize the bactericidal activity of

医药大学堂
WWW.YIYAODXT.COM

β-lactam antibiotics.

1.1 Pharmacodynamics

One major difference between eukaryotic and prokaryotic cell is the cell wall made from peptidoglycan layers. The cell wall is a rigid outer layer that surrounds the cytoplasmic membrane, maintains cell integrity, and prevents cell lysis from high osmotic pressure. PBPs catalyze formation of cross-links between peptidoglycan chains. β-lactam antibiotics mainly inhibit bacteria growth by binding to PBPs and interfering with the transpeptidation reaction of bacterial cell wall synthesis (Figure 33-2). β-lactam antibiotics kill rapidly growing bacteria when they are synthesizing cell wall.

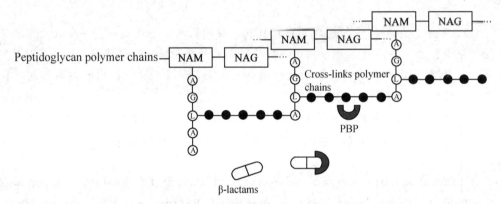

Figure 33-2   β-lactams inhibit bacterial cell wall synthesis

Cell wall synthesis starts in the cytoplasm with the synthesis of NAM and NAG. After peptidoglycans form long chains, the final step is cross linking. Cross linking of peptidoglycan residues of neighboring strands needs cleavage of terminal D-alanine (D-Ala) and transpeptidation with the chain of 5 glycine residues. This cross-linking increases stability and rigidity of the cell wall. β-lactams inhibit transpeptidation by targeting PBPs

1.2 Resistance

Resistance to β-lactam antibiotics is due to one of four general mechanisms: ①β-lactamases catalyze enzymatic hydrolysis of the β-lactam ring leading to inactivation of β-lactam antibiotics. It is a major mechanism of resistance in most *Staphylococci* (葡萄球菌) and Gram-negative bacteria. ②Structure modified PBPs have a lower affinity for β-lactam antibiotics and are responsible for methicillin resistance in staphylococci and for resistance to penicillin G in pneumococci. ③Decreased penetration of β-lactam antibiotics through the outer cell wall membrane impedes the access of drugs to PBPs and is responsible for resistance in Gram-negative bacteria. ④Producing an efflux pump can reduce the concentration of intracellular antibiotics. These general mechanisms for drug resistance to β-lactam antibiotics are summarized in Figure 33-3.

1.3 Penicillins

All penicillins are derivatives of 6-aminopenicillanic acid (6-APA), comprised of a thiazolidine

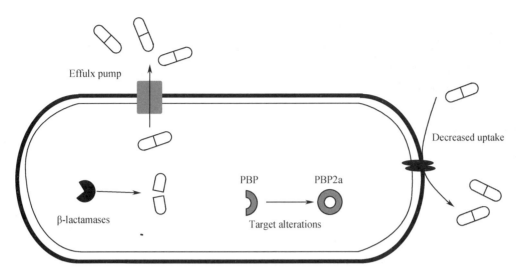

Figure 33-3 The major mechanisms of acquired resistance in microbes to β-lactam antibiotics

Penicillinase is a narrow spectrum β-lactamase mainly inactivating penicillins. Namely, penicillinase in these microorganisms can successfully destroy penicillins. Some resistant bacteria are penicillin tolerant. For an example, MRSA has PBP2a instead of PBP. Most Gram-negative bacteria have "porin" channels for β-lactams, and the loss or alteration of porin channels help them to develop drug resistance. Many bacteria can produce efflux pumps to decrease drug concentration, easily resulting in cross resistance

attached to a β-lactam ring (β-内酰胺环), shown in Figure 33-4. Penicillins are excreted in the urine. Probenecid blocks the renal tubular secretion of penicillin. This interaction may be used therapeutically to produce higher and more prolonged blood concentrations of penicillin. Penicillins and aminoglycosides are commonly used in combination to treat a variety of infections. However, concomitant use of the extended-spectrum penicillin anti-microbials may result in inactivation of the aminoglycosides.

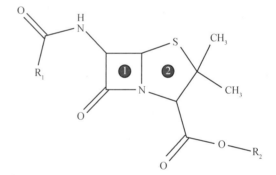

Figure 33-4 Chemical structure of penicillins

The representative structures of pencillins include: ①β-lactam ring. ②Thiazolidine ring

1.3.1 Penicillin G(青霉素G)

【Pharmacokinetics】Penicillin G is not stable to gastric acid (胃酸) with low oral bioavailability, so penicillin G is administered intramuscularly and intravenously for clinical use. Intravenous administration of penicillin G is preferred to the intramuscular route because of irritation and local pain from intramuscular injection of large doses. The normal half-life of penicillin G is approximately 30 minutes. Penicillin G is mainly excreted by the kidneys and can cross the blood-brain barrier with active inflammation in the meninges.

【Pharmacodynamics】Penicillin G is a bactericidal drug, with a limited spectrum of antibacterial activity. Penicillin G is active against Gram-positive cocci (球菌), Gram-positive bacilli (杆菌), Gram-negative cocci, non-β-lactamase-producing anaerobes (厌氧菌), spirochetes (螺旋体) and *Actinomyces* (放线菌).

【Clinical indications】Penicillin G is a choice for therapy of infections caused by susceptible *Streptococci*, *Meningococci* (脑膜炎双球菌), *Enterococci* (肠球菌), and *Pneumococci* (肺炎链球菌), including pneumonia (肺炎), meningitis (脑膜炎), enterocolitis (小肠结肠炎), etc. Activity against

Enterococci is increased by the combination with aminoglycosides (氨基糖苷类). Penicillin G remains the drug of choice for some Gram-positive *Corynebacterium* (棒状杆菌), *Clostridium* (梭状杆菌), *Actinomyces* and spirochetes infections, including diphtheria (白喉), tetanus (破伤风), syphilis (梅毒), etc.

【Adverse reactions】

(1) Hypersensitivity Allergic reactions are the most common adverse effect of penicillin G, including fever, dermatitis (皮炎), etc. Anaphylactic shock (过敏性休克) is the most serious allergy induced by penicillin G. Antigenic determinants include degradation products of penicillin G such as penicilloic acid. Penicillin skin testing must be used for prophylaxis of allergic reactions before treatment. Most patients allergic to penicillins can be treated with alternative drugs.

(2) Herxheimer reaction (赫氏反应) A spirochetal patient injected by penicillin G may exert shivering (寒战), fever, myalgia (肌痛), and even exacerbation of lesions (症状加剧), because of sudden release of spirochetal lytic products after penicillin G treatment.

(3) Others Pain and inflammation at the injection site are common when administered intramuscularly. Penicillin G treatment may also produce hyperkalemia (高钾血症), hypernatremia (高钠血症), etc.

1.3.2 Semisynthetic penicillins

Penicillin subclasses with semisynthetic chemical substituents confer unique antibacterial activities and different pharmacokinetic profiles, such as spectrum, susceptibility to acid and resistance to enzymatic hydrolysis.

(1) Acid-resistant penicillins Penicillin V is gastric acid stable and can be given orally. The antibacterial spectrum of penicillin V is similar to penicillin G, but much less active against *Neisseria* (奈瑟菌), other Gram-negative bacteria and anaerobes. Thus, penicillin V is mainly used to treat infections caused by susceptible microorganism through oral administration.

(2) Penicillinase-resistant penicillins These drugs, including methicillin (甲氧西林), oxacillin (苯唑西林), cloxacillin (氯唑西林) and dicloxacillin (双氯西林), have side chains that prevent the β-lactam ring from attacking by penicillinases. Oxacillin, dicloxacillin, and cloxacillin are eliminated by kidney and bile. They are active against penicillinase-producing staphylococci, but they are much less active against non-penicillinase-producing microorganisms. They cannot be against MRSA and methicillin-resistant *Staphylococci epidermidis* (MRSE). Their primary use is in the treatment for susceptible penicillinase-producing staphylococci infections. For the adverse reactions, oxacillin can cause hepatitis; Methicillin commonly causes interstitial nephritis. Methicillin is the first antistaphylococcal penicillin to be developed and is no longer used clinically due to high rates of adverse reactions.

(3) Broad-spectrum penicillins These drugs, including ampicillin (氨苄西林) and amoxicillin (阿莫西林), retain the antibacterial spectrum of penicillin G and are also active against Gram-negative cocci. They are acid-resistant, but they are inactivated by penicillinases. Particularly, they could not be used to treat *Pseudomonas aeruginosa* (铜绿假单胞菌) infections. They are not degraded by gastric acid. The extended-spectrum penicillins are secreted more slowly than penicillin G and have a half-life of 1 hour. Oral administration of these drugs could treat susceptible microorganism infections, especially respiratory and urinary tract infections. Food interferes with the absorption of ampicillin. Amoxicillin is partly excreted in bile, so ampicillin is a good drug for cholecystitis (胆囊炎). Diarrhoea (腹泻) is frequent after oral administration of ampicillin. Food does not interfere with absorption of amoxicillin. Incidence of diarrhoea after oral padmministration of amoxicillin is lower than ampicillin.

(4) Antipseudomonal penicillins These drugs, including carbenicillin (羧苄西林), piperacillin (哌拉西林) and ticarcillin (替卡西林), are used for serious infections with Gram-negative bacteria, especially *Pseudomonas aeruginosa*. These drugs are not acid-resistant and penicillinase-resistant. Carbenicillin is inactive orally and is excreted rapidly in urine with a half-life of 1 hour. The use for carbenicillin is serious infections caused by *Pseudomonas* or *Proteus*, e.g., burns, urinary tract infection, and septicaemia. Ticarcillin is susceptible to penicillinases and often used in combination with penicillinase inhibitors [e.g., clavulanic acid (克拉维酸)] to enhance the activity. Most drugs in this subgroup exert synergistic reactions with aminoglycosides. Piperacillin-tazobactam, when combined with vancomycin, has been associated with greater incidence of acute kidney injury compared to alternate β-lactam agents. The antipseudomonal activity of piperacillin is about 8 times more active than carbenicillin with a half-life of 1 hour.

1.4 Cephalosporins

The cephalosporins are derivatives of 7-aminocephalosporanic acid (7-ACA), containing a β-lactam ring (Figure 33-5). Cephalosporins also bind to PBPs, inhibiting bacterial cell wall synthesis. Structural differences from penicillins make them less susceptible to penicillinases, but some bacteria can produce other β-lactamases, resulting in the resistance to cephalosporins. Patients allergic to penicillins can take cephalosporins instead. Local pain occurs after intramuscular injection. Some of them have

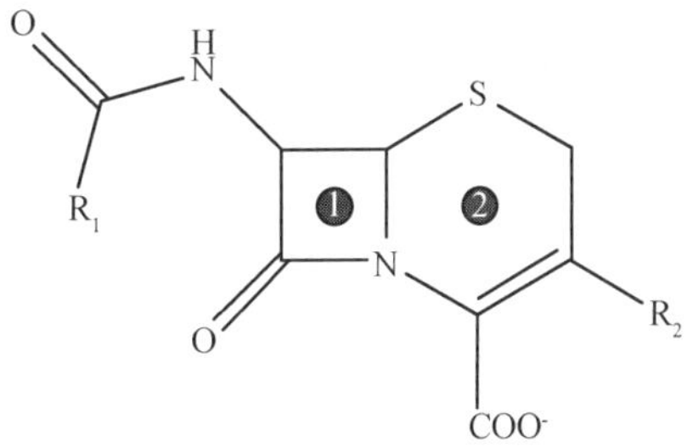

Figure 33-5 Chemical structure of cephalosporins
The representative structures of cephalosporins include: ①β-lactam ring. ②Hydrothiazine ring

nephrotoxicity. Cephalosporins vary in their antibacterial activity and have traditionally been classified into five major generations, depending mainly on the order of their introduction into clinical use.

1.4.1 First-generation cephalosporins

These drugs, including cefazolin (头孢唑啉), cephalexin (头孢氨苄), cefadroxil (头孢羟氨苄), cephalothin and cephradine (头孢拉定), are very active against Gram-positive cocci, such as *Staphylococcus* and *Streptococcus*, and have minimal activity against Gram-negative bacteria. Excretion is mainly by glomerular filtration and tubular secretion into the urine. These drugs exert obvious nephrotoxicity. Cephalexin is the oral first-generation cephalosporin, and cefazolin is the only parenteral first-generation cephalosporin still in general use. Oral cephalosporins are mostly used for skin and soft tissue infections. The antibacterial activity of cefadroxil is similar to cefazolin, with a half-life of 1 hour. It is excreted unchanged in urine. Cefazolin penetrates well into most tissues and is mostly used for infections caused by Gram-positive bacteria requiring intravenous therapy. Cefazolin does not penetrate the central nervous system and cannot be used to treat meningitis. It has a half-life of 2 hours.

1.4.2 Second-generation cephalosporins

These drugs, including cefaclor (头孢克洛), cefamandole (头孢孟多), cefonicid (头孢西尼), cefuroxime (头孢呋辛) and cefuroxime axetil (酯), are more active against Gram-negative bacteria, and have slightly less activity against Gram-positive bacteria than first-generation cephalosporins. The nephrotoxicity of these drugs decreases compared to first-generation cephalosporins. They can inhibit some anaerobes. The oral second-generation cephalosporins are active against β-lactamase-producing *Moraxella catarrhalis* and have been used primarily to treat sinusitis, otitis, and lower respiratory tract infections. Among them, cefuroxime axetil is effective orally, though absorption is incomplete. Cefaclor has a significant activity by the oral uptake. Cefuroxime is resistant to most β-lactamases produced by Gram-negative bacteria. It is sometimes used to treat community-acquired pneumonia.

1.4.3　Third-generation cephalosporins

These drugs, including cefoperazone (头孢哌酮), cefotaxime (头孢噻肟), ceftazidime (头孢他啶), ceftriaxone (头孢曲松), and cefixime (头孢克肟), have highly augmented activity against Gram-negative bacteria and are less active on Gram-positive bacteria than second-generation cephalosporins. Additionally, third generation cephalosporins have a high activity against *Pseudomonas aeruginosa* and increased activity against β-lactamases, but they are not resistant to extended-spectrum β-lactamases. These drugs are not nephrotoxic. Most of them, except cefoperazone and cefixime, can penetrate the blood-brain barrier. Cefixime is an orally active third-generation cephalosporin and is resistant to many β-lactamases. After 1g intravenous infusion of a parenteral third-generation cephalosporin, serum levels are 60-140μg/ml. Ceftazidime and cefoperazone have stronger activity against *Pseudomonas aeruginosa* than other third-generation cephalosporins. Ceftriaxone has a longer duration of action differing from others. Cefotaxime is not active on anaerobes, while cefoperazone is active on anaerobes. Ceftriaxone and cefotaxime can be used to treat serious infections caused by pencillin-non-susceptible strains.

1.4.4　Fourth-generation cephalosporins

These drugs, including cefepime (头孢吡肟) and cefpirome (头孢匹罗), are more resistant to hydrolysis by chromosomal β-lactamases. However, they are not resistant to extended-spectrum β-lactamases. They are often used for hospital-acquired infections. They are more potent against Gram-positive and some Gram-negative bacteria than third-generation cephalosporins. They can also inhibit *Pseudomonas aeruginosa*. Cefepime has good activity against Enterobacteriaceae, methicillin-susceptible *S. aureus*, and *S. pneumoniae*. Cefepime penetrates well into cerebrospinal fluid. Cefepime is exerted by the kidneys and has a half-life of 2 hours.

1.4.5　Fifth-generation cephalosporins

These drugs include ceftobiprole (头孢比罗) and ceftaroline (头孢洛林). They have a good inhibition on PBP2a, suggesting the use for MRSA infections in clinical. Ceftobiprole has anti-pseudomonal activity and is more resistant to β-lactamases. Ceftaroline has activity against MRSA, with no effect on *Pseudomonas aeruginosa* or vancomycin-resistant enterococci. Ceftaroline is not active against AmpC or extended-pectrum β-lactamase-producing organisms.

1.5　Other β-lactams

1.5.1　Monobactams

Monobactams are drugs with a monocyclic β-lactam ring, mainly inhibiting Gram-negative bacteria. Unlike other β-lactam antibiotics, their antibacterial spectrum includes none of Gram-positive bacteria or anaerobes. Aztreonam (氨曲南) is the mainly prescribed in their family. It is excerted unchanged in urine with a half-life of 1.8 hours. Penicillin-allergic patients tolerate aztreonam without reaction. It preferentially binds to PBP3 and is synergistic with aminoglycosides. It is stable to many β-lactamases including AmpC β-lactamases and extended-spectrum β-lactamases. It penetrates well into the cerebrospinal fluid. It could be used for penicillin-allergic patients with serious infections such as pneumonia, meningitis, and sepsis caused by susceptible Gram-negative bacteria. The main use of aztreonam is hospital acquired infections originating from urinary, biliary, gastrointestinal and female genital tracts.

1.5.2   Carbapenems

These drugs, including doripenem (多尼培南), ertapenem (厄他培南), imipenem (亚胺培南), and meropenem (美罗培南), are structurally containing the β-lactam ring with low susceptibility to β-lactamases. These drugs have a wide spectrum with good activity against most Gram-positive bacteria and Gram-negative bacteria. Thus, they are frequently used for infections caused by drug-resistant bacteria, except MRSA. Imipenem is the first drug of this class. It is resistant to most β-lactamases. It inhibits penicillinase producing staphylococci, but it is not used to treat MRSA infections in clinical. Meanwhile, it is not resistant to carbapenemases or metallo-β-lactamases. It is easily inactivated by dehydropeptidases (DHP) in renal tubules. Consequently, imipenem must be co-administrated with cilastatin, a DHP-I inhibitor, for clinical use. Imipenem and cilastatin have a half-life of 1 hour. Common adverse reactions include nausea, vomiting, diarrhea, skin rashes, and reactions at the infusion sites. Imipenem-cilastatin can even cause renal impairing and induce seizures. Additionally, it is partial cross-allergenicity with the penicillins. Doripenem and meropenem are similar to imipenem but have slightly greater activity against Gram-negative aerobes and slightly less activity against Gram-positive bacteria. Moreover, they are not significantly degraded by renal dehydropeptidase, so they do not require an inhibitor for clinical use. Meropenem is used for the treatment of serious nosocomial infections like septicaemia, febrile neutropenia, intraabdominal and pelvic infections, etc. caused by cephalosporin-resistant bacteria.

1.5.3   Cephamycins

The cephamycins are structurally similar to the cephalosporins, with an additional 7-α-methoxyl group, resulting in the high resistance to β-lactamases. Cephamycins have been shown to be stable against extended-spectrum β-lactamase producing organisms. Cephamycins can be against a broad spectrum of bacteria, including anaerobes. They improve the activity against Gram-negative bacteria and Gram-positive bacteria comparing to second-generation cephalosporins. Cefoxitin (头孢西丁) is the first semisynthetic cephamycin and almost resistant to all β-lactamases. Cefoxitin is bactericidal and can be used to treat *Bacteroides fragilis* (脆弱类杆菌属) infection. Cefoxitin is mainly used for infections by a mixture of aerobic and anaerobic pathogens in clinical.

1.5.4   Oxacephem(氧头孢烯类)

Oxacephem is a derivative of cephem, with an oxygen substituted for the sulfur. These drugs are broad-spectrum β-lactam antibiotics, including latamoxef (拉氧头孢) and flomoxef (氧氟头孢). They can inhibit Gram-positive bacteria, Gram-negative bacteria and anaerobic bacteria. Latamoxef can be used for meningitides with the ability to pass the blood-brain barrier. Flomoxef can be used for urinary tract infection.

1.5.5   β-lactamase inhibitors

β-lactamase inhibitors, e.g., clavulanic acid, sulbactam (舒巴坦), and tazobactam (他唑巴坦), resemble β-lactam molecules. These drugs can inhibit most bacterial β-lactamases and can prevent the β-lactam ring of other β-lactams from hydrolysis by these enzymes. They are most active against plasmid-encoded β-lactamases and have no activity against chromosomal β-lactamase. These drugs are often used with other β-lactams. Clavulanic acid has a β-lactam ring, with no antibacterial activity. The binding with β-lactamase is reversible. Clavulanic acid has a good oral bioavailability and can also be injected, with a half-life of 1 hour. Clavulanic acid is eliminated mainly by glomerular filtration and its excretion is not affected by probenecid. Addition of clavulanic acid enhance the activity of amoxicillin/ticarcillin against β-lactamase producing resistant bacteria. Sulbactam is a semisynthetic β-lactamase inhibitor. Oral absorption of sulbactam is inconsistent. Therefore, it is preferably given parenterally. Sulbactam has been combined with ampicillin, cefoperazone and ceftriaxone. Tazobactam has been combined with piperacillin and ceftriaxone. Its pharmacokinetics matches with piperacillin.

2. Other inhibitors of cell wall synthesis

2.1 Fosfomycin

Fosfomycin is an analog of phosphoenolpyruvate and it's structure is unrelated to any other antimicrobial agent. Fosfomycin is a bactericidal drug and inhibits a very early stage of bacterial cell wall synthesis by preventing the formation of UDP-N-acetylmuramic acid. The oral bioavailability is approximately 40%, with a half-life of approximately 4 hours. Fosfomycin has a broad spectrum of antibacterial activity, active against both Gram-positive and Gram-negative bacteria. Fosfomycin is used for susceptible strains infections, especially uncomplicated urinary tract infections. Fosfomycin is eliminated by the kidney with a low incidence of serious side effects. Resistance is due to inadequate transport of drug into the cell.

2.2 Cycloserine

Cycloserine is an analog of the amino acid D-alanine. Cycloserine interferes with an early step in bacterial cell wall synthesis in the cytoplasm by competitive inhibition of L-alanine racemase and D-alanylalanine synthetase. Cycloserine is a broad-spectrum antibiotic and active against Gram-positive and Gram-negative bacteria. Cycloserine is widely distributed in tissues. Most of the drug is excreted in active form into the urine. It has a half-life of 10 hours. It is used almost exclusively to treat tuberculosis caused by bacteria resistant to first-line agents.

2.3 Bacitracin

Bacitracin is a cyclic peptide mixture first obtained from *Bacillus subtilis*. Bacitracin is active against Gram-positive bacteria. It inhibits cell wall formation by interfering with dephosphorylation in cycling of the lipid carrier that transfers peptidoglycan subunits to the growing cell wall. Bacitracin is poorly absorbed. Bacitracin is highly nephrotoxic. It is often used to treat skin and eye infections.

2.4 Glycopeptides

Vancomycin and teicoplanin (替考拉宁) are glycopeptides. Vancomycin can primarily kill Gram-positive bacteria and is hard to penetrate through Gram-negative cell membranes due to its large molecular weight and size. Vancomycin is used for serious infections caused by susceptible microorganisms, mainly restricted to serious MRSA infections. Oral vancomycin is used to treat colitis caused by *Clostridium difficile*. Vancomycin binds to the D-Ala-D-Ala terminal of nascent peptidoglycan pentapeptide and inhibits the transglycosylase (转糖酶), affecting cell wall synthesis. The antibacterial action and spectrum of teicoplanin is similar to vancomycin. Adverse reactions of vancomycin include chills, fever, phlebitis, ototoxicity (耳毒性), and nephrotoxicity (肾毒性). Particularly, rapid intravenous infusion may cause "red man syndrome". It is the most common toxicity of vancomycin therapy and typical symptom is the reddening of the skin. The ototoxicity and nephrotoxicity of teicoplanin are less than vancomycin.

2.5 Daptomycin

Daptomycin is a novel cyclic lipopeptide fermentation product of *Streptomyces roseosporus*. Daptomycin is a bactericidal drug for treating infections caused by drug-resistant Gram-positive bacteria, especially vancomycin-resistant strains, so daptomycin is an alternative to vancomycin in some cases. The precise pharmacodynamics is not fully understood. Daptomycin could induce depolarization of the cell membrane, inhibit synthesis of DNA, RNA and protein, and suppress peptidoglycan synthesis. Daptomycin is eliminated by the kidney. The approved doses of daptomycin are 4mg/kg per dose for treatment of skin and soft tissue infections and 6mg/kg per dose for treatment of bacteremia and endocarditis once daily in patients with normal renal function.

重 点 小 结

药物	抗菌作用	临床应用	不良反应
β-内酰胺类抗生素	抑制细菌转肽酶、青霉素结合蛋白 PBP，抑制转肽过程，从而抑制细菌细胞壁的合成	详见青霉素类与头孢类	详见青霉素类与头孢类
青霉素 G	繁殖期杀菌药，主要抑制革兰阳性菌、革兰阴性球菌、部分厌氧菌、放线菌以及致病螺旋体	敏感菌引起的感染，如溶血性链球菌所致的败血症、草绿色链球菌所致的心内膜炎、气性坏疽、梅毒以及回归热	过敏反应、赫氏反应、局部反应、高血钠、高血钾
第一代头孢菌素	繁殖期杀菌药，抗菌谱与广谱青霉素相似，对革兰阴性菌作用差。对青霉素酶稳定，但易被头孢菌素酶分解	敏感菌引起的感染，如耐青霉素金黄色葡萄球菌感染	有一定的肾毒性
第二代头孢菌素	繁殖期杀菌药，抗革兰阳性菌作用弱于第一代，抗革兰阴性菌作用强于第一代，对厌氧菌有一定作用。对β-内酰胺酶稳定性增高	敏感菌引起的肺炎、胆道感染、菌血症、尿路感染等	肾毒性弱于第一代

续表

药物	抗菌作用	临床应用	不良反应
第三代头孢菌素	繁殖期杀菌药，抗革兰阳性菌作用弱于第一代、第二代，抗革兰阴性菌作用强于第一代、第二代，抗菌谱增宽，对厌氧菌和铜绿假单胞菌有一定作用。对大部分 β-内酰胺酶稳定	敏感菌所致的严重全身感染	基本没有肾毒性
第四代头孢菌素	繁殖期杀菌药，抗菌谱较第三代更宽，对革兰阳性球菌较第三代强，对多数耐药菌有效，但对 MRSA 和 MRSE 无效。极低的 β-内酰胺酶亲和性及诱导性	敏感菌所致的严重感染，如呼吸道感染、尿路生殖道感染、皮肤软组织感染	无肾毒性
第五代头孢菌素	繁殖期杀菌药，抗菌谱宽，主要针对 MRSA 和 MRSE	MRSA 或耐万古霉素 VRSA 引起的感染	无肾毒性
万古霉素	与细菌细胞壁前体 D-Ala-D-Ala 结合，干扰转糖作用与转肽作用，抑制细菌细胞壁合成。繁殖期杀菌药，对革兰阳性球菌有强大杀灭作用，特别是 MRSA 和 MRSE，对厌氧菌、革兰阴性菌无效	MRSA 与 MRSE 所致的严重感染。与氨基糖苷类联用可治疗肠球菌所致的心内膜炎症。口服可用于治疗难辨梭状芽孢杆菌结肠炎	副作用严重，如耳毒性、肾毒性、过敏反应、红人综合征
达托霉素	与细菌细胞壁前体 D-Ala-D-Ala 结合，干扰转糖作用与转肽作用，抑制细菌细胞壁合成。快速杀菌、窄谱抗菌药，对需氧革兰阳性菌有强杀灭作用，包括 MRSA 和 PRSP	敏感菌所致的皮肤及组织感染，MRSA 引起的心内膜炎	便秘、恶心、头痛、失眠
磷霉素	干扰黏肽合成的第一步，抑制细胞壁的合成。快速杀菌、广谱抗菌药，对革兰阳性菌、革兰阴性菌、MRSA、铜绿假单胞菌、部分厌氧菌均有良好抗菌作用	单用适用于敏感菌所致的轻中度感染	轻度胃肠道反应

题库

目 标 检 测

一、选择题

（一）单项选择题

1. β-内酰胺类抗生素的作用靶位是（　　）
   A. 细菌核蛋白体 50S 亚基　　　B. 青霉素结合蛋白 PBP
   C. 二氢叶酸还原酶　　　　　　　D. DNA 回旋酶
   E. 麦角固醇

2. 青霉素类最严重的不良反应是（　　）
   A. 电解质紊乱　　　　　　　　　B. 赫氏反应
   C. 菌群失调　　　　　　　　　　D. 过敏性休克
   E. 红人综合征

3. 对青霉素 G 的描述下列哪项错误（　　）

　　A. 不耐酸、不耐酶　　　　　　　　B. 其母核为 6-APA

　　C. 抗菌谱广　　　　　　　　　　　D. 对繁殖期的细菌有杀灭作用

　　E. 可能引起赫氏反应

4. 第一代头孢菌素与第三代头孢菌素相比叙述错误的是（　　）

　　A. 肾毒性大　　　　　　　　　　　B. 对革兰阳性菌作用强

　　C. 对 β- 内酰胺酶稳定性差　　　　　D. 对 MRSA 作用强

　　E. 对厌氧菌无效

5. 第一代头孢菌素主要用于（　　）

　　A. 耐药金黄色葡萄球菌感染　　　　B. 铜绿假单胞菌感染

　　C. 伤寒杆菌感染　　　　　　　　　D. 假丝酵母病

　　E. 耐药肠杆菌感染

（二）多项选择题

6. 青霉素 G 的抗菌谱包括（　　）

　　A. 脑膜炎球菌　　　　　B. 肺炎球菌　　　　　　　C. 白喉杆菌

　　D. 伤寒杆菌　　　　　　E. 钩端螺旋体

7. 头孢哌酮抗菌作用的特点是（　　）

　　A. 对铜绿假单胞菌有较强的作用　　B. 对厌氧菌有较强的作用

　　C. 对 β- 内酰胺酶稳定性差　　　　　D. 对金黄色葡萄球菌抗菌作用强

　　E. 对肾基本无毒性

二、思考题

试从 β- 内酰胺类抗生素的作用机制解释其耐药机制。

（彭　芙）

PPT

Chapter 34   Aminoglycosides

 学习目标

    1.掌握 氨基糖苷的抗菌作用机制、常见不良反应机制及症状。

    2.熟悉 链霉素、庆大霉素、妥布霉素、阿米卡星和依替米星的主要药理作用和临床应用。

    3.了解 氨基糖苷的化学结构、来源、临床抗菌谱。

Aminoglycosides (氨基糖苷) are polycationic compounds, all actions of which are linked to the glycoside chain by a cyclic alcohol ring containing an amino group. Because it has a glycosyl group, pharmacokinetics exhibits the characteristics of polar compounds, such as difficult absorption by oral administration, poor blood barrier permeability, and faster renal excretion. Aminoglycosides are derived from actinomycetes (放线菌属) in the soil, such as Streptomyces and Micromonas. Amikacin (阿米卡星) was obtained after artificial modification of the chemical kanamycin, and etimicin (依替米星) was obtained after the modification of sisomicin.

1. Common properties of aminoglycosides

【Pharmacodynamics】Aminoglycosides can destroy the integrity of cell membranes through ion adsorption. Aminoglycosides enter the cytoplasm (胞质) through water channels formed by the outer membrane pores of Gram-negative bacteria (革兰阴性菌). Because the cation or hypertonicity can reduce the membrane's transport ability, the antibacterial activity of aminoglycoside is significantly reduced when abscesses (脓肿) or hypertonic acidic urine(Figure 34-1).

Aminoglycosides mainly affect the initiation, extension and termination of bacterial protein synthesis. This effect works by binding to the target protein on the 30S small subunit of the bacterial ribosome. If this protein is mutated, the bacterium becomes resistant to aminoglycosides.

Aminoglycoside has a rapid bactericidal effect (杀菌作用), and its concentration dependence is more significant. Aminoglycosides have significant post-antibacterial effects (抗菌后效应). Therefore, it is usually administered once a day.

【Antibacterial spectrum】Aminoglycosides have no antibacterial activity against anaerobic microorganisms (厌氧微生物) and facultative bacteria (兼性细菌) living under anaerobic conditions.

医药大学堂
WWW.YIYAODXT.COM

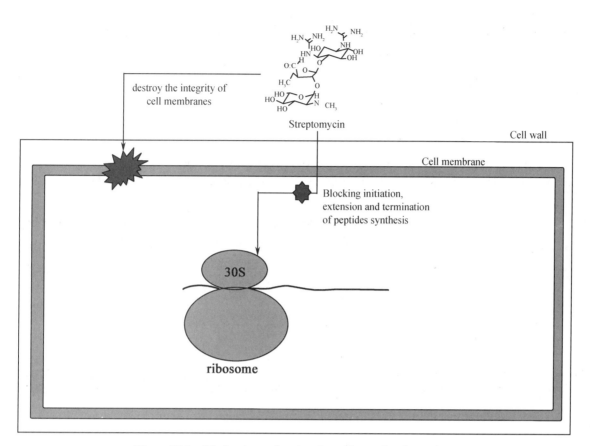

Figure 34-1　Mechanisms of aminoglycosides against bacterium

Aminoglycosides have very limited effects on Gram-positive bacteria (革兰阳性菌). Aminoglycosides are mainly used for infections caused by aerobic Gram-negative bacteria (需氧革兰阴性细菌), such as *Citrobacter* (枸橼酸杆菌), *Enterobacter* (肠杆菌属), *Pneumococcus* (肺炎杆菌), *Staphylococcus aureus* (金黄色葡萄球菌), *Enterococcus faecalis* (粪肠球菌), *Serratia* (沙雷菌属), etc. Gentamycin, tobramycin, etifloxacin, and amikacin have a broad spectrum of action, while kanamycin and streptomycin have a smaller antibacterial spectrum and cannot be used for *Serratia* and *Pseudomonas aeruginosa* (铜绿假单胞菌).

【Resistance】There are three main reasons for the resistance of microorganisms to aminoglycosides, including the reduction of aminoglycoside permeability due to the variation of cell membrane water proteins, the decrease of ribosome protein variation and the binding force, and the production of aminoglycoside inactivated enzymes.

【Adverse reactions】Aminoglycosides are more severely toxic, with nephrotoxicity and ototoxicity being the most dangerous.

(1) **Nephrotoxicity (肾毒性)**   Aminoglycosides are prone to accumulate in the proximal tubules (近端肾小管), resulting in a decrease in renal concentrating function, proteinuria (蛋白尿) and granular tubular urine (颗粒管型尿). The patient's plasma creatinine (肌酐) will increase slightly. Due to the remodeling function of proximal tubule cells, this toxic effect is often reversible. Neomycin (新霉素) is relatively nephrotoxic, and its systemic administration is forbidden clinically. In general, nephrotoxic drugs should be avoided in combination to avoid more significant renal toxicity, such as furosemide (呋塞米).

(2) **Ototoxicity (耳毒性)**   Aminoglycosides accumulate in the lymph (淋巴) of the inner ear,

273

destroying sensory cells in the vestibule (前庭) and cochlea (耳蜗). This cellular damage is often irreversible. Toxic effects are manifested by vestibular dysfunction and deafness. Vestibular dysfunction manifests as headache, nausea (恶心), vomiting, orthostatic vertigo (直立性眩晕), and ataxia (共济失调). Cochlear toxicity is early manifested as treble tinnitus (高音耳鸣). If continuing to use the medicine after cell damage, permanent deafness will occur. In general, hearing loss in older people is more pronounced than in younger people.

Hearing tests should be strengthened when clinical use of aminoglycosides, but it should also be noted that very few patients will develop deafness even after stopping the drug after long-term or high-dose use.

(3) Neuromuscular blockade (神经肌肉阻滞) Neuromuscular blockade may occur after high-dose aminoglycoside injections, with neomycin being the most common. This side effect occurs more frequently in patients with myasthenia gravis (重症肌无力) when using aminoglycosides.

(4) Other adverse reactions Allergic reactions (过敏反应) are rare, so as the flora disorders (菌群失调症).

2. Drugs in common use

Streptomycin (链霉素)

Streptomycin was the first aminoglycoside to be used clinically and is now relatively rare. Streptomycin has a weaker effect on aerobic Gram-negative bacteria than other aminoglycosides. Intramuscular injection is often used, and clinical attention may be given to the formation of induration at the injection site. Streptomycin is the most effective drug in the treatment of pestilence (鼠疫). Streptomycin can also be used in the treatment of tuberculosis (结核) , but it is generally required to be combined. Streptomycin has significant ototoxicity, and the effect of early vestibular function is obvious. Once deafness occurs, it is more irreversible.

Gentamicin (庆大霉素)

Gentamicin is mainly used intramuscularly or intravenously. Although its efficacy is exact, it is severely and highly toxic due to ototoxicity and nephrotoxicity, and is therefore strictly restricted for use in critical infections. Gentamicin is commonly used clinically for pneumonia (肺炎), urinary tract infection, and peritonitis (腹膜炎) caused by *Pneumococcus*, *Enterobacter*, *Serratia* and *Pseudomonas aeruginosa*. It is often used clinically as the antibiotic of choice for *Serratia*. Gentamicin can also be applied topically, often using creams or oils, and can be used in burn patients.

Tobramycin (妥布霉素)

Tobramycin can be administered intramuscularly or intravenously. Tobramycin is commonly used clinically for pneumonia, urinary tract infection, and peritonitis caused by *Pneumoniae*, *Enterobacter*, *Serratia* and *Pseudomonas aeruginosa*. In particular, tobramycin has a strong antibacterial effect on

Pseudomonas aeruginosa. Ophthalmology is also common by using eye drops of tobramycin.

Amikacin (阿米卡星)

Amikacin has a therapeutic effect on gentamicin and tobramycin resistant bacteria. Amikacin is usually used intramuscularly and intravenously. Amikacin is effective against gentamicin and tobramycin-resistant *Pneumococci*, *Enterobacteria*, and *E. coli*.

Kanamycin (卡那霉素)

It is relatively toxic and not commonly used. It is currently used clinically for the treatment of drug-resistant bacteria.

Etimicin (依替米星)

It is obtained by modifying sisomicin. Etimicin has a broad antibacterial spectrum and strong antibacterial activity. Etimicin toxicity is the lowest among aminoglycosides. Etimicin still retains antibacterial activity against some gentamicin-resistant bacteria. It is commonly used in adults for urinary tract infections caused by sensitive bacteria, and can also be used for a variety of infectious diseases in pediatrics.

重 点 小 结

分项	内容
作用机制	通过离子吸附作用破坏细胞膜的完整性；与细菌核糖体的 30S 小亚基上的靶蛋白结合，影响细菌蛋白质合成的始动、延伸和终止 3 个过程
抗菌谱和耐药性	主要用于需氧革兰阴性细菌引起的感染；对厌氧微生物和生活在厌氧条件下的兼性细菌没有抗菌活性；对革兰阳性菌作用极为有限。微生物对氨基糖苷具耐药性主要有三种原因：细胞膜水蛋白的变异导致氨基糖苷渗透力降低、核糖体蛋白变异而结合力降低和产生氨基糖苷的灭活酶
不良反应	具有较为严重的毒性，尤以肾毒性和耳毒性最为危险。易在近端肾小管蓄积，出现蛋白尿、颗粒管型尿。在内耳的淋巴中蓄积，破坏前庭和耳蜗内的感觉细胞，常不可逆，表现为前庭功能失调和耳聋

目 标 检 测

题库

一、选择题

（一）单项选择题

1. 氨基糖苷类抗生素的抗菌机制是（　　　）
   A. 抑制黏肽的合成而使细胞壁缺损
   B. 抑制叶酸的合成
   C. 离子吸附影响细胞膜的通透性
   D. 干扰核酸的合成
   E. 抑制细菌蛋白质的合成而杀菌

2. 氨基糖苷类药物的不良反应不含（　　　）

    A. 耳毒性　　　　　　　　　　　B. 肝毒性　　　　　　　　C. 肾毒性

    D. 神经肌肉阻断作用　　　　　　E. 过敏反应

3. 治疗鼠疫的首选药物是（　　　）

    A. 氯霉素　　　　　　　　　　　B. 四环素　　　　　　　　C. 罗红霉素

    D. 链霉素　　　　　　　　　　　E. 头孢他啶

4. 氨基糖苷类抗生素对哪类细菌无效（　　　）

    A. 需氧革兰阴性菌　　　　　　　B. 耐甲氧西林金黄色葡萄球菌　　C. 沙门菌属

    D. 厌氧菌和肠球菌　　　　　　　E. 革兰阳性菌

（二）多项选择题

5. 关于氨基糖苷类引起肾毒性叙述正确的是（　　　）

    A. 与药物主要经肾排泄并在肾蓄积有关

    B. 肾皮质内药物浓度蓄积越高，对肾毒性越大

    C. 主要影响肾小球

    D. 与其他肾毒性药物合用时易发生肾功能损害

    E. 与药物和血浆蛋白结合导致排泄慢有关

6. 关于氨基糖苷类抗生素叙述错误的是（　　　）

    A. 口服在胃肠道不吸收，用于胃肠道消毒

    B. 属杀菌药且对繁殖期细菌作用较强

    C. 肾皮质内药物浓度高于血药浓度

    D. 不能进入内耳外淋巴液

    E. 在体内不被代谢，多以原型经排出

二、思考题

氨基糖苷类抗生素主要有哪些不良反应？

（王　平）

Chapter 35　Synthetic antibacterial drugs

PPT

 学习目标

　　1. **掌握**　喹诺酮类、磺胺类和甲氧苄啶的抗菌作用机制、常见不良反应机制及症状。

　　2. **熟悉**　诺氟沙星、氧氟沙星、环丙沙星、莫西沙星和磺胺的主要药理作用和临床应用。

　　3. **了解**　喹诺酮、磺胺和甲氧苄啶的产生历史、临床抗菌谱。

Antibacterial drugs produced by chemical synthesis methods are called artificial antibacterial drugs. Common synthetic antibacterial drugs include quinolone (喹诺酮类) and sulfonamide (磺胺). Quinolones have a broad antibacterial spectrum and good pharmacokinetics (药物代谢动力学) properties. Sulfonamide is one of the earliest antibacterial drugs used clinically, but it has been used less frequently, due to its many adverse reactions (不良反应).

1. Quinolone

Quinolone has a 4-pyridone-3-carboxylic acid (4-吡啶酮-3-羧酸) in its chemical structure. The first and second generation quinolones are derived from the by-products of chloroquine (氯喹) synthesis and have been withdrawn from the clinic due to their relatively high toxicity. The third-generation quinolone has a fluoro group substitution at the 6-position of 4-pyridone-3carboxylic acid, so it is also called fluoroquinolone (氟喹诺酮). The safety of fluoroquinolones has been significantly improved, and it is currently widely used. Common fluoroquinolones include norfloxacin (诺氟沙星), ofloxacin, levofloxacin (左氧氟沙星), pefloxacin (培氟沙星), enoxacin (依诺沙星), ciprofloxacin (环丙沙星), etc. The fluoroquinolones are further modified to enhance the effects on anaerobic and Gram-positive bacteria, and fourth-generation quinolones are obtained, such as gatifloxacin, travafloxacin, clinfloxacin, and moxifloxacin.

1.1　Common properties of quinolone

【Pharmacokinetics】The third or fourth generation of quinolones are better absorbed orally,

医药大学堂
WWW.YIYAODXT.COM

277

and some varieties can also be administered intravenously (静脉给药). Fluoroquinolones are widely distributed and high in concentration. Fluoroquinolones have a longer plasma half-life (血浆半衰期), a lower plasma protein binding rate, and most are excreted in the urine. Because ciprofloxacin, levofloxacin, moxifloxacin have higher concentrations in the lung tissue, they are also known as respiratory quinolone (呼吸喹诺酮).

【Pharmacodynamics】Quinolones can inhibit the DNA gyrase (促旋酶) of Gram-negative bacteria, prevent the DNA double helix structure of the uncoiling bacteria, thereby reducing bacterial replication. Quinolones can also interfere with the isomerases (异构酶) of Gram-positive bacteria. First, second, and third generation quinolones have good antibacterial activity against Gram-negative bacteria such as *Escherichia coli* (大肠埃希菌), *Shigella* (痢疾杆菌), *Klebsiella* (克雷伯杆菌), a small number of *Proteus*, *Enterobacter*, *Citrobacter*, *Pseudomonas aeruginosa*, *Serratia*, etc. Third generation quinolone-fluoroquinolone also has a good effect on Gram-positive bacteria such as *Staphylococcus*, *Chlamydia*, *Mycoplasma*, *Legionella* and *Mycobacterium*. The fourth generation quinolone further enhanced the effects of anaerobic bacteria (厌氧菌) such as fragile bacteria. The bacteria changed the structure of DNA gyrase through chromosome mutation (突变), which caused drug resistance（Figure 35-1）.

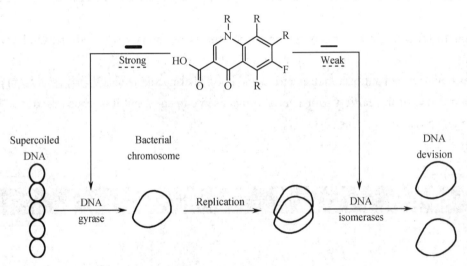

Figure 35-1　Mechanisms of quinolones against bacterium

【Adverse reactions】

(1) **Gastrointestinal reactions**　nausea, vomiting, etc. It is the most common adverse reaction of quinolone.

(2) **Central reactions**　headache, dizziness, poor sleep, etc.

Quinolone can inhibit γ-aminobutyric acid (γ-氨基丁酸), so it can induce epilepsy (癫痫). Quinolone can affect cartilage development (软骨发育). Therefore, pregnant women and underage children should be used with caution.Quinolone can cause photosensitivity reactions (光过敏反应).Quinolone can produce crystalline urine (结晶尿). Large doses or long-term application of quinolone can cause liver damage and cardiotoxicity (心脏毒性).

1.2   Drugs in common use

Norfloxacin (诺氟沙星)

Norfloxacin is the first fluoroquinolone. Norfloxacin has good antibacterial activity against Gram-positive and negative bacteria, including *Pseudomonas aeruginosa*. Norfloxacin is orally absorbed by about 35% to 45%, but is easily affected by food. Norfloxacin has 2-3 times higher blood levels on an empty stomach than after taking a meal with Plasma protein binding rate is 14%, widely distributed in the body with high tissue concentration, and drug elimination half-life is 3 to 4 hours. Mainly used for urinary tract and intestinal infections.

Levofloxacin (左氧氟沙星)

Levofloxacin has a strong effect on Gram-positive bacteria and Gram-negative bacteria, including *Pseudomonas aeruginosa*; it also has certain activity on *Mycoplasma* pneumoniae, *Neisseria* disease, anaerobic bacteria, and *Tuberculosis bacteria*. Oral absorption is fast and complete, high blood concentration and long-lasting, plasma elimination half-life is 5-7 hours, the drug is widely distributed in the body, especially in high sputum concentration, 70% to 90% of the drug is excreted by the kidney, 48 hours of urine drug. The concentration can still reach the level of sterilization of sensitive bacteria, and the drug concentration in bile is about 7 times the blood concentration.

Ciprofloxacin (环丙沙星)

The antibacterial activity of ciprofloxacin *in vitro* is currently the strongest among quinolone in clinical application. Ciprofloxacin is effective against drug-resistant *Pseudomonas aeruginosa*, MRSA, penicillin-producing *Neisseria gonorrhoeae*, enzyme-producing influenza bacilli, *Legionella pneumoniae*, and *Campylobacter*. Some Gram-negative and positive bacteria that are resistant to aminoglycosides and third generation cephalosporins are still sensitive to ciprofloxacin. After oral administration, the bioavailability of this product is 38% to 60%, and the blood concentration is low. Intravenous infusion can make up for this shortcoming. The half-life is 3.3 to 5.8 hours, and it is widely distributed in the body after drug absorption.

Moxifloxacin (莫西沙星)

Moxifloxacin is a fourth generation quinolone antibacterial. Moxifloxacin has strong antibacterial activity against *Streptococcus pneumoniae*, *Haemophilus influenzae*, *Moraxella catarrhalis*, and *Staphylococcus aureus*. Clinically used to treat acute sinusitis, community-acquired pneumonia, and uncomplicated skin infections and skin and soft tissue infections. Moxifloxacin has almost no photosensitivity, has good tissue penetration, and can reach high concentrations in lung tissues. It is a good drug for treating respiratory infections.

2. Sulfonamides and trimethoprim

Sulfonamides are derivatives with p-aminobenzenesulfonamide (对氨基苯磺酰胺) as the basic structure. In 1932, prontosil was found to fight the infection of *Streptococcus* (链球菌). In 1935, sulfonamides was used clinically. Trimethoprim (甲氧苄啶) was discovered in 1969, forming a compound preparation in combination with sulfonamide. The use of this compound enhances the effects of sulfonamide and increases its range of treatment.

【Pharmacodynamics】 Sulfonamide can bind dihydrofolate synthase (二氢叶酸合成酶), which affects the bacterial dihydrofolate synthesis, and thus inhibits the growth and reproduction of bacteria. Trimethoprim can affect dihydrofolate reductase (二氢叶酸还原酶). The combination of the two can systematically affect the production of tetrahydrofolate required by bacteria. Sulfamethoxazole and trimethoprim are made into compound at a ratio of 5 : 1, and the antibacterial effect can be multiplied to dozens of times.

Sulfonamide is effective against Gram-positive *Streptococcus* and *Pneumococcus* (肺炎球菌). Among the Gram-negative bacteria, *Meningococcus*, *E. coli*, *Proteus*, *Dysentery bacillus*, and *Plague bacillus* are sensitive to sulfonamide. Bacteria can develop resistance to sulfonamide by changing the metabolic pathway of folic acid.

【Classification】

(1) Intestinal easily absorbed sulfonamide drugs (肠道易吸收的磺胺药)   Mainly used for systemic infections, such as sepsis, urinary tract infections, typhoid fever, osteomyelitis, etc. The short-acting class absorbs quickly in the intestine and excretes quickly. The half-life is 5 to 6 hours. It needs to be taken 4 times a day, such as sulfamethazine (SM2) and sulfisoxazole (SIZ). The median-acting class, take medication twice daily, such as sulfadiazine (SD), sulfamethoxazole (SMZ). The long-acting half-life is more than 24 hours, such as sulfadiazine (SMD), sulfadiazine (SDM) and so on.

(2) Digestive sulfa drugs (肠道难吸收的磺胺药)   It maintains high drug concentration in the intestine. It is mainly used for intestinal infections, such as bacillary dysentery, enteritis, phthalazamide (PST), etc.

(3) Topical sulfa drugs (外用磺胺药)   Mainly used for burn infections, purulent wound infections, ophthalmic diseases, such as sulfacetamide (SA), silver sulfadiazine (SD-Ag), and mesosulfur purulent (SML).

【Clinical indications】 The first dose of sulfonamides is often doubled. Clinically, it is mainly used in the following aspects. ①Epidemic cerebrospinal meningitis (流行性脑脊髓膜炎). The highest concentration of sulfadiazine penetrated into the cerebrospinal fluid. Therefore, when treating meningitis, sulfadiazine is preferred. ②Urinary tract infection. Generally, a sulfa drug with a large solubility and a large amount excreted from the urine is selected. Commonly used SIZ, SMZ. ③Respiratory and pharynx infections. Acute upper and lower respiratory tract infections caused by bacteria. SMZ + TMP is commonly used in clinical practice. ④Intestinal infection. Generally, sulfa drugs that are difficult to absorb in the gastrointestinal tract are used. ⑤Local infection. Select topical sulfa drugs.

【Adverse reactions】

(1) Allergic reactions   The most common are rashes (皮疹) and fevers, especially common in children. There is cross-allergy between sulfa drugs.

(2) Kidney damage   Sulfonamide has low solubility, especially when urine is acidic, and crystals are easily precipitated in renal tubules. The following measures can be taken to prevent: add bicarbonate (碳酸氢盐)or citrate (柠檬酸) to alkalinize urine and increase the solubility of excretion; drink plenty of water and increase urine output.

(3) Impact of the hematopoietic system   Sulfonamides can inhibit bone marrow leukocyte (白细胞) formation and cause leukopenia. Occasionally, agranulocytosis can be recovered after drug withdrawal. Hematology should be checked for long-term application of sulfa drugs. It can cause hemolytic anemia for those who are congenitally lacking 6-phosphate glucose dehydrogenase. Sulfonamides can enter the fetal circulation through the mother's body, competing with free bilirubin (胆红素) for plasma protein binding sites, increasing the concentration of free bilirubin and causing jaundice (黄疸). Sulfonamides are not suitable for pregnant women, newborns, especially premature babies.

(4) Central nervous system and gastrointestinal reactions   They are mostly due to the high amount of sulfonamides.

重 点 小 结

药物	分项	内容
喹诺酮类	作用机制	可抑制革兰阴性菌的DNA促旋酶，干扰革兰阳性菌的局部异构酶
	抗菌谱和耐药性	一、二和三代喹诺酮对革兰阴性菌均具有良好的抗菌活性。三代喹诺酮——氟喹诺酮等对葡萄球菌等革兰阳性菌、衣原体、支原体、军团菌及分枝杆菌也有较好的作用。四代喹诺酮对脆弱拟杆菌等厌氧菌作用进一步增强。敏感菌通过染色体突变，使DNA促旋酶结构发生变化从而出现了耐药现象
	不良反应	胃肠道反应是喹诺酮最为常见的不良反应；可致中枢反应；可抑制γ-氨基丁酸，因此可诱发癫痫；可影响软骨发育；可致光过敏反应；可产生结晶尿；大剂量或长期使用可致肝损害和心脏毒性
磺胺类	作用机制	磺胺可结合二氢叶酸合成酶，从而影响细菌的二氢叶酸合成；甲氧苄啶可影响二氢叶酸还原酶。二者合用，可系统影响细菌所需四氢叶酸的生成
	分类	①肠道易吸收的磺胺药：如磺胺嘧啶(SD)和磺胺甲恶唑(SMZ)。②肠道难吸收的磺胺药。③外用磺胺药
	临床应用	流行性脑脊髓膜炎(SD在磺胺中最为常用)；尿道感染；呼吸道及咽部感染；肠道感染；局部感染
	不良反应	过敏反应；肾脏损害；影响造血系统；中枢神经系统和胃肠道反应

目 标 检 测

一、选择题

（一）单项选择题

1. 喹诺酮类药物抗菌作用机制是（　　　）
   A. 抑制细菌二氢叶酸合成酶　　　　B. 抑制细菌二氢叶酸还原酶
   C. 抑制细菌蛋白质合成　　　　　　D. 抑制细菌 DNA 促旋酶
   E. 抑制细菌转肽酶

2. 磺胺类药的抗菌机制是（　　　）
   A. 抑制细菌二氢叶酸合成酶　　　　B. 抑制细菌二氢叶酸还原酶
   C. 抑制细菌蛋白质合成　　　　　　D. 抑制细菌 DNA 促旋酶
   E. 抑制细菌转肽酶

3. 治疗暴发型流行性脑脊髓膜炎应首选（　　　）
   A. 氯霉素 + 磺胺嘧啶 (SD) 口服　　B. 四环素 + 青霉素静脉注射
   C. 罗红霉素 + 青霉素鞘内注射　　　D. 链霉素口服
   E. 氯霉素口服

4. 下列药物中，体外抗菌活性最强的是（　　　）
   A. 氧氟沙星　　　B. 诺氟沙星　　　C. 洛美沙星　　　D. 环丙沙星　　　E. 氟罗沙星

（二）多项选择题

5. 喹诺酮类药物常见的不良反应有（　　　）
   A. 胃肠道反应　　　　　　B. 变态反应　　　　　　C. 神经系统反应
   D. 肾损伤　　　　　　　　E. 肌肉疼痛、无力

6. 细菌对喹诺酮类药物耐药的机制是（　　　）
   A. 细菌 DNA 促旋酶改变　　　　　B. 细菌细胞膜孔蛋白通道改变或缺失
   C. 耐药菌株基因突变　　　　　　　D. 细菌产生钝化酶
   E. 细菌产生水解酶

二、思考题

分析三代喹诺酮类药物的抗菌作用特点及临床应用。

（王　平）

Chapter 36　Macrolides, clindamycin and polypeptide antibiotics

PPT

　学习目标

1. **掌握**　大环内酯类抗生素的抗菌作用机制、特点、抗菌谱及临床应用。
2. **熟悉**　林可霉素类抗生素的特点、主要临床应用及不良反应。
3. **了解**　多肽类抗生素的特点及临床应用。

1.　Macrolides

Macrolides (大环内酯类) are a group of closely related compounds characterized by a macrocyclic lactone ring (usually containing 14 or 16 atoms) to which deoxy sugars are attached. The prototype drug, erythromycin, which consists of two sugar moieties attached to a 14-atom lactone ring, was obtained in 1952 from *Streptomyces erythreus* (链霉菌属). Clarithromycin and azithromycin (克拉霉素和阿奇霉素) are semisynthetic derivatives of erythromycin.

Erythromycin (红霉素)

【Antimicrobial activity】Erythromycin is effective against Gram-positive organisms, especially *Pneumococci*, *Streptococci*, *Staphylococci*, and *Corynebacteria*(棒状杆菌), in plasma concentrations of 0.02-2μg/ml. *Mycoplasma*, *Legionella*, *Chlamydia trachomatis*, *C psittaci*, *C pneumoniae*, *Helicobacter*, *Listeria*, and certain mycobacteria (*Mycobacterium kansasii*, *Mycobacterium scrofidaceum*) are also susceptible. Gram-negative organisms such as neisseria species, *Bordetella pertussis*, *Bartonella henselae*, and *B quintana* (etiologic agents of cat scratch disease and bacillary angiomatosis), some rickettsia species, *Treponema pallidum* (梅毒螺旋体), and *Campylobacter* species are susceptible. *Haemophilus influenzae* (流感嗜血杆菌)is somewhat less susceptible.

The antibacterial action of erythromycin may be inhibitory or bactericidal, particularly at higher concentrations, for susceptible organisms. Activity is enhanced at alkaline pH. Inhibition of protein synthesis occurs via binding to the 50S ribosomal RNA. Protein synthesis is inhibited because aminoacyl translocation reactions and the formation of initiation complexes are blocked (Figure 36-1).

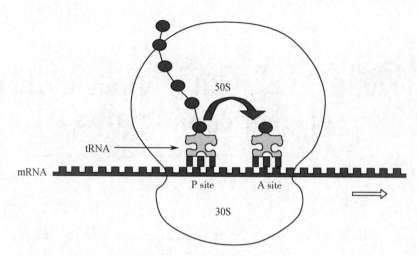

Figure 36-1   Steps in bacterial protein synthesis and targets of chloramphenicol, macrolides, clindamycin (50S); and tetracyclines (30S)

The 70S ribosomal mRNA complex is shown with its 50S and 30S subunits. The peptidyl tRNA at the donor site donates the growing peptide chain to the aminoacyl tRNA at the acceptor site in a reaction catalyzed by peptidyl transferase. The tRNA, discharged of its peptide, is released from the donor site to make way for translocation of the newly formed peptidyl tRNA. The acceptor site is then free to be occupied by the next charged M aminoacyl tRNA.

【Resistance】 Resistance to erythromycin is usually plasmid-encoded. Three mechanisms have been identified. ①Reduced permeability of the cell membrane or active efflux. ②Production (by *Enterobacteriaceae*) of esterases that hydrolyze macrolides. ③Modification of the ribosomal binding site (so-called ribosomal protection) by chromosomal mutation or by a macrolide-inducible or constitutive methylase (甲基化酶). Efflux and methylase production account for the vast majority of cases of resistance in Gram-positive organisms. Cross-resistance is complete between erythromycin and the other macrolides. Constitutive methylase production also confers resistance to structurally unrelated but mechanistically similar compounds such as clindamycin and streptogramin B (so-called macrolide-lincosamide-streptogramin, or MLS type B, resistance), which share the same ribosomal binding site.

【Pharmacokinetics】 Erythromycin base is destroyed by stomach acid and must be administered with enteric coating. Food interferes with absorption. Stearates and esters are fairly acid resistant and somewhat better absorbed. However, only the base is microbiologically active, and its concentration tends to be similar regardless of the formulation.

Absorbed drug is distributed widely except to the brain and cerebrospinal fluid. Erythromycin is taken up by polymorphonuclear (多形核的) leukocytes and macrophages. It traverses the placenta and reaches the fetus. Large amounts of the administered dose is excreted in the bile and lost in feces, and only 5% is excreted in the urine. Therefore, adjustment for renal failure is not necessary.

【Clinical indications】 An erythromycin is the drug of choice in coryne-bacterial infections [diphtheria (白喉), corynebacterial sepsis (脓毒症), erythrasma(红癣)]; in respiratory, neonatal, ocular, or genital chlamydial infections; and in treatment of community-acquired pneumonia because its spectrum of activity includes the pneumococcus, mycoplasma, and legionella. Erythromycin is also useful as a penicillin substitute in penicillin-allergic individuals with infections caused by *Staphylococci* (assuming that the isolate is susceptible), *Streptococci*, or *Pneumococci*. Emergence of erythromycin resistance in strains of group *Streptococci* and *Pneumococci* (penicillin-resistant *Pneumococci* in particular) has made macrolides less attractive as the first-line agents for treatment of pharyngitis, skin and soft tissue infections, and pneumonia. Erythromycin has been recommended as prophylaxis against endocarditis during dental procedures in individuals with valvular (瓣膜) heart disease, though clindamycin, which is better tolerated, has largely replaced it. Although erythromycin estolate is the best-absorbed salt, it imposes the greatest risk of adverse reactions. Therefore, the stearate or succinate salt may be preferred.

Oral erythromycin base (1g) is sometimes combined with oral neomycin or kanamycin for preoperative preparation of the colon. The higher and intravenous dosage of erythromycin gluceptate (葡萄糖酸盐) or lactobionate is recommended when treating pneumonia caused by legionella species.

【Adverse reactions】

(1) Gastrointestinal effects　Anorexia, nausea, vomiting, and diarrhea, which due to the direct stimulation of gut motility, occasionally accompany oral administration.

(2) Liver toxicity　Erythromycins, particularly the estolate, can produce acute cholestatic (胆汁郁积) hepatitis (fever, jaundice, impaired liver function), probably as the hypersensitivity reaction. Most patients will recover, but hepatitis recurs if the drug is read ministered. Other allergic reactions include fever, eosinophilia, and rashes.

Clarithromycin (克拉霉素)

Clarithromycin is derived from erythromycin by addition of a methyl group and has improved acid stability and oral absorption compared with erythromycin. Its mechanism of action is the same as that of erythromycin. Clarithromycin and erythromycin are virtually identical with respect to antibacterial activity except that clarithromycin is more active against *Mycobacterium avium* (结核分枝杆菌) complex. Clarithromycin also has activity against *M leprae* and *Toxoplasma gondii*.

The longer half-life of clarithromycin (6 hours) compared with erythromycin permits twice-daily dosing. Clarithromycin penetrates most tissues well, with concentrations equal to or exceeding serum concentrations.

Clarithromycin is metabolized in the liver. The major metabolite is 14-hydroxyclarithromycin (14羟基克拉霉素), which also has antibacterial activity. A portion of active drug and this major metabolite is eliminated in urine, and dosage reduction is recommended for patients with creatinine clearances less than 30ml/min. Clarithromycin has drug interactions similar to those described for erythromycin.

The advantages of clarithromycin compared with erythromycin are lower frequency of gastrointestinal intolerance and less frequent closing.

Azithromycin (阿奇霉素)

Azithromycin, a 15-atom lactone macrolide ring compound, is derived from erythromycin by addition of a methylated nitrogen (甲基化氮) into the lactone ring of erythromycin.

Its spectrum of activity and clinical uses are virtually identical to those of clarithromycin. Azithromycin is active against *M avium* complex and *T gondii*. Azithromycin is slightly less active than erythromycin and clarithromycin when against *Staphylococci* and *Streptococci* and slightly more active against *H influenzae*. Azithromycin is highly active against chlamydia. Azithromycin differs from erythromycin and clarithromycin mainly in pharmacokinetic properties. A 500mg dose of azithromycin produces relatively low serum concentrations of approximately 0.4g/ml. However, azithromycin penetrates into most tissues (except cerebrospinal fluid) and phagocytic cells extremely well, with tissue concentrations exceeding serum concentrations by 10-fold to 100-fold. The drug is slowly released from tissues (tissue half-life of 2-4 days) to produce an elimination half-life approaching 3 days. These unique properties permit once-daily dosing and shortening of the duration of treatment in many cases.

Azithromycin is rapidly absorbed and well tolerated orally. It should be administered 1 hour before or 2 hours after meals. Aluminum and magnesium antacids do not alter bioavailability but delay absorption and reduce peak serum concentrations. Because it has a 15-member (not 14-member) lactone ring, azithromycin does not inactivate cytochrome P450 enzymes and therefore is free of the drug interactions that occur with erythromycin and clarithromycin.

2. Clindamycin

Clindamycin (克林霉素)

Clindamycin is a chlorine-substituted derivative of lincomycin, which is an antibiotic that is elaborated by *Streptomyces lincolnensis* (波塞链霉菌). Lincomycin, although structurally distinct, resembles erythromycin in activity, but it is toxic and no longer used.

【Antibacterial activity】*Streptococci*, *Staphylococci*, and *Pneumococci* are inhibited by clindamycin. *Enterococci* and Gram-negative aerobic organisms are resistant (in contrast to their susceptibility to erythromycin). Bacteroides species and other anaerobes, both Gram-positive and Gram-negative, are usually susceptible. *Clostridium difficile* (艰难梭菌), an important cause of pseudomembranous colitis, is resistant. Clindamycin, like erythromycin, inhibits protein synthesis by interfering with the formation of initiation complexes and with aminoacyl translocation reactions. The binding site for clindamycin on the 50S subunit of the bacterial ribosome is identical with that for erythromycin.

【Clinical indications】Clindamycin is indicated for treatment of severe anaerobic infection caused by bacteroides and other anaerobes that often participate in mixed infections. Clindamycin, sometimes in combination with an aminoglycoside or cephalosporin, is used to treat penetrating wounds of the abdomen and the gut; infections originating in the female genital tract, e.g., septic abortion and pelvic abscesses; or aspiration pneumonia. Clindamycin is now recommended instead of erythromycin for prophylaxis of endocarditis in patients with valvular heart disease who are undergoing certain dental procedures. Clindamycin plus primaquine (伯氨喹) is an effective alternative to trimethoprim-sulfamethoxazole for moderate to moderately severe *Pneumocystis carinii* (卡氏肺孢菌) pneumonia in AIDS patients. It is also used in combination with pyrimethamine for AIDS- related toxoplasmosis of the brain.

【Adverse reactions】Common adverse effects are diarrhea, nausea, and skin rashes. Impaired liver function (with or without jaundice) and neutropenia sometimes occurs. Severe diarrhea and enterocolitis have followed clindamycin administration. Antibiotic-associated colitis that has followed administration of clindamycin and other drugs is caused by toxigenic *C difficile*. This potentially fatal complication must be recognized promptly and treated with metronidazole or vancomycin. Relapse may occur. Variations in the local prevalence of *C difficile* may account for the great differences in incidence of antibiotic-associated colitis. For unknown reasons, neonates given clindamycin may become colonized with toxigenic *C difficile* but do not develop colitis.

3. Polypeptide antibiotics

Vancomycin (万古霉素)

Vancomycin is an antibiotic produced by *Streptococcus orientalis* (东方型鼠疫耶尔森菌), an actinomycete isolated from soil samples obtained in Indonesia and India. It is a complex and unusual tricyclic glycopeptide with a molecular mass of about 1500 daltons.

【 Antimicrobial activity 】 Vancomycin is primarily active against Gram-positive bacteria. Strains are considered susceptible at MICs of 4pLg/ml. *S. aureus* and *S. epidermidis* (金黄色葡萄球菌和表皮葡萄球菌), including strains resistant to methicillin, usually are inhibited by concentrations of 1.0 to 4.0ig/ml. Strains of *Enterococci* were also once uniformly susceptible to vancomycin.

Vancomycin resistance determinants in *E. aecium* and *E. faecalis* (大肠埃希菌和粪肠杆菌) are located on a transposon, which is itself part of a conjugative plasmid, rendering it readily transferable among *Enterococci* and potentially other Gram-positive bacteria. These strains typically are resistant to multiple antibiotics, including streptomycin, Gentamicin, and ampicillin, which effectively eliminating these as alternative therapeutic agents. Essentially all species of Gram-negative bacilli and mycobacteria are resistant to vancomycin.

Vancomycin inhibits the synthesis of the cell wall in sensitive bacteria by binding with high affinity to the D-alanyl-D-alanine (D-丙氨酰-D-丙氨酸) terminus of cell wall precursor units. The drug is bactericidal for dividing microorganisms.

【 Pharmacokinetics 】 Vancomycin is poorly absorbed after oral administration, and large quantities are excreted in the stool. For parenteral therapy, the drug should be administered intravenously, never intramuscularly. A single intravenous dose of 1g in adults produces plasma concentrations of 15 to 30ig/ml 1 hour after a 1-2-hour infusion. The drug has a serum elimination half-life of about 6 hours. Approximately 30% of vancomycin is bound to plasma protein. Vancomycin appears in various body fluids, including the CSF when the meninges are inflamed (7% to 30%); bile; and pleural, pericardial, synovial, and ascetic fluids. About 90% of an injected dose is excreted by glomerular filtration. The drug accumulates if renal function is impaired, and dosage adjustments must be made under these circumstances.

【 Clinical indications 】 Vancomycin hydrochloride (盐酸万古霉素) is marketed for intravenous use as a sterile powder for solution. It should be diluted and infused over at least a 60-minute period to avoid infusion-related adverse effects. A higher dose, 60mg/kg per day in 4 divided doses, is recommended for meningitis. This regimen will yield an average steady-state concentration of 15xg/ml in patients with normal renal function. Alteration of dosage is required for patients with impaired renal function. The drug has been used effectively in functionally anephric patients (who are being dialyzed).

Vancomycin can be administered orally to patients with pseudomembranous colitis, although metronidazole is preferred. Vancomycin hydrochloride for oral solution is available for this purpose, as are capsules. Vancomycin should be employed only to treat serious infections and is particularly useful in the management of infections due to methicillin-resistant staphylococci, including pneumonia, empyema, endocarditis, osteomyelitis, and soft-tissue abscesses and in severe staphylococcal infections in patients who are allergic to penicillins and cephalosporins (青霉素和头孢菌素). However, vancomycin is less rapidly bactericidal than any of the antistaphylococcal 3-lactams (抗葡萄球菌3-内酰胺类药物) (e.g., nafcillin or cefazolin), and therefore may be less efficacious clinically.

Treatment with vancomycin is effective and convenient when there is disseminated staphylococcal infection or localized infection of a shunt in patients with irreversible renal disease who is being maintained by hemodialysis or peritoneal dialysis, because the drug can be administered once weekly or in the dialysis fluid. Intraventricular administration of vancomycin (via a shunt or reservoir) has been necessary in a few cases of CNS infections due to susceptible microorganisms that did not respond to intravenous therapy alone. Administration of vancomycin is an effective alternative for the treatment of endocarditis caused by viridans *Streptococci* in patients who are allergic to penicillin. In combination with an aminoglycoside, it may be used for entero-coccal endocarditis in patients with serious penicillin allergy. Vancomycin is also effective for the treatment of infections caused by *Flavobaderium* and *Corynebacterium* spp (黄杆菌属和棒状杆菌属). Vancomycin has become an important antibiotic in the management of known or suspected penicillin-resistant pneumococcal infections.

【Adverse reactions】Hypersensitivity reactions produced by vancomycin are macular skin rashes and anaphylaxis. Phlebitis and pain at the site of intravenous injection are relatively uncommon. Chills, rash, and fever may occur. Rapid intravenous infusion may cause a variety of symptoms, including erythematous or urticarial reactions, flushing, tachycardia, and hypotension. The extreme flushing that can occur is sometimes called "red neck" or "red man" syndrome. Ototoxicity is associated with excessively high concentrations of the drug in plasma (60 to 100xg/ml). Nephrotoxicity, formerly quite common probably because of less pure concentrations of the drug, has become an unusual side effect when appropriate doses are used, as judged by renal function and determinations of the concentration of the antibiotic in blood.

Teicoplanin (替考拉宁)

Teicoplanin is a glycopeptide antibiotic produced by *Actinoplanes teichomyetius* (游动放线菌属). It is similar to vancomycin in chemical structure, mechanism of action, spectrum of activity, and route of elimination (e.g., primarily renal).

【Antimicrobial activity】Teicoplanin, like vancomycin, is an inhibitor of cell-wall synthesis, and it is active only against Gram-positive bacteria. It is reliably bactericidal against susceptible strains, except for *Enterococci*. It is active against methicillin-susceptible and methicillin-resistant staphylococci, which typically have minimal inhibitory concentrations of < 4jxg/ml. Minimal inhibitory concentrations for *Listeria monocytogenes* (单核增生李斯特菌), *Corynebacterium* spp. (棒状杆菌), *Clostridium* spp. (梭状芽孢杆菌), and anaerobic Gram-positive cocci range from 0.25 to 2.0jjLg/ml. Non-viridans and viridans streptococci, *S. pneumoniae*, and *Enterococci* are inhibited by concentrations ranging from 0.01 to 1.0xg/ml. Some strains of *Staphylococci*, both coagulase-positive and coagulase-negative, as well as *Enterococci* and other organisms that are intrinsically resistant to vancomycin [e.g., *Lactobacillus* spp. and *Leuconostoc* spp. (乳酸菌属和白串珠菌属)] are resistant to teicoplanin.

【Pharmacokinetics】The primary differences between vancomycin and teicoplanin are that teicoplanin can be administered safely by intramuscular injection; it is highly bound by plasma proteins (90% to 95%); it has an extremely long serum elimination half-life (up to 100 hours in patients with normal renal function). As with vancomycin, teicoplanin doses must be adjusted in patients with renal insufficiency. For functionally anephric (无肾脏) patients, administration once weekly has been appropriate, but serum drug concentrations should be monitored to determine that the therapeutic range has been maintained (e.g., trough concentration of 15-20xg/ml).

【Clinical indications】Teicoplanin has been used to treat a wide variety of infections, including osteomyelitis and endocarditis, caused by methicillin-resistant and methicillin-susceptible *Staphylococci*, *Streptococci*, and *Enterococci*. Teicoplanin has been found to be comparable to vancomycin in efficacy, except for treatment failures from low doses used to treat serious infections, such as endocarditis. Teicoplanin is not as efficacious as antistaphylococcal penicillins for treating bacteremia and endocarditis caused by methicillin-susceptible *S. aureus*, with teicoplanin cure rates of 60% to 70% versus 85% to 90% for the penicillins. The efficacy of teicoplanin against *S. aureus* may be improved by the addition of an aminoglycoside to provide a synergistic effect. Strains of *Streptococci* are uniformly susceptible to teicoplanin. This drug has been very effective in a once-daily regimen for patients with streptococcal osteomyelitis or endocarditis. Teicoplanin is among the most active drugs against *Enterococci*. Limited experience indicates that it is effective, although only bacteriostatic, for serious enterococcal infections. It should be combined with gentamicin to achieve a bactericidal effect in the treatment of enterococcal endocarditis.

【Adverse reactions】The main side effect reported for teicoplanin is skin rash, which is more common in higher dosages. Hypersensitivity reactions, drug fever, and neutropenia also have been reported. Ototoxicity has occurred rarely.

Polymyxin B (多黏菌素B) and polymyxin E (多黏菌素E)

The polymyxins, discovered in 1947, are a group of closely related antibiotic substances elaborated by various strains of *Bacillus polymyxa* (芽孢杆菌), an aerobic spore-forming rod found in soil. Polymyxin E (colistin) is produced by *Bacillus (Aerobacillus) colistinus*, a microorganism isolated from a soil sample obtained from Fukushima Prefecture, Japan. These drugs, which are cationic detergents, are relatively simple, basic peptides with molecular masses of about 1000 daltons.

【Antimicrobial activity】The antimicrobial activities of polymyxin B and colistin are similar and are restricted to Gram-negative bacteria, including *Enterobacter* (肠杆菌属), *E.coli* (大肠埃希菌), *Klebsiella* (克雷伯菌), *Salmonella* (沙门菌), *Pasteurella* (巴斯德杆菌), *Bordetella* (博德特杆菌), and *Shigella* (志贺杆菌), which usually are sensitive to concentrations of 0.05 to 2.0ig/ml. Most strains of *P. aeruginosa* are inhibited by less than 8xg/ml *in vitro*.

Polymyxins are surface-active, amphipathic agents [containing both lipophilic (亲脂的) and lipophobic (亲水的) groups within the molecule]. They interact strongly with phospholipids and penetrate into and disrupt the structure of cell membranes. The permeability of the bacterial membrane changes immediately on contact with the drug. Sensitivity to polymyxin B apparently is related to the phospholipid content of the cell wall-membrane complex. The cell wall of certain resistant bacteria may prevent access of the drug to the cell membrane.

【Pharmacokinetics】Neither polymyxin B nor colistin is absorbed when given orally. They are also poorly absorbed from mucous membranes and the surface of large bums.

【Clinical indications】Polymyxin B sulfate is available for ophthalmic, otic, and topical use in combination with a variety of other compounds. Although parenteral preparations are still marketed, they are not recommended. Infections of the skin, mucous membranes, eye, and ear due to polymyxin B-sensitive microorganisms (微生物) respond to local application of the antibiotic in solution or ointment. External otitis, frequently due to *Pseudomonas* (假单胞菌), may be cured by the topical use of the drug. *P. aeruginosa* (铜绿假单胞菌), which is a common cause of infection of corneal ulcers; local application or subconjunctival injection of polymyxin B is often curative.

【Adverse reactions】Polymyxin B applied to intact or denuded skin or mucous membranes producing no systemic reactions because of its almost complete lack of absorption from these sites. Hypersensitization (超敏) is uncommon with topical application.

重 点 小 结

药物	抗菌机制	抗菌谱	临床应用	不良反应
红霉素	与细菌核糖体50S亚基结合，抑制细菌蛋白质合成	革兰阳性菌、部分革兰阴性菌，厌氧菌、支原体、衣原体、军团菌	败血症、肠炎、支原体肺炎、婴儿肺炎、白喉	胃肠道反应、肝损伤、耳毒性、过敏反应、神经症状
林可霉素	与细菌核糖体50S亚基结合，抑制细菌蛋白质合成	厌氧菌、革兰阳性菌、革兰阴性球菌、支原体、沙眼衣原体、恶性疟原虫、弓形体	是金黄色葡萄球菌所致的急慢性骨髓炎及关节感染的首选药	胃肠道反应，二重感染
多黏菌素B	增加细菌细胞膜通透性，使菌体内容物外漏死亡	革兰阴性需氧杆菌	败血症、泌尿道感染、烧伤创伤感染	肾脏毒性以及神经毒性
万古霉素	抑制细菌细胞壁合成	窄谱，革兰阳性菌（金黄色葡萄球菌、溶血性链球菌、肺炎球菌、棒状杆菌）	败血症、心内膜炎、骨髓炎、呼吸道感染	肾脏损伤

目 标 检 测

一、选择题

（一）单项选择题

1. 军团菌感染首选药是（　　　）
   A. 头孢氨苄　　　B. 青霉素　　　　C. 红霉素　　　　D. 磺胺类　　　　E. 林可霉素

2. 林可霉素的特点是（　　　）
   A. 脑组织中浓度高　　　　　　B. 胆汁中浓度高　　　　　　C. 血中浓度高
   D. 骨组织中浓度高　　　　　　E. 肝中浓度高

题库

医药大学堂
WWW.YIYAODXT.COM

3. 克林霉素引起的伪膜性肠炎可用何种药物治疗（　　）

    A. 四环素　　　　　　　　　　B. 万古霉素和甲硝唑　　　　　C. 氯霉素

    D. 青霉素　　　　　　　　　　E. 红霉素

4. 大环内酯类抗生素中对肺炎支原体作用最强的是（　　）

    A. 红霉素　　　　B. 吉他霉素　　　C. 阿奇霉素　　　D. 克拉霉素　　　E. 交沙霉素

5. 红霉素对下列哪类感染无效（　　）

    A. 革兰阳性菌　　　　　　　　B. 革兰阴性球菌　　　　　　　C. 大肠埃希菌

    D. 军团菌　　　　　　　　　　E. 支原体

6. 在骨组织中药物浓度高，常用于金黄色葡萄球菌所致的骨髓炎的药物是（　　）

    A. 红霉素　　　B. 万古霉素　　　C. 四环素　　　D. 林可霉素　　　E. 氯霉素

（二）多项选择题

7. 克林霉素的应用范围比林可霉素广是由于前者的（　　）

    A. 抗菌谱比林可霉素广　　　　B. 口服吸收较林可霉素好　　　C. 较易透过血脑屏障

    D. 毒性较林可霉素小　　　　　E. 抗菌作用强于林可霉素

8. 大环内酯类抗生素的特点有（　　）

    A. 抗菌谱窄，但比青霉素略广

    B. 在碱性环境中抗菌作用增强

    C. 容易透过血脑屏障

    D. 主要经胆汁排泄，并进行肝肠循环

    E. 细菌对本类各药间不产生交叉耐药性

9. 大环内酯类抗生素对下列哪些细菌有抑制作用（　　）

    A. 需氧革兰阳性和阴性菌　　　B. 厌氧菌　　　　　　　　　　C. 军团菌

    D. 淋病奈瑟菌　　　　　　　　E. 衣原体和支原体

二、思考题

阿奇霉素与红霉素比较具有哪些特点？

（吕　莹）

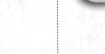
PPT

Chapter 37 Tetracyclines and chloramphenicol

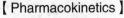
学习目标

1. 掌握 四环素类药物及氯霉素的抗菌谱、抗菌作用机制、临床应用及不良反应。
2. 熟悉 多西环素和米诺环素的药理特点。
3. 了解 四环素类和氯霉素的体内过程。

Tetracyclines (四环素类) and chloramphenicol are broad-spectrum antibiotics and have strong inhibitory effects on Gram-positive and Gram-negative bacteria as well as Rickettsia (立克次体), Mycoplasma (衣原体) and Chlamydia (支原体). Tetracyclines can also inhibit some Spirochetes and Protozoa (原虫).

1. Tetracyclines

Tetracyclines are a group of compounds with the basic structure of phenanthrene (菲), which are amphoteric substance (两性物质) and stable in acid solution, but easy to be destroyed in alkaline solution. There are two classes of tetracyclines, one is natural tetracyclines and another is semi-synthetic tetracyclines. Tetracycline, terramycin (土霉素), chlortetracycline (金霉素) and demeclocycline (去甲环素) are natural tetracyclines, while metacycline (美他环素), doxycycline (多西环素) and minocycline (米诺环素) are semi-synthetic tetracyclines, also known as the second generation of tetracycline antibiotics. Both natural tetracyclines and semi-synthetic tetracyclines have similar antibacterial mechanism, with differences slightly in their clinical efficacy.

Tetracyclines are bacteriostatic antibiotics and just show bactericidal effect at extremely high concentration. They exert inhibitory effects on a wide range of aerobic and anaerobic Gram-positive and Gram-negative bacteria as well as some other microorganisms, such as Richettsia, Mycoplasma pneumoniae (肺炎支原体), Chlamydia and *Legionella* (军团菌). The inhibition of tetracyclines on Gram-positive bacteria is stronger than that on Gram-negative bacteria, but still is not as good as penicillins and cephalosporins, and the effect on Gram-negative bacteria is also not as good as aminoglycosides and chloramphenicol. Tetracyclines have no effect on *Typhoid bacillus* (伤寒杆菌), *Paratyphoid bacillus* (副伤寒杆菌), *Pseudomonas aeruginosa*, *Mycobacterium tuberculosis* (结核分枝杆菌), fungi and viruses.

【 Pharmacokinetics 】

(1) Absorption All tetracyclines are adequately, yet incompletely absorbed after oral

医药大学堂
WWW.YIYAODXT.COM

administration. Its absorption is promoted by acid drugs such as vitamin C, but impaired by the concurrent ingestion of foods or drugs with Fe^{2+}, Ca^{2+}, mg^{2+} or Al^{3+} due to the formation of nonabsorbable chelates of the tetracyclines with divalent or trivalent cations. Therefore, when used with iron, basic drugs, H_2 receptor blockers or antacids, the interval should be 2-3 hours.

(2) Distribution Tetracyclines are distributed widely throughout the body tissues and fluids. They concentrate in the liver, kidney, spleen, bone marrow, and deposit in the newly formed teeth and bones. Relative high concentrations of these drugs are also found in breast milk. All tetracyclines cross the placenta barrier and blood-brain barrier and enter the cerebrospinal fluid. However, they are usually ineffective for central nervous system infection.

(3) Elimination Tetracyclines are metabolized in the liver and concentrated in the bile where concentrations can be up to 10-20 times than those in the plasma. Most tetracyclines are reabsorbed in the intestine via the enterohepatic circulation. Doxycycline, minocycline, and chlortetracycline are excreted primarily in the feces. The other tetracyclines are eliminated primarily in the urine by glomerular filtration and their excretion can be increased by alkalized urine.

【Pharmacodynamics】Tetracyclines bind specifically to the A site of ribosome 30S subunit to prevent aminoacyl-tRNA (氨酰 tRNA) from entering the A site, thereby inhibit peptide chain extension and protein synthesis. Drugs can also change the permeability of bacterial cell membrane, leading to the leakage of nucleotides and other important components in bacteria, thus inhibiting bacterial DNA replication (Figure 37-1).

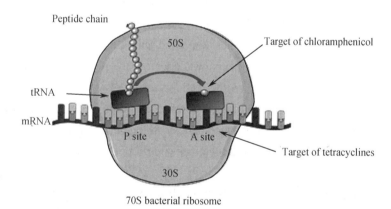

Figure 37-1　Schematic diagram of the action site of tetracyclines and chloramphenicol on inhibiting bacterial protein synthesis

【Resistance】Cross-resistance (交叉耐药性) within the group is significant. Usually, tetracycline, terramycin and aureomycin are completely cross resistant, but bacteria resistant to natural tetracyclines may still be sensitive to semi-synthetic tetracyclines. Resistance is related largely to decreased intracellular concentration of drug due to decreased penetration in some bacteria and a resultant increased efflux from the cell by an energy-dependent mechanism. Other mechanisms, such as production of proteins that interfere with tetracycline binding to ribosomes and enzymatic inactivation of the drug, have been reported.

【Clinical indications】Tetracyclines are still the drugs of choice to treat Rickettsia infection [typhus (斑疹伤寒), Q fever (Q热), scrub typhus (丛林斑疹伤寒), etc.], mycoplasma infection [mycoplasma pneumonia, urogenital system infection (泌尿生殖系统感染), etc.], chlamydia infection [psittacosis (鹦鹉热), trachoma (沙眼) and venereal lymphogranuloma (性病淋巴肉芽肿), etc.] and some spirochete infection [relapsing fever (回归热), etc.]. Tetracyclines can also be effective to treat plague, brucellosis (布鲁菌病), cholera, peptic ulcer caused by *Helicobacter pylori* infection (幽门螺杆菌感染), groin granuloma (腹股沟肉芽肿) caused by Chlamydia granuloma infection (肉芽肿衣原体感染) and periodontitis (牙周炎) caused by *Porphyromonas gingivalis* (牙龈卟啉单胞菌). Among of them, doxycycline is the first choice when using this kind of drugs.

【Adverse reactions 】

(1) **Gastric discomfort** Oral administration of tetracyclines can cause nausea, vomiting, diarrhea, epigastric burning, stomatitis, and glossitis. Drug administration after meal can reduce the stimulation symptoms, but also decrease drug absorption. Intramuscular injection is highly irritating and forbidden, and intravenous injection can cause phlebitis.

(2) **Superinfection** When chronic using of tetracyclines or other broad-spectrum antibiotics, the normal intestinal flora may be altered in which sensitive bacteria are inhibited, while non-sensitive bacteria multiply in large numbers, resulting in new infection, which is called superinfection or double infection or bacterial alternation. Two kinds of superinfection are very common. One is fungal infection caused by *Candida albicans* (白念珠菌), which is characterized by thrush and enteritis (鹅口疮和肠炎), and usually needs cessation of tetracycline treatment immediately and antifungal treatment at the same time. The other is pseudomembranous colitis (伪膜性肠炎) caused by overgrowth of *Clostridium difficile* (艰难梭菌) resistant to tetracycline, which is characterized by severe diarrhea, necrosis of intestinal wall, exudation of body fluid or even shock, and usually resolved by stop using of tetracycline immediately and treatment with vancomycin or metronidazole (甲硝唑). Superinfection is more common for infants, the elderly and the weak patient who received tetracyclines combined with glucocorticoids or anticancer drugs.

(3) **Effects on calcified tissues** Tetracyclines deposit in the primary dentition where combine with hydroxyapatite crystal (羟基磷灰石晶体) in the teeth to form tetracycline calcium phosphate complex, causing permanent brown discoloration of teeth (commonly known as yellow staining of teeth), and incomplete enamel development. The drugs also deposit in the skeleton which may depress bone growth in fetus and premature infant. Therefore, tetracyclines should not be used for pregnant women, lactating women and children under 8 years old.

(4) **Others** Hepatic and renal toxicity typically develop in patients who received high doses or long term of tetracyclines, which is more common in pregnant women, especially in those with renal impairment. Occasionally, anaphylaxis and cross anaphylaxis (过敏反应与交叉过敏反应) were observed. It can also cause photosensitive reactions and vestibular problems such as dizziness, nausea, vomiting, etc.

2. Commonly used tetracyclines

Doxycycline (多西环素) and minocycline (米诺环素)

Both doxycycline and minocycline are the long-acting semi-synthetic tetracycline and have higher antibacterial activity than that of tetracycline. They are effective to treat rosacea (酒渣鼻), acne (痤疮), prostatitis (前列腺炎) and respiratory tract infections such as chronic tracheitis (慢性气管炎) and pneumonia. Among tetracyclines, doxycycline is the drug of choice for those diseases. Due to the high incidence of dose-related unique vestibular side effects (nausea, vomiting, dizziness, dyskinesia and other symptoms), minocycline is usually not used as the drug of choice for those infections.

3.　Chloramphenicol

Chloramphenicol, an antibiotic produced by *Streptomyces venezuelae* (威尼斯链霉菌), was introduced into clinic practice in 1948. However, in 1950, it was found to cause fatal adverse reactions, which limits greatly its application in clinic. Nowadays, chloramphenicol is just restricted to life-threatening infections for which no alternatives exist. Only levorotatory form is biologically effective in the clinic.

Chloramphenicol is a broad-spectrum antibiotic and has stronger antibacterial activity not only against aerobic bacteria, but also against anaerobes and other microorganisms, such as Rickettsia. However, *Pseudomonas aeruginosa* is not affected, nor are the Chlamydiae. For most species, chloramphenicol is bacteriostatic drug, but it has a killing effect on *Haemophilus influenza* (流感嗜血杆菌), *Neisseria meningitides* (脑膜炎奈瑟菌) and *Streptococcus pneumoniae* (肺炎链球菌). Its antibacterial activity on Gram-negative bacteria is better than positive bacteria, but is still not as good as aminoglycosides and its antibacterial activity on Gram-positive bacteria is also not as good as penicillin and tetracycline. Chloramphenicol has no effect on *Mycobacterium tuberculosis*, fungi and protozoa.

【Pharmacokinetics】Chloramphenicol may be administered either intravenously or orally, and is widely distributed throughout the body. It can be present in the bile, milk and placental fluid, and readily reaches the therapeutic concentration in CSF. *In vivo*, 90% of the drugs are inactivated by binding to glucuronic acid in the liver, and only 10% of the prototype drugs are excreted by the kidney, which can also reach an effective antibacterial concentration in the urinary system.

【Pharmacodynamics】By binding reversibly to 50S subunit of bacterial ribosome, chloramphenicol inhibits the peptidyl transferase reaction, thus preventing the extension of the peptide chain and hindering the protein synthesis. Because the binding sites of chloramphenicol are very close to the action sites of macrolides and clindamycin. The combined application of these drugs may produce antagonistic effects by competing with targets.

【Drug resistance】Resistance to chloramphenicol usually is caused by a plasmid-encoded acetyltransferase that inactivates the drug. Another mechanism for resistance is associated with decreased outer membrane permeability to chloramphenicol, which may be the basis of multidrug resistance.

【Clinical indications】Therapy with chloramphenicol must be limited to infections for which the benefits of the drug outweighs the risks of the potential toxicities. Chloramphenicol should never be used when other antibiotics can be used, or the cause of infection is unknown.

(1) Serious infection induced by drug-resistant bacteria　Chloramphenicol remains an alternative drug for the treatment of the serious and life-threatening infections such as meningitis induced by drug-resistant *H. influenzae*, *N. meningitides* and *S. pneumoniae* in patients who are allergic to β-lactams.

(2) **Typhoid fever (伤寒)**　Quinolones or the third generation cephalosporins are the drugs of choice for the treatment of typhoid fever, due to their quick acting, low toxicity, less recurrence and no bacteria after recovery. Because of low cost, chloramphenicol is still used to treat typhoid fever in some countries and regions. In addition, chloramphenicol is still effective for the treatment of recurrent cases.

(3) **Severe rickettsia infection**　Chloramphenicol may be used for pregnant women with severe Rickettsia infection (Typhus, Q fever and tsutsugamushi disease), children under 8 years old, and people allergic to tetracycline.

(4) **Others**　Combined with other antibiotics, chloramphenicol may be used to treat anaerobic bacteria infection in abdominal cavity or pelvic cavity. It can also be used topically for ophthalmology to treat intraocular infection, whole eyeball infection, trachoma and conjunctivitis caused by sensitive bacteria.

【Adverse reactions】

(1) **Hematotoxicity (血液系统毒性)**　①Reversible hemocytopenia (可逆性血细胞减少)：It is common and dose-related toxicity manifested by anemia (贫血), leukopenia (白细胞减少症) or thrombocytopenia (血小板减少症), which occurs concomitantly with the large dose or prolonged therapy of chloramphenicol. The probably reason for reversible erythroid suppression is that high dose of chloramphenicol can inhibit the ribosome 70 subunit of the mitochondria in bone marrow hematopoietic cells, which reduces the activity of the host mitochondrial iron chelate enzyme and the synthesis of hemoglobin, and also cause damage to other blood cells. Reversible hemocytopenia can be recovered if the drug is stopped in time, but may progressed to fatal aplastic anemia or acute myelogenous leukemia if treatment is continued. ②Aplastic anemia (再生障碍性贫血)：Aplastic anemia accounts for approximately 70% of the cases of blood dyscrasias due to chloramphenicol. It is dose-independent and may occur after once treatment or several weeks or months of drug withdrawal. The incidence is rare (1 / 30 000), but usually fatal and the incidence of female is 2-3 times higher than that of male. There is a high probability that the survivors will develop into leukemia in the future.

(2) **Gray baby syndrome (灰婴综合征)**　Neonates or premature infants have a poor detoxification ability to chloramphenicol due to the lack of glucuronosyl transferase in the liver and the inadequate renal excretion function. When exposed to excessive dose of chloramphenicol, they may develop a serious illness termed gray baby syndrome, which is manifested as circulatory exhaustion, dyspnea, progressive blood pressure drop, pale skin and cyanosis. Usually, it occurs on the second to the ninth day after treatment, and the mortality rate can be as high as 40% within two days after symptoms appear. Adults who have received very high doses of the drug can also exhibit this toxicity.

(3) **Others**　Nausea, vomiting, diarrhea and other symptoms may follow the oral administration of chloramphenicol. A few patients have allergic reactions such as rash, drug fever, angioneuroedema, optic neuritis, visual impairment, etc. Hemolytic anemia (溶血性贫血) (patients with glucose-6-phosphate dehydrogenase deficiency) and superinfection may also occur. Chloramphenicol should not be used in patients with liver and renal damage, glucose-6-phosphate dehydrogenase deficiency, newborns, premature infants, pregnant and lactating women.

重 点 小 结

药物	药理作用	临床应用	不良反应
四环素类	特异性地与细菌核糖体 30S 亚基的 A 位置结合，抑制肽链增长和蛋白质合成；广谱抗菌作用	斑疹伤寒、鹦鹉热等	胃肠道反应、二重感染、骨牙生长等
氯霉素类	可逆地与 50S 亚基肽酰转移酶作用位点结合，阻止肽链增长；广谱抗菌作用	对青霉素过敏患者的细菌性脑膜炎治疗等	骨髓造血功能抑制、灰婴综合征、二重感染等

目 标 检 测

一、选择题

（一）单项选择题

1. 易引起灰婴综合征的药物是（　　　）
　　A. 四环素　　　　B. 土霉素　　　　　　C. 呋喃妥因　　　　D. 多西环素　　　　E. 氯霉素

2. 某男，因伤寒服用氯霉素，一周后查血象发现有严重贫血和白细胞、血小板减少，这种现象发生的原因是（　　　）
　　A. 氯霉素破坏了红细胞
　　B. 氯霉素缩短了红细胞的寿命
　　C. 氯霉素抑制了线粒体铁螯合酶的活性
　　D. 氯霉素抑制了高尔基体的功能
　　E. 氯霉素加强了吞噬细胞的功能

3. 服用四环素引起假膜性肠炎，应如何抢救（　　　）
　　A. 服用头孢菌素　　　　　　　　B. 服用林可霉素　　　　　　　　C. 服用土霉素
　　D. 服用万古霉素　　　　　　　　E. 服用青霉素

4. 对青霉素过敏的细菌性脑膜炎患者，可选用（　　　）
　　A. 卡那霉素　　　B. 氯霉素　　　C. 多黏菌素　　　D. 头孢氨苄　　　E. 大观霉素

（二）多项选择题

5. 四环素的抗菌谱包括（　　　）
　　A. 立克次体　　　　　　　　B. 支原体　　　　　　C. 破伤风杆菌
　　D. 铜绿假单胞菌　　　　　　E. 真菌

二、思考题

简述四环素的不良反应及预防措施。

（张海宁）

Chapter 38　Antiparasitic drugs

 学习目标

1. **掌握** 疟疾、血吸虫病、阿米巴病的常用治疗药物。
2. **熟悉** 疟疾、血吸虫病、阿米巴病的药物治疗原则和药物治疗方法。
3. **了解** 疟疾、血吸虫病、阿米巴病的病因、发病机制和临床表现。

Protozoan infections are parasitic diseases caused by organisms classified in the Kingdom Protozoa. Examples include *Entamoeba histolytica*, *Plasmodium* (some of which cause malaria) etc. Malaria (疟疾), amebiasis (阿米巴病) and leishmaniasis (利什曼病) are common parasitic diseases in China.

Malaria is the most important parasitic disease of humans in tropical area and causes hundreds of millions of illnesses per year. There are four species of plasmodium (疟原虫) causing human malaria: *Plasmodium falciparum*, *P.vivax*, *P. malariae,* and *P. ovale*. An anopheline (按蚊的)mosquito inoculates plasmodium (疟原虫) sporozoites (孢子体) to cause human infection. Sporozoites in blood rapidly invade liver cells, and exoerythrocytic (红细胞外的) stage tissue schizonts mature in the liver. After that, merozoites (裂殖子) are released from the liver and invade erythroeytes (红细胞).

Parasites in clinical medicine include protozoa and helminthes (寄生虫). Ideal antiparasitic drugs should target structures and biochemical pathway only present or accessible in parasites.

1. Drugs that disrupt parasitic membrane structure

Artemisinin (青蒿素) and its derivatives (衍生物)

Artemisinin is a sesquiterpene lactone endoperoxide (倍半萜内酯内过氧化物) and is an active component of an herbal medicine that has been used as an antipyretic in China for over 2000 years.

【Pharmacokinetics】This compound is insoluble and can only be used orally. Artemisinin and the derivatives are rapidly metabolized to the active metabolite dihydroartemisinin. Blood drug levels appear to decrease after a number of days of therapy.

【Antimalarial action and mechanism】Artemisinin and its analogs are very rapidly acting blood schizonticides against all human malaria parasites. The mechanism of artemisinins is the result from the production of free radicals from cleavage of the drugs' endoperoxide bridge by heme iron in the parasite food vacuole or from inhibition of a parasite calcium ATPase. These agents may also covalently bind to and damage specific malarial proteins.

【Therapeutic uses】Artemisinin-based combination therapy is now the standard regimens for treatment of uncomplicated falciparum malaria in nearly all areas endemic for falciparum malaria. Artemisinins (青蒿素类) have also been proved to have outstanding efficacy in the treatment of complicated falciparum malaria.

【Adverse reactions and resistance】Artemisinins are generally very well tolerated. The most commonly reported adverse reactions are nausea vomiting, diarrhea, and dizziness. These adverse effects may be due to underlying malaria rather than the medications. Rare serious toxicities include anemia, hemolysis, neutropenia, elevated liver enzymes, and allergic reactions.

2. Drugs that inhibit heme polymerase

Chloroquine (氯喹)

Chloroquine has been the drug of choice for both treatment and prevention of malaria since the 1940s.

【Pharmacokinetics】Chloroquine is a synthetic 4-aminoquinoline formulated as the phosphate salt for oral use. It is rapidly and almost completely absorbed from the gastrointestinal tract, reaches maximum plasma concentrations in 3h, and rapidly distributes to the tissues. Chloroquine is mainly excreted in the urine with an initial half-life of 3-5d, and with a much longer terminal elimination half-life of 1-2 months.

【Pharmacodynamics】Chloroquine is a highly effective blood schizonticide and is moderately effective against gametocytes of *P. vivax*, *P.ovale* and *P malariae*. The drug is not effective against *P. falciparum* and not against liver stage parasites.

【Clinical indications】

(1) Acute attack of malaria　Chloroquine is the drug of choice in the treatment of falciparum malaria. It can rapidly terminate fever (in 24-48h) and clear parasitemia (in 48-72h) caused by sensitive parasites.

(2) Chemoprophylaxis　Chloroquine is the preferred chemoprophylactic (化学预防的) agent in the regions without resistant falciparum malaria. To eradicate *P. vivax* and *P. ovale*, a combination with primaquine is needed to clear hepatic stages.

(3) Amebic liver abscess　Chloroquine can reach very high liver concentration and may be used for amebic abscesses that fail in initial therapy with metronidazole (甲硝唑).

【Adverse reactions】Pruritus is often seen and abdominal pain headache. anorexia. malaise, blurring of vision, and urticaria are uncommon. The long-term administration of high doses of chloroquine for rheumatologic diseases may cause irreversible ototoxicity (耳毒性), retinopathy (视网膜病变), myopathy (肌病), and peripheral neuropathy (外周神经病变).

Quinine (奎宁)

【Pharmacokinetics】Quinine is derived from the bark of the cinchona tree, a traditional remedy for intermittent fevers from South America. After oral administration, quinine is rapidly absorbed, reaches peak plasma levels in 1-3h, and is widely distributed in body tissues.

【Pharmacodynamics】Quinine is still an important drug for falciparum malaria, especially severe cases although toxicity may complicate therapy. This drug is also gametocidal against *P. vivax* and *P. ovale*. It is not active against liver stage parasites.

【Clinical indications】

(1) **Parenteral treatment of severe falciparum malaria**　Intravenous artesunate now provides an alternative for this indication.

(2) **Oral treatment of falciparum malaria**　Quinine sulfate is suitable therapy for uncomplicated falciparum malaria. Quinine is less effective than chloroquine against other human malarias and is more toxic.

【Adverse reactions】Therapeutic doses of quinine commonly cause tinnitus (耳鸣), headache, nausea, dizziness, flushing, and visual disturbances the symptoms termed cinchonism.

3. Drugs that alter mitochondrial function

Primaquine (伯氨喹)

Primaquine is principally used for the eradication of dormant liver forms of *P.vivax* and *P. ovale*, and can also be used for chemoprophylaxis against all malarial species.

【Pharmacokinetics】Primaquine is a synthetic 8-aminoquinoline. This drug may be well absorbed orally, reaching peak plasma levels in 1-2h. The plasma half-life is 3-8h. It is widely distributed to the tissues and is rapidly metabolized and excreted in the urine. Three major metabolites appear to have less antimalarial activity but more potential for inducing hemolysis than the parent compound.

【Pharmacodynamics】Primaquine is active against hepatic stages of all human malaria parasites. It is the only available agent active against the dormant hypnozoite stages of *P. vivax* and *P.ovale*. It is also gametocidal against the four human malaria species. Primaquine is effective against erythrocytic stage parasites, but this activity is too weak to play an important role.

【Clinical indications】

(1) **Therapy of acute *P. Vivax* and *P. Ovale* malaria**　Standard therapy for these infections firstly is the use of chloroquine to eradicate erythrocytic forms and then, primaquine to eradicate liver hypnozoites and prevent a subsequent relapse.

(2) **Terminal prophylaxis of *P. Vivax* and *P. Ovale* malaria**　The chemoprophylaxis cannot prevent alapse of tina or orale malaria because the hypnozolte forms of these parasites cannot be eradicated by chloroquine or other available blood schizonticide agents.

(3) **Chemoprophylaxis of malaria**　Primaquine has been reported as a daily agent to provide good

levels of protection against *Plasmodium falciparum* and *P. vivax* malaria.

(4) **Gametocidal action**   A single dose of primaquine can be used as a control measure to render *Plasmodium falciparum* gametocytes noninfective to mosquitoes.

【Adverse reactions】Primaquine is usually well tolerated. Nausea, epigastric pain (上腹痛), abdominal cramps (腹痛), and headache are uncommon if the dose is not high. Serious effects are leukopenia, agranulocytosis, leukocytosis, and cardiac arrhythmias (心律失常).

【Contraindications and cautions】Primaquine should be avoided in patients with a history of granulocytopenia. It is never given parenterally because it may induce marked hypotension. Patients should be tested for G-6-PD deficiency before primaquine is prescribed.

4. Inhibitor of folate synthesis

Pyrimethamine (乙胺嘧啶)

【Pharmacokinetics】Pyrdimethane is a 2, 4-diaminopyrimidine related to trimethoprim. The drug is slowly absorbed from the gastrointestinal tract, reaches peak plasma levels 2-6h after oral administration, binds to plasma proteins, and has an elimination half-life of about 3.5 days. It is extensively metabolized before excretion.

【Pharmacodynamics】Pyrimethamine is active against erythrocytic forms of susceptible strains of all four human malaria species and is not gametocidal or effective against the persistent liver stages of *P. vivax* or *P. ovale.*

【Clinical indications】

(1) Chemoprophylaxis with single folate antagonists is no longer recommended because of frequent resistance. A number of agents are used in combination regimens, for example, trimethopeim-sultamethoxazole.

(2) A new strategy for malaria control is intermittent preventive therapy, in which high-risk patients receive intermittent treatment for malaria, regardless of their infection status.

(3) Treatment of chloroquine-resistant Falciparum malaria.

【Adverse reactions】Most patients tolerate pyrimethamine well. Gastrointestinal symptoms, skin rashes, and itching are rare. Folate supements should be routinely administered during pregnancy.

5. Chemotherapy for amebiasis

Amebiasis is infection with *Entamoeba histolytica*. This organism can cause asymptomatic intestinal intection, mild to moderate colitis, severe intestinal infection (dysentery), ameboma (阿米巴瘤), liver abscess, and other extraintestinal infections. The choice of drugs for amebiasis depends on the clinical presentation.

Metronidazole (甲硝唑)

Metronidazole, a nitroimidazole, is used in the treatment of extraluminal amebiasis. It kills trophozoites but not cysts of *E. histolytica* and effectively eradicates intestinal and extraintestinal tissue infections.

【Pharmacokinetics】Oral metronidazole is easily absorbed and permeates all tissues by simple diffusion. Intracellular concentrations rapidly approach extracellular levels. Peak plasma concentrations reach in 1-3h. Protein binding of the drug is low and the half-life of unchanged drug is 7.5h for metronidazole.

【Pharmacodynamics】As for the mechanism of metronidazole, the nitrogroup of metronidazole is chemically reduced in anaerobic bacteria and sensitive protozoans and reactive reduction products are responsible for antimicrobial activity.

【Clinical indications】

(1) **Amebiasis** Metronidazole is the drug of choice in the treatment of all tissue infections with *E.histolytica*. The drug is not effective against luminal parasites and therefore must be used with a luminal ameicide to ensure eradication of the infection.

(2) **Trichomoniasis** Metronidazole is the treatment of choice.

(3) **Giardiasis** Metronidazole is the very useful treatment of giardiasis. The dosage for giardiasis is much lower, resulting in less and mild side effects. Efficacy after a single treatment is about 90%.

【Adverse reactions】Nausea, headache, dry mouth, and a metallic taste in the mouth are common side effects. Uncommon adverse reactions include vomiting, diarrhea, insomnia, weakness, dizziness, thrush rash, dysuria, dark urine, vertigo (眩晕), paresthesias (皮肤感觉异常), and neutropenia. Taking the drug with meals lessens gastrointestinal irritation.

6. Drugs for the treatment of schistosomiasis praziquantel

【Pharmacokinetics】Praziquantel (吡喹酮) is a synthetic isoquinoline-pyrazine derivative. It is rapidly absorbed with a bioavailability of 80% after oral administration. Peak serum concentrations reach after 1-3h administration. The half life is 0.5-1.5h. Renal excretion accounts for 60%-80% and bile, for 15%-35%.

【Clinical indications】

(1) **Schistosomiasis** Praziquantel is effective in the treatment of schistosome infections of all species and lost other trematode and cestode infection cysticercosis.

(2) **Clonorchiasis, opisthorchiasis, and paragonimiasis** Standard dosing is 25mg/kg three times daily for 2 days for each of these fluke infections.

(3) **Taeniasis** A single dose of praziquantel results in almost 100% cure rates for *T. saginata*, *T. solium*, and *D. latum* infections.

Mild and transient adverse reactions are common. Most common are headache, dizziness, drowsiness, and lassitude (疲乏) and others include nausea vomiting abdominal pain, loose stools, pruritus, urticaria, arthralgia, myalgia and low-grade fever.

7. Drug for intestinal worm infections

Albendazole (阿苯达唑)

Albendazole is a broad-spectrum oral antihelminthic, and used in the treatment of pinworm(蛲虫) and hookworm (钩虫) infections, ascariasis (蛔虫病), trichuriasis (鞭虫病), and strongyloidiasis (类圆线虫病). It is also used for treatment of hydatid disease (包虫病) and cysticercosis (囊尾幼虫病).

【Pharmacokinetics】Albendazole is a benzimidazole carbamate (苯并咪唑氨基甲酸酯). After oral administration, it is irregularly absorbed and undergoes first-pass metabolism in the liver to the active metabolite albendazole sulfoxide (阿苯达唑亚砜). The plasma half-life is 8-12h. Its metabolites are excreted in the urine.

【Pharmacodynamics】Albendazole act against nematodes by inhibiting microtubule synthesis. It also has larvicidal effects (杀幼虫作用) in hydatid disease, cysticercosis, ascariasis, and hookworm infection and ovicidal effects in ascariasis, ancylostomasis, and trichuriasis.

【Clinical indications】

(1) Ascariasis, trichuriasis, hookworm and pinworm infection.

(2) **Hydatid disease**　Albendazole is the treatment of choice for the disease and is a useful adjunct to surgical removal or aspiration of cysts. It is more active against *Echinococcus granulosus* than against *E. multilocularis*.

(3) **Neurocysticercosis**　This drug therapy may be appropriate for symptomatic parenchymal or intraventricular cysts (症状性实质性或脑室内囊肿). Corticosteroids (类固醇) are commonly given with the antihelminthic drug (驱肠虫药) to decrease inflammation.

【Adverse reactions】Albendazole is nearly free of significant adverse reactions when taken shortly, Mild and transient epigastric distress, diarrhea, headache, nausea, dizziness, lassitude, and insomnia can be seen during treatment.

重 点 小 结

药物	药理作用	临床应用	不良反应
氯喹、奎宁	抑制疟原虫 DNA 转录	杀灭红细胞内疟原虫，控制疟疾症状；对肠外阿米巴病有较好疗效	奎宁会引起金鸡纳反应、溶血和过敏反应
青蒿素及其衍生物	通过产生自由基，对恶性疟原虫红内期的生物膜产生破坏作用，或与原虫蛋白结合，使之死亡	用于控制间日疟的症状以及耐氯喹虫株的治疗	偶见头晕、恶心、食欲缺乏、腹痛、耳鸣、睡眠不佳、皮肤瘙痒等不良反应

续表

药物	药理作用	临床应用	不良反应
伯氨喹	可能与疟原虫的活性氧产生或干扰其线粒体电子转运有关	对良性的红细胞外期级各型疟原虫的配子体均有效,是控制疟原虫复发和阻止疟疾传播的首选药	毒性较大,少数特异质患者可发生急性溶血性贫血和高铁血红蛋白血症
甲硝唑、替硝唑	可能与影响病原虫的能量代谢有关	治疗阿米巴病、滴虫病、贾第鞭毛虫病的首选药物,对厌氧菌引起的感染有良好的疗效	可见恶心、呕吐、食欲缺乏、腹痛等消化系统症状

题库

目 标 检 测

一、单项选择题

1. 广谱驱肠虫药是（　　）
　　A. 哌嗪　　　　B. 吡喹酮　　　　C. 乙胺嗪　　　　D. 氯硝柳胺　　　　E. 阿苯达唑

2. 某患者,近期出现腹痛、腹泻、粪便有脓血,粪检见阿米巴滋养体,甲硝唑治疗后症状消失,为防止复发应选用的药物是（　　）
　　A. 甲硝唑　　　B. 替硝唑　　　　C. 二氯尼特　　　D. 氯喹　　　　E. 依米丁

3. 某大学毕业生拟计划去非洲氯喹耐药高发区工作一年,为了进行适当的疟疾预防,他应该服用的抗疟药是（　　）
　　A. 伯氨喹　　　B. 多西环素　　　C. 甲氟喹　　　D. 乙胺嘧啶　　　E. 奎宁

4. 治疗肠内外阿米巴病常选用（　　）
　　A. 氯喹　　　　B. 甲硝唑　　　　C. 依米丁　　　D. 链霉素　　　　E. 巴龙霉素

二、多项选择题

5. 某疟疾患者突然昏迷,给予二盐酸奎宁静脉滴注抢救,抢救过程中,患者又出现寒战、高热,他不应该服用的抗疟药是（　　）
　　A. 氯喹　　　　B. 甲氟喹　　　　C. 伯氨喹　　　D. 乙胺嘧啶　　　E. 青蒿素

（辛晓明）

医药大学堂
WWW.YIYAODXT.COM

Chapter 39   Antifungal drugs

PPT

学习目标

1. **掌握** 多烯类、唑类、烯丙胺类的药理作用及机制、临床应用和不良反应。
2. **熟悉** 氟胞嘧啶的主要药理作用、临床应用及不良反应。
3. **了解** 卡泊芬净的药理作用、临床应用及不良反应。

Fungal infection can be divided into superficial fungal infection and deep fungal infection. The superficial fungal infection is caused by fungus that intrude the skin, hair and nail with the high incidence and low mortality. The deep fungal infection is caused by fungus that intrude people internal organs with the low incidence and high mortality. Antifungal agents (抗真菌药) have the ability to inhibit or kill the growth and breed of fungi. According to the difference of the resources, antifungal drugs can be divided into two main classes of antifungal drugs: antifungal antibiotic (抗真菌抗生素) and synthetic antifungal agents.

1. Antifungal antibiotic-polyene macrolides

The amphotericin B, which is a drug of polyene macrolides (多烯类抗生素) and with the antibacterial activity to almost fungus, is a broad-spectrum antifungal agent. Amphotericin B has a strong effect of bacteriostasis especially to the *Cryptococcus* (隐球菌属), *Candida albicans* (白念珠菌), *Blastomyces* (芽生菌属), *Ajellomyces capsulate* (荚膜组织胞浆菌) and *Coccidioides immitis* (粗球孢子菌). It also has a bactericidal effect at a high concentration.

【Pharmacodynamics】Amphotericin B can selectivity junctures with ergosterol (麦角固醇) in the fungal cell, forming micropore or access to increase membrane permeability and causing the molecular substance and electrolyte, especially K^+ ion that in the fungal cell, exosmosis (外渗). Finally, fungus will growth arrest or die.

【Clinical indications】

(1) Fungal infection   Intravenous drip the amphotericin B can use to treat the deep part of infection fungal. It can just use to cure infection fungal of intestines by oral. Local application can be used to treat superficial part of infection fungal such as the skin, tunica mucosa (黏膜) and cornea (角膜).

(2) Fungal meningitis (真菌性脑膜炎)   Amphotericin B is sometimes used in the treat of fungal

医药大学堂
WWW.YIYAODXT.COM

305

meningitis by the ways of intravenous drip and intrathecal injections in the meantime.

【Adverse reactions】This kinds of drug may cause a fever, headache, vomiting, anorexia (食欲缺乏), low blood pressure, thrombophlebitis (血栓性静脉炎) and even renal functional lesion.

2. Synthetic antifungal agents

2.1 Antifungal azoles (唑类抗真菌药)

There are two kinds of antifungal azoles drugs: imidazoles and triazoles (三唑类). Ketoconazole (酮康唑), miconazole (咪康唑), econazole(益康唑), clotrimazole (克霉唑) are four major drugs of imidazoles. Ketoconazole is the drug of first choice to cure superficial part fungal infection and is also the first broad spectrum antifungal agents by oral. Ketoconazole has an effect on the cure of deep part or subcutaneous and superficial appearance that has been infected by fungi. Itraconazole (伊曲康唑), fluconazole (氟康唑) and voriconazole (伏立康唑) are three major drugs of triazoles, and those are the drug of first choice to cure deep part fungal infection.

【Pharmacodynamics】Imidazole can selectivity restrain the cytochrome P450 dependency enzyme (细胞色素P450依赖酶) of fungi and inhibit biosynthesis of ergosterol in fungal cell, making the fungal membrane become deletion and leading the membrane permeability increase. Finally, several intra-cellular important materials leak and then fungus die. Imidazole can also inhibit fungal biosynthesis of triglyceride and phospholipid, and restrain the activity of oxidase and katalase (过氧化氢酶), causing the peroxid (过氧化氢) accumulate, and making cellular submicrostructure degeneration (细胞亚微结构变性) and cellular necrosis.

【Clinical indications】

(1) **Deep mycosis**   Miconazole can through the way of intravenous drip cure various deep mycosis. However, the miconazole has lots of adverse reactions, so it is just used as the substitute when the amphotericin B is useless or not tolerant to patients.

(2) **The infection of dermatophytes (皮肤癣菌)**   The bifonazole (联苯苄唑) can restrain 2,4-methylenedihydrogen lanosterol (2,4-甲烯二氢羊毛固醇)translate to demethylated sterol (脱甲基固醇) and also inhibit methylol glutaryl-coenzyme A (羟甲基戊二酰辅酶A) translate to mevalonic acid (甲羟戊酸). Then double cut-out the synthesis of ergosterol, making the antibacterial activity of bifonazole obviously stronger than other imidazole antifungal agents, having broad spectrum and high performance in antibacterial activity.

(3) **Fungal infection**   Miconazole which is a broad spectrum antifungal agents, taking it by the oral intake will have a very low bioavailability (生物利用度低). Now, miconazole is a major drug to cure fungal infection of vagina (阴道), skin and nail by using it in some local part. The skin and mucous membrane (黏膜) are unable to absorb this drug, therefore, the miconazole has no obviously adverse reactions.

(4) **To cure rare fungal infection**   Itraconazole has a wider antibiogram than ketoconazole, the antifungal activity are better than ketoconazole. Therefore, the deep part, subcutaneous (皮下) and simple fungal infection can be treated in effect. Itraconazole has been the choice drug to cure the rare fungal

infection such as tissue hyalomitome (透明质) bacterium infection and blastomyces infection (芽生菌感染).

【Adverse reactions】Contact dermatitis(接触性皮炎), burning sensation (灼烧感), gargalesthesia (瘙痒) and skin crack.

2.2　Allylamine (烯丙胺类抗真菌药)

Terbinafine (特比萘芬) is one of the most usual allylamine antifungal agents in clinical at the moment, with the high activity, low toxicity and oral bioactivity. Terbinafine also has a better antibacterial activity to aspergillus, fusarium and other filamentous fungus (丝状真菌).

【Pharmacodynamics】The squalene epoxidase (角鲨烯环氧化酶) can be inhibited by terbinafine, which can restrain the way that use squalene (角鲨烯) to make ergosterol by the key enzyme catalysis, and then the dyssynthesis (合成障碍) of ergosterol fungal cell wall will occur.

【Clinical indications】Terbinafine has the ability to cure onychomycosis and some superficial fungal infection by the ways of external or oral. It also be used with amphotericin B to cure deep fungus infection such as the aspergillus infection (曲霉菌感染), candida infection and cryptococcosis of lung (肺隐球菌感染).

【Adverse reactions】Terbinafine has little adverse reaction. Gastrointestinal tract (胃肠道反应) is common and the reaction of hepatitis and rash are rare.

2.3　Miazines (嘧啶类抗真菌药)

Flucytosine (氟胞嘧啶)

【Pharmacodynamics】Flucytosine can deaminate and form the 5-fluorouracil which is a kind of antimetabolite, and then transform from the uridine-5-phosphoric acid pyrophosphorylase (尿苷-5-磷酸焦磷酸化酶)to 5-fluorodeoxyuridine to inhibit thymidine synthetase (胸腺嘧啶核苷合成酶) and to block the uracil deoxynucleoside (尿嘧啶脱氧核苷) becoming thymidine. Finally, flucytosine affects DNA synthesis.

【Clinical indications】

(1) Cryptococcus infection (隐球菌感染)　The major use of flucytosine is to cure some infection of cryptococcus, candida(念珠菌) and pigmented fungi (色素真菌), but it is not as good as the effect of amphotericin B.

(2) Meningitis (脑膜炎)　Flucytosine is usually used with amphotericin B, resulting in that flucytosine has a better cure effect on meningitis that infected by cryptococcus, because it can through the blood-brain barrier easily.

【Adverse reactions】Vomiting, diarrhea (腹泻), emerging rash, fever and transaminase rising.

重 点 小 结

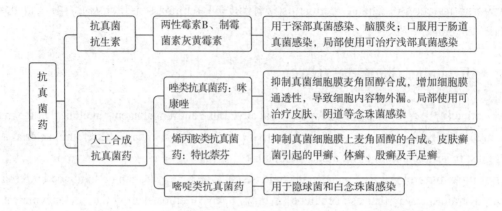

目 标 检 测

单项选择题

1. 唑类抗真菌的作用机制是（　　）
   A. 竞争性抑制鸟嘌呤进入 DNA 分子，干扰 DNA 合成
   B. 替代尿嘧啶进入 DNA 分子中，阻断核酸合成
   C. 抑制以 DNA 为模板的 RNA 聚合酶，阻碍 mRNA 合成
   D. 选择性与细胞膜的麦角固醇结合，增加膜的通透性
   E. 选择性抑制细胞色素 P450 依赖性的 14-α 脱甲基酶

2. 两性霉素 B 抗真菌的作用机制是（　　）
   A. 竞争性抑制鸟嘌呤进入 DNA 分子，干扰 DNA 合成
   B. 替代尿嘧啶进入 DNA 分子中，阻断核酸合成
   C. 抑制以 DNA 为模板的 RNA 聚合酶，阻碍 mRNA 合成
   D. 选择性与细胞膜的麦角固醇结合，增加膜的通透性
   E. 选择性抑制细胞色素 P450 依赖性的 14-α 脱甲基酶

3. 氟胞嘧啶抗真菌的作用机制是（　　）
   A. 竞争性抑制鸟嘌呤进入 DNA 分子，干扰 DNA 合成
   B. 替代尿嘧啶进入 DNA 分子中，阻断核酸合成
   C. 抑制以 DNA 为模板的 RNA 聚合酶，阻碍 mRNA 合成
   D. 选择性与细胞膜的麦角固醇结合，增加膜的通透性
   E. 选择性抑制细胞色素 P450 依赖性的 14-α 脱甲基酶

（白　莉）

PPT

Chapter 40　Antitubercular drugs

Tuberculosis (结核病) is a chronic infectious disease caused by *Mycobacterium tuberculosis* (结核分枝杆菌), which can invade many organs of the body, especially the lungs. Tuberculosis can be divided into two groups: phthisis (肺结核) and extrapulmonary tuberculosis(肺外结核). Antitubercular drugs (抗结核药) currently have two groups. ①First-line antitubercular drugs with high efficacy and few adverse reactions, such as isoniazid, rifampicin (利福平), ethambutol (乙胺丁醇), streptomycin and pyrazinamide (吡嗪酰胺). These drugs are recognized as choice drugs. ②Second-line antitubercular drugs with higher toxicity, poorer efficacy and resistance against first-line antituberculous drugs, including para-aminosalicylic acid (对氨基水杨酸), ethionamide (乙硫异烟胺) and capreomycin (卷曲霉素). In addition, rifandine (利福定) and roxithromycin (罗红霉素) represent a new generation antituberculous drugs.

1. First-line antitubercular drugs

Isoniazid (INH,异烟肼)

【Pharmacokinetics】Isoniazid is easily absorbed orally or by injection. After oral administration, the blood concentration reached a peak value of 1-2h. In clinic, people are divided into two groups based on the acetylation rate of isoniazid *in vivo*: extensive metabolizers ($t_{1/2}$ = 70min), poor metabolizers ($t_{1/2}$ = 3h).

【Pharmacodynamics】Isoniazid has a bactericidal effect on bacteria in breeding period and an inhibitory effect on mycobacterium tuberculosis in quiescent period. It has high selectivity to mycobacterium tuberculosis and strong anti-mycobacterium tuberculosis ability on both inside and outside the cell. The actions of isoniazid have two views. ① Mycolic acid (分枝菌酸) is an important component of the cell wall of mycobacterium tuberculosis. Isoniazid suppresses the biosynthesis of mycolic acid and blocks the extension of long chain fatty acids of mycotic acid precursors, resulting in the mycobacterium tuberculosis cell wall synthesis stopping and dying. ② Isoniazid inhibits DNA synthesis

医药大学堂
WWW.YIYAODXT.COM

of mycobacterium tuberculosis to exert antibacterial action. ③Isoniazid could bind to an enzyme in mycobacterium tuberculosis to cause metabolic disorders.

【Clinical indications】Isoniazid is the first-line drug for the treatment of various types of tuberculosis, which can be used alone for early mild tuberculosis or prophylactic drugs, and must be used in combination with other first-line drugs for standardized treatment. Acute miliary tuberculosis (粟粒性肺结核) and tuberculous meningitis (结核性脑膜炎) should be used increased dose and duration of treatment, if necessary, intravenous drip administration.

【Adverse reactions】

(1) **Nervous system**   The common reaction is peripheral neuritis, which is manifested as numbness in hands and feet, muscle tremor and gait instability. Large dose can cause headache, dizziness, excitement and optic neuritis. It is necessary to timely supplement vitamin B_6 when isoniazid administration.

(2) **Hepatotoxicity**   Isoniazid can induce liver cells injury and increase aminotransferase. A few patients appear jaundice. If severe, it can cause liver lobule necrosis. The patient using isoniazid should check liver function regularly. In addition, patients with rapid metabolism and liver dysfunction should be with caution, when using isoniazid.

(3) **Others**   It can also cause various rashes, fever, gastrointestinal reactions (胃肠道反应), granulocytopenia (粒细胞减少), thrombocytopenia (血小板减少) and hemolytic anemia (溶血性贫血).

Rifampicin (利福平)

【Pharmacokinetics】Oral absorption of rifampicin is rapid and complete, and the blood concentration reaches the peak at 2-4h. It has a half-life of 4h. The effective serum concentration can be maintained for 8-12h.

【Pharmacodynamics】Rifampicin can specifically inhibit the enzyme activity of DNA-dependent RNA polymerase in bacteria and block mRNA synthesis, but has no effect on RNA polymerase in animal cells. Rifampicin has a broad spectrum of antibacterial effects. It has not only a strong antibacterial effect on mycobacterium tuberculosis, leprosy bacillus (麻风杆菌), Gram-positive coccus and drug-resistant staphylococcus aureus, but also has inhibitory effects on Gram-negative bacteria, some viruses and mycoplasma trachomatis (沙眼衣原体). It has bacteriostasis at low concentration and sterilization at high concentration. It is effective to tuberculosis bacillus both inside and outside the cell.

【Clinical indications】Rifampicin is one of the most effective drugs to treat tuberculosis. It is easy to develop drug resistance when used alone. It is often combined with isoniazid in the treatment of severe patients, and combined with ethambutol and pyrazinamide to patients with retreatment. Topical use can treat trachoma (沙眼), acute conjunctivitis (急性结膜炎), and viral keratitis (病毒性角膜炎).

【Adverse reactions】The common adverse reactions are nausea, vomiting, anorexia, abdominal pain and diarrhea (腹痛腹泻). A few patients develop jaundice and hepatomegaly (肝大). It has a teratogenic effect (致畸作用) on animals. Use with caution in the first trimester of pregnancy and in patients with liver dysfunction.

Ethambutol (乙胺丁醇)

【Pharmacokinetics】Oral absorption of ethambutol is rapid, and the blood concentration reached the peak at 2-4h. It has a half-life of 3-4h. 20 % of the drugs are excreted from the stool, and 50% are excreted in the urine as a prototype.

【Pharmacodynamics】Ethambutol has a high antibacterial activity against almost all types of mycobacterium tuberculosis in the breeding period, but has no effect on other bacteria. Its antibacterial mechanism is to bind to Mg^{2+} and interfere with bacterial RNA synthesis.

【Clinical indications】Ethambutol is used in combination with isoniazid for the treatment of various types of tuberculosis, especially for patients who have failed treatment with streptomycin and isoniazid, but not for children under 5 years of age.

【Adverse reactions】It common occurs gastrointestinal reactions, rashes, thrombocytopenia, and hyperuricemia (高尿酸血症). The serious adverse reaction is optic neuritis, which usually occurs within 2-6 months after taking the medicine, showing amblyopia (弱视), reduced field of vision (视野缩小), red and green color blindness (红绿色盲), etc.

Streptomycin (链霉素)

The antituberculous effect of streptomycin is weaker than that of isoniazid and rifampicin. It has poor efficacy in the treatment of tuberculous meningitis, due to poorer penetration. Combined with other antituberculous drugs, it can be used for invasive tuberculosis, miliary tuberculosis, especially for acute exudative lesions.

Pyrazinamide (吡嗪酰胺)

Pyrazinamide has strong inhibitory and bactericidal effects on mycobacterium tuberculosis under acidic conditions. It is easy to develop drug resistance when used alone, but no cross-resistance when used with other drugs. It has a synergistic effect when used with isoniazid and rifampicin. Severe liver damage can occur when pyrazinamide is used in large quantities over a long period of time.

2.　Second-line antitubercular drugs

Para-aminosalicylic acid (对氨基水杨酸)

Para-aminosalicylic acid only has a bacteriostatic effect on extracellular mycobacterium tuberculosis, with narrow antibacterial spectrum. It can competitively inhibit dihydropteroate synthase (二氢蝶酸合酶) and block the synthesis of dihydrofolic acid (二氢叶酸), thereby stopping protein synthesis and suppressing the reproduction of mycobacterium tuberculosis. At present, it is mainly used in combination with isoniazid and streptomycin to delay the emergence of drug resistance and increase the curative effect. Para-aminosalicylic acid exists in sodium salt. Sodium salt solution is unstable, and easy to be decomposed and discolored by light. Therefore, it should be prepared fresh and used in dark conditions. Its oral absorption is rapid and good. It reaches a peak value 2h later and a half-life is 1h. The common adverse reactions are nausea, vomiting, anorexia, abdominal pain and diarrhea.

Ethionamide (乙硫异烟胺)

Ethionamide is a derivative of isoniazid. Drug resistance occurs easily when used alone. It has common adverse reactions with high incidence, such as gastrointestinal reaction. Thus, it is mainly used in patients who fail to respond to first-line antituberculous drugs and need to be combined with other drugs. It is not suitable for pregnant women and children under 12 years old.

Capreomycin (卷曲霉素)

Capreomycin is polypeptide antibiotic (多肽抗生素). Its antibacterial effect is mainly through suppressing protein synthesis. Drug resistance occurs easily when used alone, and there is cross-resistance with neomycin (新霉素) and kanamycin (卡那霉素).

3. New generation antitubercular drugs

They are shown in Table 40-1.

Table 40-1　Characteristics of new generation antitubercular drugs

Drugs	Actions	Uses	Adverse reactions
Rifandine	Antituberculosis effect is stronger than rifampicin; Effective for Gram-positive and negative bacteria	Combined with other drugs to treat tuberculosis; to treat staphylococcus aureus infections that are resistant to other antibiotics	Gastrointestinal reactions, thrombocytopenia, rash
Roxithromycin	It is the strongest antibiotics of macrolides against tuberculosis, but less effective than isoniazid	It has synergistic effects with isoniazid or rifampicin	Less adverse effects; occasionally rash, skin itching, headache, dizziness

4. Application principles of antitubercular drugs

The principle of tuberculosis treatment is early medication, drug combination, appropriate doses, regular medication in the whole process.

4.1　Early medication (早期用药)

The early stage of tuberculosis is mainly exudative inflammatory response. *Mycobacterium tuberculosis* in the tuberculous lesions grow vigorously, and is sensitive to antituberculous drugs and easy to be suppressed or killed. Moreover, there is no obstacles at local blood circulation in the early lesions, so drugs may easily to penetrate for exerting antibacterial effect. The early medication can obtain a better curative effect.

4.2　Drug combination (联合用药)

Combined use of two or more antituberculous drugs can enhance efficacy, delay the development of drug resistance and reduce toxicity.

4.3　Appropriate doses (适量)

The dosage should be appropriate. If the drug dose is insufficient, it is difficult to reach the effective concentration of the drug in the tissue, and easy to produce drug resistance. If the dose is large, it is easy to induce sever adverse reactions.

4.4　Regular medication in the whole process (坚持全程规律用药)

Tuberculosis is a relapsing disease, and early withdrawal of drugs can cause suppressed bacteria to reproduce or migrate again, leading to treatment failure. Therefore, regular use of drugs throughout the course and not to stop early are necessary. For example, mild phthisis should be continued for 9-12 months, moderate and severe phthisis for 18-24 months, or medication regimens should be adjusted depending on the patient's condition.

重 点 小 结

药物	药理作用	临床应用	不良反应
异烟肼	抑制分枝菌酸合成或结核分枝杆菌 DNA 合成而发挥杀菌或抑菌作用	各类结核病患者的首选药物	周围神经炎、肝脏毒性、皮疹、发热、胃肠道反应等
利福平	特异性抑制细菌 DNA 依赖的 RNA 聚合酶活性，阻碍 mRNA 合成	目前治疗结核病最有效的药物之一	恶心、呕吐、食欲缺乏、腹痛、腹泻，少数出现黄疸和肝大
乙胺丁醇	与 Mg^{2+} 结合，干扰菌体 RNA 的合成	适用于经链霉素和异烟肼治疗无效的结核病	胃肠道反应、皮疹、血小板减少症、高尿酸血症

目 标 检 测

题库

一、选择题

（一）单项选择题
1. 各种类型的结核病可首选（　　　　）
　　A. 利福平　　　　　　　　B. 对氨基水杨酸　　　　　　C. 链霉素
　　D. 异烟肼　　　　　　　　E. 吡嗪酰胺

2. 下列全部为一线抗结核药的是（　　　）
   A. 异烟肼、利福平、卷曲霉素　　　　　B. 异烟肼、链霉素、利福平
   C. 乙胺丁醇、对氨基水杨酸、利福平　　D. 罗红霉素、利福平、异烟肼
   E. 异烟肼、对氨基水杨酸、利福平

3. 异烟肼抗结核分枝杆菌的机制是（　　　）
   A. 抑制结核分枝杆菌蛋白质合成　　　　B. 抑制结核分枝杆菌分枝菌酸合成
   C. 抑制结核分枝杆菌核酸代谢　　　　　D. 影响结核分枝杆菌胞浆膜的通透性
   E. 抑制结核分枝杆菌细胞壁的合成

4. 下列不属于异烟肼不良反应的是（　　　）
   A. 神经肌肉接头阻滞　　　　　B. 血小板减少　　　　　C. 周围神经炎
   D. 皮疹　　　　　E. 肝损伤

5. 乙胺丁醇与利福平合用目的在于（　　　）
   A. 加快药物的排泄速度
   B. 有利于药物进入结核感染病灶
   C. 起协同作用，并能延缓耐药性的产生
   D. 延长利福平作用时间
   E. 起拮抗作用

（二）多项选择题

6. 异烟肼具有的作用是（　　　）
   A. 口服吸收快而完全　　　　　B. 主要经肝乙酰化代谢
   C. 对结核分枝杆菌有高度选择性　　D. 对细胞外的结核分枝杆菌无作用
   E. 与其他抗结核药之间无交叉耐药性

7. 抗结核病药的使用原则有（　　　）
   A. 早期用药　　　　　B. 联合用药　　　　　C. 坚持全程规律用药
   D. 适量　　　　　E. 终生用药

8. 以下为一线抗结核药的是（　　　）
   A. 异烟肼　　　　　B. 对氨基水杨酸　　　　　C. 利福平
   D. 乙胺丁醇　　　　　E. 卡那霉素

二、思考题

试述异烟肼作为治疗各型结核病首选药的药理学基础，应用时应注意哪些问题？

（程媛媛）

Chapter 41　Antiviral drugs

 学习目标

　　1. **掌握**　抗病毒药物的分类、抗病毒机制；利巴韦林、齐多夫定、阿昔洛韦的药理作用及机制、临床应用和不良反应。
　　2. **熟悉**　干扰素、奥司他韦的药理作用和临床应用。
　　3. **了解**　金刚烷胺、碘苷、阿糖腺苷的临床应用。

　　Viruses are pathogenic organisms that are too small to reproduce outside the host cell. The virus particles that can survive on their own are called virions, and viruses contain fragments of nucleic acid (RNA or DNA). The virus can absorb or penetrate into the host cell, remove the protein shell in the cell, release the infectious nucleic acid, and carry on the nucleic acid replication, transcription and the protein synthesis, the synthesized nucleic acid and the protein assemble into the progeny virus particle, from the cell in one form or another, and infect the new host cell. Viruses have caused some of the most dramatic and deadly disease pandemics in human history.

　　Antiviral drug (抗病毒药物) acts as a treatment by blocking the growth and reproduction of the virus at various stages, including: ① stop the virus from attaching to the host cell. ② Prevent the virus from entering the host cell or shedding its shell. ③ Inhibit viral nucleic acid replication, affecting DNA synthesis. ④ Inhibit the process of virus transcription, translation and assembly by enhancing the disease resistance of the host. Because the virus is strictly intracellular and depends on many functions of the host cell when it replicates, the drug may kill the normal cells of the host as well as resist the virus. In addition, the virus mutates through repeated replication errors, which limits the use of antiviral drug and reduces the effectiveness of antiviral drug.

　　Antiviral drugs are used to treat virus infection in clinic. According to the different uses of antiviral drugs, they are divided into broad-spectrum antiviral drugs (广谱抗病毒药物), anti human immunodeficiency virus (HIV) drugs (抗人类免疫缺陷病毒药物) and other antiviral drugs to treat herpes virus (疱疹病毒), influenza virus (流感病毒), hepatitis virus (肝炎病毒) and other infections.

1. Broad-spectrum antiviral drugs

Ribavirin (利巴韦林)

【Pharmacokinetics】 Ribavirin is absorbed rapidly with a bioavailability of 45% after oral

315

administration. Ribavirin can pass placenta, blood-brain barrier and enter milk. It is metabolized in the liver and excreted mainly by the kidney.

【Pharmacodynamics】The drug acts as a competitive inhibitor of virus synthetase, which inhibits creatinine monophosphate dehydrogenase, influenza virus RNA polymerase, and mRNA guanyltransferase. It can inhibit the growth of various viruses such as respiratory syncytial virus (呼吸道合胞病毒), influenza virus, hepatitis A virus (甲肝病毒) and adenovirus (腺病毒) *in vitro*.

【Clinical Indications】Ribavirin is the best treatment of RSV pneumonia and bronchitis (支气管炎). Usually, small particles of aerosols are used for the treatment of RSV pneumonia and bronchitis. Influenza is also treated by aerosols, while most other viral infections are treated by intravenous injection. It has certain curative effect on acute hepatitis A and C (急性甲型和丙型肝炎).

【Adverse reactions】The common adverse reactions are headache, diarrhea, anemia, fatigue, bilirubin rise, etc., which disappear after drug withdrawal. Teratogenic effects have been observed in animals.

Interferon (干扰素), transfer factor (转移因子), thymosin α₁ (胸腺肽α₁)

These drugs enable cells to obtain immune function, induce T cells to differentiate and mature, and regulate their functions, and has antitumor and immune regulation effects. They are being clinically used for acute viral infectious diseases such as influenza and other upper respiratory infectious diseases, viral myocarditis, mumps, Japanese encephalitis, etc. and chronic viral infections such as chronic active hepatitis, congenital and acquired immune deficiency adjuvant treatment of diseases, fungal infections and tumors.

2. Anti-AIDS drugs

AIDS is a retrovirus and has two main types: HIV-1 and HIV-2. Current anti-HIV drugs work by inhibiting reverse transcriptase or HIV protease, including nucleoside reverse transcriptase inhibitors (NRTIs), non-nucleoside reverse transcriptase inhibitors (NNRTIs) and protease inhibitors (PIs).

Zidovudine (齐多夫定)

【Pharmacokinetics】Zidovudine is rapidly absorbed orally with an absorption rate of 65% and bioavailability of 52%-75%. The drug is widely distributed throughout the body tissues and body fluids. About 18% of the drug was excreted by the kidney after combining with glucuronic acid in the liver, and some hepatic metabolites were toxic.

【Pharmacodynamics】Zidovudine inhibits the host cell DNA polymerase and show cytotoxic effects.

【Clinical indications】

AIDS It has both anti-HIV-1 activity and anti-HIV-2 activity. It can reduce the incidence of HIV infection and prolong the survival period. It can treat dementia and thrombocytopenia induced by HIV.

【Adverse reactions】Zidovudine causes myelosuppression (骨髓抑制), anemia (贫血) or neutropenia (中性粒细胞减少症). High dose can cause anxiety(焦虑), mental disorder (精神错乱) and tremor (震颤). Zidovudine should be used with caution in patients with liver dysfunction.

3. Anti-herpes virus drug

Acyclovir (阿昔洛韦),vidarabine (阿糖腺苷), ganciclovir (更昔洛韦), idoxuridine (碘苷)

【Pharmacokinetics】Acyclovir has poor oral absorption and with bioavailability of 15%-20%, which can be distributed to various tissues and organs of the whole body. The highest concentrations were found in the kidneys and small intestine, and the concentration in the cerebrospinal fluid was about 50% of that in the blood. The plasma protein binding rate of acyclovir is low. Acyclovir is mainly excreted via glomerular filtration and tubular secretion, and only 14% of the unchanged agent is excreted in the urine.

【Pharmacodynamics】Acyclovir is a broad-spectrum anti-herpes virus drug, which has the strongest effect on HSV, about 10 times stronger than iodide and about 160 times stronger than vidarabine, and also has a certain effect on hepatitis B virus. After acyclovir enters the infected cells, it is transformed into acyclovir triphosphate under the catalysis of adenosine kinase and cytokinase, which has a strong inhibitory effect on viral DNA polymerase and prevents the synthesis of viral DNA. Acyclovir has no effect on RNA virus.

【Clinical indications】Treatment of HSV infection is the first choice. It is used to prevent and treat skin and mucous membrane infection caused by HSV, such as keratitis, cutaneous mucous membrane infection, herpes simplex, herpes encephalitis, etc. It is also used to treat herpes zoster virus infection.

【Adverse reactions】Acyclovir causes gastrointestinal reactions, headaches, and rash; intravenous injections of acyclovir can cause phlebitis (静脉炎) and renal abnormalities. Ganciclovir causes myelosuppression, digestive and urinary system damage, which is contraindicated for allergy. Long-term use of idoxuridine damages the cornea, resulting in degeneration and opacification.

4. Anti-flu drugs

Amantadine (金刚烷胺)

Amantadine acts in the early stage of virus replication, prevents the influenza A virus from entering the host cell and inhibits its replication. It is not effective against influenza B virus and other viruses, and it can also resist tremor paralysis.

Oseltamivir (奥司他韦)

Oseltamivir is an antiviral neuraminidase inhibitor used for the treatment and prophylaxis of infection with influenza viruses A (including pandemic H1N1) and B.Oseltamivir exerts its antiviral activity by inhibiting the activity of the viral neuraminidase enzyme found on the surface of the virus, which prevents budding from the host cell, viral replication, and infectivity.

5. Anti-hepatitis virus drugs

Hepatitis virus is divided into five types: A, B, C, D, and E. Hepatitis C is more common in western countries, and hepatitis B is mainly prevalent in China. In clinical practice, interferon and ribavirin are often used in combination to treat chronic viral hepatitis and acute hepatitis C.

重 点 小 结

药物	药理作用	临床应用	不良反应
广谱抗病毒药：利巴韦林	改变病毒核酸合成所需的核苷酸或干扰病毒 mRNA 的合成	呼吸道合胞病毒性肺炎、急性甲型和丙型肝炎	贫血、乏力
抗 HIV 药：齐多夫定	与病毒 DNA 聚合酶结合，阻止病毒复制；抑制 HIV	减少 HIV 从感染孕妇到胎儿的子宫转移发生率，治疗 HIV 诱发的痴呆和血栓性血小板减少症	骨髓抑制、贫血或中性粒细胞减少症，过大剂量引发焦虑、精神错乱和震颤
抗疱疹病毒药：阿昔洛韦	抑制病毒 DNA 聚合酶，阻滞病毒 DNA 合成	治疗 HSV 首选药物，还可用于疱疹性角膜炎、单纯疱疹和带状疱疹、单纯疱疹脑炎、生殖器疱疹	胃肠道功能紊乱、头痛和斑疹、静脉炎、可逆性肾功能紊乱、神经毒性（包括震颤和谵妄）
抗流感病毒药：奥司他韦	抑制流感病毒神经氨酸酶	流感，抗禽流感甲型 H1N1 病毒	流感，抗禽流感甲型 H1N1 病毒
抗肝炎病毒药：恩替卡韦	有效抑制 HBV 的 DNA，促进 ALT 恢复	慢性乙肝	乏力、头痛、腹泻、恶心和消化不良、肾毒性

目 标 检 测

一、选择题

（一）单项选择题

1. 下列何药有骨髓抑制作用（　　　）

　　A. 齐多夫定　　　B. 拉米夫定　　　　C. 阿昔洛韦　　　D. 奈韦拉平　　　　E. 沙奎那韦

2. 特异性抑制甲型流感病毒的是（　　　）

    A. 阿糖腺苷　　　B. 金刚烷胺　　　C. 奥司他韦　　　D. 阿昔洛韦　　　E. 碘苷

3. 奥司他韦通过抑制哪种酶发挥作用（　　　）

    A. 蛋白酶　　　　　　　　　B. RNA 聚合酶　　　　　　　C. HIV 反转录酶

    D. DNA 聚合酶　　　　　　　E. 神经氨酸酶

（二）多项选择题

4. 关于利巴韦林的作用及机制的叙述，下列哪些是正确的（　　　）

    A. 体外可抑制呼吸道合胞病毒

    B. 不改变病毒吸附、侵入和脱壳

    C. 诱导干扰素的产生

    D. 抑制肌苷单磷酸脱氢酶

    E. 损害病毒 RNA 和蛋白质合成

二、思考题

简述齐多夫定与奈韦拉平联合应用的意义。

（朱星枚）

PPT

Chapter 42　Cancer chemotherapeutic drugs

学习目标

1. **掌握** 抗恶性肿瘤药物的分类与作用机制。
2. **熟悉** 抗恶性肿瘤药物的药理作用与临床应用。
3. **了解** 抗恶性肿瘤药物的不良反应。

Malignant tumors, often called cancers, are characterized by uncontrolled growth and spread of the body's own cells. They occupy an important position in human disease spectrum and death spectrum, seriously threatening human health all over the world. Currently, there are still no satisfactory measures to prevent and treat malignant tumors. The three major therapeutic strategies are surgery, radiation therapy, and chemotherapy. Among them, chemotherapy using antineoplastic drugs still plays a pivotal role in the comprehensive managements of cancers. Although some malignant tumors, such as chorionic epithelial cancer and malignant lymphoma, may be cured by antineoplastic drugs, ideal therapeutic efficacy against solid tumors, which account for more than 90% of malignant tumors, are not achieved in clinical chemotherapy.

There are two major obstacles to the application of traditional cytotoxic antineoplastic drugs for tumor chemotherapy, that is, the toxicity of chemotherapeutic drugs and tumor resistance to chemotherapeutic drugs. Antineoplastic drugs often lack sufficient selectivity towards tumor cells, and thus may damage normal cells to different degrees. In addition, cancer cells are easy to develop resistance to chemotherapeutic drugs. During recent years, under the theoretical guidance of cell molecular biology, cell dynamics, immunology and other related disciplines, new antineoplastic agents represented by molecular targeted drugs (分子靶向药物) have been increasingly developed and used in clinical context. Encouragingly, combination therapy has significantly improved the efficacy of chemotherapy for malignant tumors and reduced the incidence of adverse reactions and drug resistance. Drugs are generally more effective in combination and may be synergistic through biochemical interactions. These interactions are useful in designing new regiments. It is more effective to use drugs that do not share common mechanisms of resistance and that do not overlap in their major toxicities.

1.　Classification and mechanism of cancer chemotherapeutic drugs

医药大学堂
WWW.YIYAODXT.COM

Cancer chemotherapeutic drugs are commonly divided into cytotoxic and non-cytotoxic drugs. The cytotoxic drugs (细胞毒类药物) are referred to the traditional chemotherapeutic drugs, which affect the structure or function of biological macromolecules such as nucleic acids and proteins in tumor cells, or directly inhibit tumor cell proliferation or induce tumor cell apoptosis. The non-cytotoxic drugs usually have novel mechanisms of targeting some key regulatory molecules in the molecular pathogenesis of tumors.

1.1 Classification based on chemical structure and source of drugs

(1) Alkylating agents (烷化剂) Nitrogen mustards (氮芥), ethyleneimines, nitrosoureas, methanesulfonates, etc.

(2) Antimetabolites Folic acid analogs, pyrimidine analogs, purine analogs, etc.

(3) Antitumor antibiotics Anthracycline antibiotics, mitomycin (丝裂霉素), bleomycins (博来霉素), actinomycins, etc.

(4) Antitumor botanicals Vinblastin (长春碱), camptothecin (喜树碱), paclitaxel, cedar alkaloids, podophyllotoxin derivatives, etc.

(5) Hormones Adrenocortical hormones, estrogen, estrogens and their antagonists.

(6) Others Platinum complexes and enzymes.

1.2 Classification based on biochemical mechanisms of drugs

(1) Drugs affecting biosynthesis of nucleic acids (DNA and RNA) Inhibitors of synthesis of pyrimidine nucleotides such as 5-fluorouracil, inhibitors of synthesis of purine nucleotides such as 6-mercaptopurine (6-MP, 巯嘌呤), dihydrofolate reductase inhibitors such as methotrexate (甲氨蝶呤), DNA polymerase inhibitors such as cytarabine (Ara-C, 阿糖胞苷), and nucleotide reductase (核苷酸还原酶) inhibitors such as hydroxyurea.

(2) Drugs affecting DNA structure and function Alkylating agents such as nitrogen mustard and cyclophosphamide (环磷酰胺), platinum compounds such as cisplatin (顺铂), antibiotics such as mitomycin C and bleomycin, and topoisomerase (Ⅰ or Ⅱ) inhibitors such as camptothecin and podophyllotoxin derivatives.

(3) Drugs affecting transcription and RNA synthesis They can be inserted between DNA and interfere with the transcription process. They are DNA intercalators, including actinomycin D (放线菌素 D), daunorubicin (柔红霉素), adriamycin, etc.

(4) Drugs affecting protein synthesis and function Tubulin inhibitors such as vinblastin and paclitaxel, ribosomal function inhibitors such as cunninghamia alkaloids, inhibitors of amino acid supply such as L-asparaginase, and drugs affecting hormone balance such as adrenal cortex hormones, androgens, estrogens and their antagonists.

1.3 Classification based on the cell cycle phase affected by drugs

Cancer cells are mainly composed of proliferating populations and non-proliferating populations. The proliferating cells can continuously divide and proliferate exponentially. The time duration from the end of one division to the end of next division of cancer cell is termed cell cycle (细胞周期), including four phases: the presynthetic phase (G_1), DNA synthesis phase (S), the postsynthetic phase (G_2), and mitosis phase (M). Antineoplastic drugs may exert cytotoxic effects on cancer cells through regulating cell cycle or inducing cell cycle arrest. According to the sensitivity of cancer cells at certain cell cycle phase, antineoplastic drugs can be generally divided into two categories (Figure 42-1).

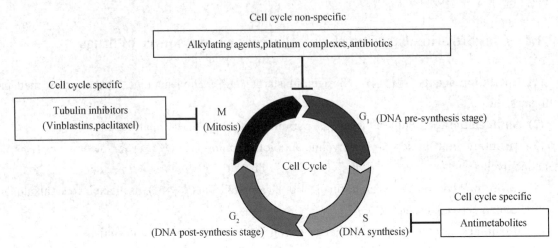

Figure 42-1   Cell cycle non-specific and specific agents

(1) Cell cycle non-specific agents (细胞周期非特异性药物)   These drugs such as alkylating agents can kill cancer cells at each cell cycle phase even at G_0 phase. Such drugs often have strong effects on malignant tumor cells in a dose-dependent manner. These drugs are particularly useful in low growth fraction solid tumors as well as in high growth fraction tumors.

(2) Cell cycle specific agents (细胞周期特异性药物)   These drugs have strong effects on cancer cells only at certain cell cycle phase. For example, the antimetabolites have a significant effect on the S phase cells, and vinblastin acts on the M phase cells. These drugs usually have relatively weak effects in a time-dependent manner, and are most effective for hematologic malignancies and solid tumors in which a relatively large proportion of the cells are proliferating or in the growth fraction.

2. Adverse reactions of cancer chemotherapeutic drugs

2.1 Short-term toxicity

(1) Myelosuppression   Most antineoplastic drugs have the adverse effect of myelosuppression to varied degrees. Peripheral blood cells, which are short-lived, are prone to be decreased. Usually, the number of white blood cells is decreased first, followed by platelets and even granulocytes, red blood cells and whole blood cells. Once myelosuppression occurs, the drug should be immediately discontinued or replaced with vincristine, bleomycin, etc., which have mild myelosuppression effects.

(2) Gastrointestinal reactions   Antineoplastic drugs can directly stimulate gastrointestinal tract, or act on medulla oblongata (延髓) vomiting center or the chemoreceptor trigger zone (催吐化学感受区),

leading to the occurrence of nausea and vomiting.

(3) Hair loss In normal human body, a majority of germinal cells are in the statues of active growth. Most antineoplastic drugs can cause hair loss, but it can be reversed after chemotherapy is halted.

(4) Damages to key organs and nervous system Adriamycin usually has cardiotoxicity. Long-term use of bleomycin at high dose may cause pulmonary fibrosis. Asparagine may induce liver injury. Cyclophosphamide at large dose may result in liver injury and bleeding cystitis. Vinblastins and cisplatin have neurotoxic effects, and cisplatin may also damage renal tubules.

(5) Allergic reactions Polypeptide or proteinaceous antineoplastic drugs such as asparaginase and bleomycin are likely to cause allergic reactions after intravenous injection.

2.2 Long-term toxicity

(1) Mutagenesis, carcinogenesis and immunosuppression Some antineoplastic agents such as alkylating agents have mutagenic, carcinogenic and immunosuppressive effects. Therefore, a secondary malignant tumor that is associated with chemotherapy may occur in some patients.

(2) Infertility and teratogenicity Some antineoplastic agents such as alkylating agents may affect reproductive system and endocrine functions, causing infertility and teratogenicity. Sometimes, the number of testicular germ cells can be reduced in male patients, leading to male infertility. Ovarian dysfunction and amenorrhea may be caused in female patients. Abortion or malformed fetus may be caused in pregnant women.

3. Common cancer chemotherapeutic drugs

3.1 Drugs affecting nucleic acid biosynthesis

These drugs are known as antimetabolites (抗代谢物). The biochemical pathways that have far proved to be most vulnerable to antimetabolites have been those relating to nucleotide and nucleic acid synthesis. The chemical structures of antimetabolites are similar to folic acid, purines, pyrimidines, etc. They can specifically interfere with nucleic acid metabolism and prevent cell division and proliferation. These drugs mainly affect the S phase, and thus are cell cycle specific drugs.

(1) Dihydrofolate reductase inhibitor Methotrexate, a folic acid antagonist, can competitively inhibit dihydrofolate reductase, leading to decreased production of tetrahydrofolate. This further inhibits deoxythymidylate synthesis and DNA synthesis in cancer cells. This drug can also prevent purine nucleotide synthesis, thereby disrupting protein synthesis. Intracellular conversion to polyglutamate metabolites is important for the therapeutic action of methotrexate. The polyglutamates of methotrexate are selectively retained within cancer cells and increase the inhibitory effects on enzymes involved in folate metabolism, making them important determinants of the duration of methotrexate action. Methotrexate is easily absorbed orally with a $t_{1/2}$ about 2 hours, and a half amount is excreted in its original form through urine. It is clinically used for children acute leukemia and chorionic epithelial cancer. The adverse reactions mainly are gastrointestinal reactions (anorexia, gastritis, diarrhea and blood in the stool) and myelosuppression (reduced leukocytes and platelets).

(2) Thymidylate synthase (胸苷酸合成酶) inhibitor　Fluorouracil is a prodrug and can be changed to be 5-fluorouracil deoxynucleotide that competitively inhibits deoxythymidylate synthetase within cells, preventing deoxyuridine methylation and DNA synthesis. 5-FU is irregularly absorbed orally and requires intravenous administration, and is highly distributed in liver and tumor tissues. 5-FU is particularly effective for digestive tract cancers (such as esophageal, gastric, and intestinal cancers) and breast cancer. It can also be used for ovarian, cervical, chorionic epithelial and bladder cancers. The earliest adverse symptoms of 5-FU are anorexia and nausea. These are followed by stomatitis and diarrhea. Myelosuppression and pigmentation also occur.

(3) Purine nucleotide interconversion inhibitor　6-MP is an adenine derivative with 6-amino substituted by a thiol group. It can be changed to be thioinosinic acid that prevents the conversion of inosinic acid into adenosine and ornithine nucleotides, thus interfering with purine metabolism and hindering nucleic acid synthesis. 6-MP has significant effects on the cancer cells at S phase and can also delay the G_1 phase. 6-MP has a slow onset of action, and is mainly used for the maintenance treatment of acute lymphoblastic leukemia. 6-MP at large doses is also effective for chorionic epithelial cancer. Myelosuppression and gastrointestinal mucosal damage are the common adverse reactions of 6-MP.

(4) Nucleotide reductase inhibitor　Hydroxycarbamide (HU, 羟基脲) via inhibition of nucleotide reductase prevents the change of cytidylic acid to be deoxycytidylic acid, and thereby inhibits DNA biosynthesis. It mainly acts on the S phase, and can enhance the sensitivity of cancer cells to chemotherapy or radiotherapy. HU has significant therapeutic effects on chronic myelogenous leukemia and can also relieve melanoma (黑色素瘤). Its main adverse reactions are myelosuppression and mild gastrointestinal reactions. Patients with renal dysfunction should use it with caution. Pregnant women should be prohibited to use HU because it can cause teratology.

(5) DNA polymerase inhibitor　Ara-C can be catalyzed by deoxycytidine kinase to be cytidine diphosphate or cytidine triphosphate, which further inhibits the activity of DNA polymerase (DNA聚合酶), thereby blocking DNA synthesis. It can also be incorporated into DNA, leading to interference with chain elongation and defective ligation of fragments of newly synthesized DNA. Ara-C has no cross-resistance with commonly used antitumor drugs. Ara-C is a cell cycle S phase specific antimetabolite, and is highly schedule-dependent and must be given either by continuous infusion or every 8-12 hours for 5-7 days. It is the first choice for acute non-lymphocytic leukemia in the clinic, particularly for adult acute non-lymphocytic leukemia. It is also used for chronic myelogenous leukemia, and head and neck cancer. Myelosuppression and gastrointestinal reactions are commonly seen. Intravenous injection can cause phlebitis and liver injury.

3.2　Drugs affecting DNA structure and function

3.2.1　Alkylating agents

Alkylating agents with active chemical properties can induce alkylation reaction of the nucleophilic groups contained in DNA, RNA or proteins, forming cross-links or depurination and leading to DNA strand breakage even cell death. Chlomethine (氮芥), cyclophosphamide and busulfan (白消安) are commonly used alkylating agents for antitumor purposes. They belong to cell cycle non-specific drugs.

Cyclophosphamide (环磷酰胺)

【Pharmacokinetics】It has good absorption when orally given with a 97% bioavailability. It can be widely distributed and has a higher drug concentration in tumor tissues than in normal tissues. Its plasma $t_{1/2}$ is about 6.5 hours, and 17%-31% of the drug is excreted in its original form through feces and 30% in its active form through urine.

【Pharmacodynamics】Cyclophosphamide is a potent bifunctional alkylating agent interfering with the functions of DNA and RNA, especially the former. It can cross-link with DNA and inhibit DNA synthesis, and significantly affect the S phase. Cyclophosphamide in its parent form does not have direct cytotoxic effects. After entering the body, it is converted by liver microsomal cytochrome P450 mixed-function oxidase system to the active metabolite aldophosphamide (醛磷酰胺) followed by nonenzymatic cleavage of aldophosphamide to phosphoramide mustard and acrolein, which have cytotoxic effects on tumor cells.

【Clinical indications】Cyclophosphamide has a broad antitumor spectrum and is one of the most commonly used alkylating agents. It has significant therapeutic effect on malignant lymphoma (恶性淋巴瘤), and is also effective for acute lymphoblastic leukemia, lung cancer, testicular cancer, ovarian cancer, breast cancer, and multiple myeloma.

【Adverse reactions】Myelosuppression, nausea, vomiting, and hair loss are commonly seen.

3.2.2　Platinum complexes

Cisplatin (顺铂)

【Pharmacokinetics】Cisplatin has a 90% plasma protein binding rate and is highly distributed in liver, kidney and bladder. It is mainly excreted in its original form through kidney.

【Pharmacodynamics】Cisplatin is an inorganic metal complex. It can cross-link with the bases on the DNA strands, thereby destroying the structure and function of DNA. It has weak inhibitory effects on RNA and protein synthesis. It kills cancer cells in all stages of the cell cycle. When used in combination regiments with vinblastin and bleomycin, or etoposide (依托泊苷) and bleomycin, cisplatin-based therapy has led to the cure of non-seminomatous testicular cancer.

【Clinical indications】Cisplatin has a broad antitumor spectrum and is effective against a variety of solid tumors, such as testicular cancer, squamous cell carcinoma, ovarian cancer, bladder cancer, and prostate cancer.

【Adverse reactions】The main adverse reactions are gastrointestinal reactions, myelosuppression, peripheral neuritis, and ototoxicity. Long-term or large dose use can cause severe renal toxicity.

3.2.3　Antibiotics

Mitomycin C is an alkylating agent that undergoes metabolic activation through an enzyme-mediated reduction to generate an alkylating agent that cross-links DNA. It is a cell cycle non-specific drug. Mitomycin C is often used in combination with fluorouracil, adriamycin, cisplatin, etc., for the treatment of gastric cancer, lung cancer, breast cancer, pancreatic cancer, chronic myelogenous leukemia, and malignant lymphoma. Mitomycin C has obvious and long-lasting myelosuppressive toxicity.

Bleomycin is a small peptide that contains a DNA-binding region and an iron-binding domain. It acts by binding to DNA, which results in single-strand and double-strand breaks following free radical formation, and inhibition of DNA biosynthesis. Bleomycin is primarily used for squamous cell carcinoma or for combination therapy against lymphoma. Combination of bleomycin with vincristine or cisplatin is often used for testicular cancer. Bleomycin may have serious pulmonary toxicity and cause pulmonary fibrosis or interstitial pneumonia.

3.2.4 Topoisomerase inhibitors

Camptothecin is an alkaloid extracted from camptotheca, a unique plant in China. Hydroxycamptothecin (羟喜树碱) is a hydroxyl derivative of camptothecin. These drugs can specifically inhibit the activity of DNA topoisomerase I and interfere with the structure and function of DNA. They are cell cycle non-specific drugs, but exert stronger effects on the S phase than the G_1 and G_2 phases. The antitumor spectrum of camptothecins includes gastric cancer, chorionic epithelial cancer, malignant hydatidiform mole, acute and chronic myelogenous leukemia, colorectal cancer, bladder cancer and liver cancer. The adverse reactions mainly include urinary tract irritation symptoms, gastrointestinal reactions, myelosuppression, and hair loss.

3.3 Drugs affecting transcription and RNA synthesis

Actinomycin D can be embedded between the adjacent guanine and cytosine base pairs in the DNA double helix, interfering with RNA polymerase-driven DNA transcription. It is a cell cycle non-specific drug, and has strong effects on the G_1 phase. This drug has a narrow antitumor spectrum including malignant hydatidiform mole, chorionic epithelial cancer, Hodgkin's disease, lymphoma, and nephroblastoma. Adverse reactions mainly include myelosuppression, gastrointestinal reactions, hair loss, dermatitis, and teratology.

Doxorubicin (多柔比星) also known as adriamycin (阿霉素) can be embedded between DNA base pairs to prevent RNA transcription and DNA replication. It is a cell cycle non-specific agent, and has strong effects on the S phase. This drug has a broad antitumor spectrum and high efficacy. It is mainly used for acute lymphoblastic leukemia or myeloid leukemia that is resistant to commonly used chemotherapeutic drugs, and preferentially used as an alternative drug for malignant lymphoma. It also has therapeutic effects against breast cancer, ovarian cancer, small cell lung cancer, gastric cancer, liver cancer and bladder cancer. Cardiotoxicity is the most serious adverse reaction manifested by the early symptoms of arrhythmia and large dose-caused myocardial degeneration and myocardial interstitial edema. Other adverse reactions include myelosuppression, gastrointestinal reactions, skin pigmentation, and hair loss.

3.4 Drugs affecting protein synthesis and function

(1) Tubulin inhibitors Vinblastin and vincristine (长春新碱) are natural alkaloids. Vindesine (长春地辛) and vinorelbine (长春瑞滨) are semisynthetic derivatives of vinblastin. Vinblastins can bind to tubulin proteins and inhibit microtubule assembly and spindle formation, resulting in mitotic arrest in tumor cells. They belong to M phase specific drugs and have no cross resistance between them. These drugs have diverse antitumor spectrum. Vinblastin combined with cisplatin and bleomycin is preferentially used for the treatment of testicular cancer. Vincristine is primarily used for acute lymphocytic leukemia, Hodgkin's disease and malignant lymphoma. Vinorelbine can be concentrated in lung and thus is effective for non-small cell lung cancer. Myelosuppression is the major adverse effect of these drugs. Vincristine also has neurotoxicity.

Paclitaxel (紫杉醇) is another alkaloid compound inhibiting tubulin function. It can promote microtubule assembly in the absence of microtubule-associated proteins and guanosine triphosphate, resulting in inhibition of mitosis and cell division. Paclitaxel has significant activity against a wide variety of solid tumors, including ovarian cancer, breast cancer, non-small cell or small cell lung cancer, head and neck cancer, esophageal cancer, prostate cancer, bladder cancer and AIDS-related Kaposi's sarcoma. Paclitaxel may cause myelosuppression, neurotoxicity and cardiac toxicity.

(2) Ribosome function inhibitors　Harringtonine (三尖杉酯碱) and homoharringtonine (高三尖杉酯碱) are natural alkaloids that can halt the initial stage of protein synthesis, decompose ribosomes, and inhibit mitosis. They are cell cycle non-specific drugs. They have good therapeutic efficacy against acute myeloid leukemia, and can also be used for acute mononuclear leukemia and chronic myelogenous leukemia, malignant lymphoma, lung cancer, and choriocarcinoma. Adverse reactions include myelosuppression, gastrointestinal reactions, and hair loss.

(3) Inhibitors of amino acid supply　L-asparaginase (L-门冬酰胺酶) hydrolyzes asparagine in serum, cutting off asparagine supply for cancer cells. This may block protein synthesis, inhibit cell growth, and cause cancer cell death. This agent is mainly used for acute lymphoblastic leukemia often in combination with methotrexate, doxorubicin, vincristine or prednisone. It leads to mild myelosuppression and gastrointestinal reactions. Urticarial and anaphylactic shock are commonly seen.

3.5　Drugs affecting hormonal balance

Androgen agents such as dimethyltestosterone and testosterone propionate can inhibit follicle-stimulating hormone secretion from anterior pituitary gland, and thus reduce estrogen secretion from ovaries and counteract the effects of estrogen. They have good therapeutic benefits for advanced breast cancer patients with bone metastases.

Estrogen agent diethylstilbestrol can inhibit the secretion of interstitial cell stimulating hormone from pituitary gland, and thus reduce androgen secretion from testicular interstitial cells and adrenal cortex. It can counteract the growth-promoting effects of estrogen on prostate cancer, and thus is mainly used for the treatment of prostate cancer.

Tamoxifen is a synthetic non-steroidal compound functioning as a competitive partial agonist-inhibitor of estrogen. It can inhibit the growth of hormone-dependent breast cancer cells, and thus is mainly used to treat advanced breast cancer with positive estrogen receptor. It is also the drug of choice for advanced breast cancer after menopause. It is also effective for solid tumors such as advanced ovarian and cervical cancer. Tamoxifen is well tolerated, and its side effects are generally mild, mainly including nausea, vomiting, transient leukopenia and thrombocytopenia.

重 点 小 结

类别		代表药物
干扰核酸生物合成的药物	二氢叶酸还原酶抑制剂	甲氨蝶呤
	胸苷酸合成酶抑制剂	氟尿嘧啶
	嘌呤核苷酸互变抑制剂	巯嘌呤
	核苷酸还原酶抑制剂	羟基脲
	DNA 聚合酶抑制剂	氮芥、环磷酰胺
直接影响 DNA 结构和功能的药物	烷化剂	顺铂、卡铂
	破坏 DNA 的铂类配合物	丝裂霉素 C、博来霉素
	破坏 DNA 的抗生素	喜树碱类
	拓扑异构酶抑制剂	丝裂霉素 C、博来霉素
干扰转录过程、阻止 RNA 合成的药物		放线菌素 D、多柔比星
抑制蛋白质合成和功能的药物	微管蛋白活性抑制剂	长春碱类、紫杉醇
	干扰核蛋白体功能的药物	三尖杉生物碱类
	影响氨基酸供应的药物	L-门冬酰胺酶
调节激素平衡的药物	甾体类激素	雌激素、雄激素
	激素拮抗剂	他莫昔芬

目 标 检 测

题库

一、选择题

（一）单项选择题

1. 体外无药理活性，需经体内生物转化后才具有抗肿瘤活性的药物是（　　　）
   　　A. 长春碱　　　　　　　　　　B. 高三尖杉酯碱　　　　　　　　C. 环磷酰胺
   　　D. L-门冬酰胺酶　　　　　　　E. 博来霉素

2. 甲氨蝶呤的抗肿瘤作用机制是（　　　）
   　　A. 抑制嘧啶碱基的合成　　　　　　　B. 抑制嘌呤碱基的合成
   　　C. 抑制二氢叶酸还原酶　　　　　　　D. 抑制二氢叶酸合成酶
   　　E. 直接破坏 DNA 的结构和功能

3. 主要作用于 S 期的抗肿瘤药物类别是（　　　）
   　　A. 烷化剂　　　　　　　　　　B. 抗肿瘤抗生素　　　　　　　　C. 抗代谢药
   　　D. 长春碱类　　　　　　　　　E. 激素类

4. 主要作用于 M 期的抗肿瘤药物是（　　　）
   　　A. 氟尿嘧啶　　　B. 长春新碱　　　C. 环磷酰胺　　　D. 泼尼松龙　　　E. 放线菌素 D

5. 环磷酰胺对何种恶性肿瘤疗效较显著（　　）

    A. 多发性骨髓瘤　　　　　　　　　B. 急性淋巴细胞性白血病　　　　C. 卵巢癌

    D. 乳腺癌　　　　　　　　　　　　E. 恶性淋巴瘤

6. 没有明显骨髓抑制不良反应的抗肿瘤药物类型是（　　）

    A. 激素类　　　　　　　　　　　　B. 烷化剂　　　　　　　　　　　C. 长春碱类

    D. 抗代谢药　　　　　　　　　　　E. 抗肿瘤抗生素

（二）多项选择题

7. 属于烷化剂的抗肿瘤药物是（　　）

    A. 巯嘌呤　　　　B. 甲氨蝶呤　　　　C. 氮芥　　　　　　D. 环磷酰胺　　　　E. 放线菌素 D

8. 属于细胞周期非特异性的抗肿瘤药物是（　　）

    A. 喜树碱　　　　B. 多柔比星　　　　C. 氮芥　　　　　　D. 环磷酰胺　　　　E. 丝裂霉素 C

9. 直接破坏 DNA 并阻止其复制的抗肿瘤抗生素是（　　）

    A. 放线菌素 D　　　　　　　　　　B. 丝裂霉素 C　　　　　　　　　C. 柔红霉素

    D. 博来霉素　　　　　　　　　　　E. 阿霉素

二、思考题

细胞周期非特异性和特异性抗恶性肿瘤药物各自有何特点？代表药是什么？

（张　峰）

Chapter 43　Immunomodulators

1. **掌握**　他克莫司、干扰素、左旋咪唑的药理作用及机制、临床应用和不良反应。
2. **熟悉**　免疫系统的功能。
3. **了解**　免疫系统的组成。

Strategies of avoidance, resistance, and tolerance represent different ways to deal with pathogens. Anatomic barriers and various chemical barriers such as complement and antimicrobial proteins (抗微生物蛋白) may be considered a primitive form of avoidance, and they are the first line of defense against entry of pathogens into host tissues. If these barriers are broken, the immune system starts to work. The immune system has three functions, namely, immune defense (免疫防御), immune surveillance (免疫监视) and immune homeostasis (免疫内环境稳定).

The immune system is the general designation of various cells, tissues and organs involved in the immune response, including thymus, bone marrow, lymph nodes, spleen, tonsil, lymphocytes and plasma cells. Immune responses are initiated in several peripheral lymphoid tissues (外周淋巴组织). The spleen serves as a filter for blood-borne infections. Lymph nodes and the mucosal and gut-associated lymphoid tissues (MALT and GALT, 黏膜相关淋巴组织和肠相关淋巴组织) are organized into specific zones where immune cells such as T and B lymphocytes can be activated efficiently. On the contrary, the abnormality of any factor in the immune system can lead to immune dysfunction.

1. Immune response and immunopathology

1.1　Immune response

The immune system defends the host against infection. There are two types of immunity: innate immunity (先天性免疫) and adaptive immunity (适应性免疫). Innate immunity including phagocytes (吞噬细胞), complements, interferon (干扰素), etc., is involved in phagocytosis, removal of foreign bodies, and mediates and participates in the immune response of specific immunity. Innate immunity provides the first defense barrier, but lacks the ability to recognize certain pathogens and to provide the specific protective immunity that prevents reinfection.

Adaptive immunity is initiated when an innate immune response fails to eliminate a new infection and activated antigen-presenting cells (抗原提呈细胞) that bear antigens from pathogens. Adaptive immunity includes cellular immunity and humoral immunity, which are mediated by T cells and B cells, respectively, and are involved in many cytokines related to the immune system. B cells mature in the bone marrow and are the source of circulating antibodies. T cells mature in the thymus and recognize peptides from pathogens presented by MHC molecules on infected cells or antigen-presenting cells. The immune response could artificially separate into three stages: recognition stage, stage of activation, proliferation and differentiation, and effect stage.

Innate immune responses occur rapidly, and in contrast, the adaptive immune responses take days rather than hours to induce. Nevertheless, the adaptive immune system could eliminate infections more efficiently because of exquisite specificity of antigen recognition by its lymphocytes. In contrast to a limited repertoire of receptors (受体库) expressed by innate immune cells, lymphocytes express highly specialized antigen receptors that collectively possess a vast repertoire of specificity. This enables the adaptive immune system to respond to virtually any pathogen and effectively focus resources to eliminate pathogens that have evaded or overwhelmed innate immunity. See Table 43-1.

1.2　Immunopathology

When the immune function of the organism is abnormal, the body may produce immunopathological reactions, including allergic reactions, autoimmune diseases, immune deficiency diseases and immunoproliferative diseases (免疫增生病). The clinical manifestations are low immune function or excessive enhancement of immune function, which can even lead to death. Immunomodulatory drugs can ward off and treat diseases caused by abnormal immune function through one or more mechanisms (Table 43-1).

Table 43-1　Phases of the immune response

	Response	Typical time after infection to start of response	Duration of response
Innate immune response	Inflammation, complement activation, phagocytosis, and destruction of pathogen	Minutes	Days
	Interaction between antigen-presenting dendritic cells and antigen-specific T cells: recognition of antigen, adhesion, co-stimulation, T-cell proliferation and differentiation	Hours	Days
Adaptive immune response	Activation of antigen-specific B cells	Hours	Days
	Formation of effector and memory T cells	Days	Weeks
	Interaction of T cells with B cells, formation of germinal centers, Formation of effector B cells (plasma cells) and memory B cells. Production of antibody	Days	Weeks
	Emigration of effector lymphocytes from peripheral lymphoid organs	A few days	Weeks
Immunological memory	Elimination of pathogen by effector cells and antibody maintenance of memory B cells and T cells and high serum or mucosal antibody levels	A few days	Weeks
	Protection against reinfection	Days to weeks	Can be lifelong

(Kenneth Murphy, Casey Weaver. Janeway's Immunobiology. 9th ed)

2. Immunosuppressants

Cyclosporine (环孢素)

This fungal antibiotic is one of many cyclosporins with a narrow spectrum of antibiotic activity, but with obviously immunosuppressive effects on immune response after transplantation and on delayed-type hypersensitivity. It has a remarkably specific affinity for lymphocytes, affecting both T cells and B cells in humans.

【Pharmacodynamics】Cyclosporine is an immunosuppressive drug with strong effects, small toxicity and high selectivity, that selectively acts on T cells, in particularly, in the stage of T cell activation. The general dose of cyclosporine has no obvious effect on B cell, but the high dose also inhibits B cell and the production of antibody. Cyclosporine inhibits monocyte/macrophage function indirectly. Cyclosporine inhibit T-cell activation by inhibiting the activity of calcineurin (钙调磷酸酶) and then inhibiting the expression of IL-2 and IL-2 receptor in helper T cells. Cyclosporine also increase expression of transforming growth factor β (TGF-β), a potent inhibitor of IL-2 stimulated T-cell proliferation and generation of cytotoxic T lymphocytes (CTLs).

【Therapeutic uses】Cyclosporine has been used broadly in organ transplantation and the treatment of autoimmune diseases.

【Adverse reactions】The most common side effect of cyclosporine is nephrotoxicity (肾毒性), which can increase mostly reversibly the levels of serum creatinine (血肌酐) and urea nitrogen (尿素氮). Other side effects include transient liver damage, anorexia (食欲缺乏), lethargy (倦怠), nausea (恶心), diarrhea(腹泻), etc.

Tacrolimus (他克莫司)

Tacrolimus is a macrolide antibiotic produced by *Streptomyces tsukubaensis* (筑波山土壤链霉菌属). Similar to cyclosporine, tacrolimus inhibits T cell activation by inhibiting calcineurin Firstly, tacrolimus binds to an intracellular immunophilin FK-binding protein (FKBP, 免疫亲和性FK结合蛋白) and forms a complex. Then, the complex inhibits the activity of calcineurin and the expression of IL-2 and IL-2 receptor in helper T cells. Thus, cyclosporine and tacrolimus target the same pathway for immunosuppression, despite the intracellular receptors are different. Tacrolimus is mainly used to prevent and treat the immune rejection of transplantation of liver, kidney and bone marrow. Large dose of tacrolimus can produce nephrotoxicity, neurotoxicity and reproductive toxicity (生殖毒性).

Adrenocortical steroids (糖皮质激素类)

Glucocorticoids exert their immunosuppressive effects by inducing the redistribution (再分布) of lymphocytes and hence resulting in a rapid and transient decrease in peripheral blood lymphocytes counts. The intracellular mechanism of glucocorticoids is that they bind to glucocorticoid receptors, which are transcription factors, and then regulate (activate or inhibit) transcription of target gene, depending on the cell types.

Glucocorticoids could be used for prevention and treatment transplant rejection, and be used to treat autoimmune disorders, e.g., rheumatoid arthritis (类风湿关节炎), and systemic lupus erythematosus (系统性红斑狼疮).

3. Immunostimulants

Levamisole (左旋咪唑)

This drug is an anthelminthic agent (驱虫药), however, which show potentiated effects on immune responses in animals and humans. It is an imidazole derivate and it is thought to act by inhibiting the function of T suppressor cells.

Levamisole can be used to reduce the incidence and severity of infection in immunocompromised patients, restore the immune function of immunocompromised patients and enhance their resistance to disease, and can be used as adjuvant therapy (辅助治疗) for tumors.

The incidence of adverse reactions of levamisole is relatively low, mainly including gastrointestinal reactions, nervous system reactions and allergies. Administrated levamisole continuously and secularly may produce granulocytopenia (粒细胞减少), which can be recovered after discontinuation. Occasionally, liver function was abnormal by levamisole.

Interferons (干扰素)

Interferons are a group of glycoproteins, which first identified as active substances possessing inhibitory effects on intracellular viral replication. To date, there are three major classes of interferons-α, β, and γ. Interferons have been produced by stimulation of lymphocyte or fibroblast precursors, and now interferon-α is available through recombinant DNA technology. Interferon-α is derived from human lymphoblasts and interferon-β from human fibroblasts. Interferon-γ is also referred to as immune interferon.

【Pharmacodynamics 】

(1) Immune regulation   Interferon can promote the change of quality and quantity of molecules (such as surface receptor and surface antigen molecules) on cell membrane of lymphocyte (淋巴细胞) and monocyte macrophage (单核巨噬细胞), and then regulate the immune function.

(2) Antiviral effects   Interferon destroys the replication cycle of virus through interferon receptor on cell membrane.

(3) Antitumor activity   Interferon can inhibit the proliferation and division of tumor cells, enhance the immune monitoring function of the body and kill tumor cells.

【Therapeutic uses 】

(1) Viral diseases   Acute and chronic viral infectious diseases, local medication for condyloma acuminatum (尖锐湿疣) and so on.

(2) Adjuvant therapy for tumors   The treatment of cancers, such as multiple myeloma, chronic myelogenous leukemia, hairy cell leukemia, and malignant melanoma.

(3) Organ transplantation　Preventing virus infection after using immunosuppressant and help to inhibit rejection of allografts (移植排斥).

(4) Other diseases　Rheumatoid arthritis, multiple sclerosis (多发性硬化), etc.

【Adverse reactions】Interferon could produce transient fever, nausea (恶心), vomiting (呕吐), tiredness, limb numbness (肢体麻木), occasional myelosuppression.

重 点 小 结

类别	药物	药理作用	临床应用	不良反应
免疫抑制剂	环孢素	选择性抑制 T 淋巴细胞活化	器官或组织移植后排异反应，自身免疫性疾病	肝肾损害
	他克莫司	类似但作用强于环孢素	器官移植后排异反应	肾、神经、胃肠和心血管毒性
	糖皮质激素类	多环节抑制各类型免疫反应	自身免疫性疾病，排异反应	类肾上腺皮质功能亢进症，诱发或加重感染
免疫增强剂	左旋咪唑	促进受抑的 T 淋巴细胞和巨噬细胞功能恢复正常	免疫低下或缺陷者感染，类风湿关节炎等自身免疫性疾病，肿瘤辅助治疗	胃肠道反应、头晕、失眠、粒细胞减少
	干扰素	广谱抗病毒，抑制细胞增生，调节免疫，抗肿瘤	病毒感染性疾病，恶性肿瘤	发热、畏寒、头痛、恶心等，大剂量可引起白细胞减少

目 标 检 测

一、选择题

（一）单项选择题

1. 临床常用的免疫增强剂不包括（　　）
    A. 左旋咪唑　　　　　　　　B. 环孢素　　　　　　　　C. 转移因子
    D. 白细胞介素　　　　　　　E. 干扰素
2. 器官移植后最常用的免疫抑制剂是（　　）
    A. 环磷酰胺　　　　　　　　B. 硫唑嘌呤　　　　　　　C. 泼尼松
    D. 环孢素　　　　　　　　　E. C 和 D
    E. 干扰素

（二）多项选择题

3. 免疫增强剂常用于（　　）
    A. 免疫缺陷疾病　　　　　　B. 器官移植　　　　　　　C. 慢性感染
    D. 难治性病毒感染　　　　　E. 恶性肿瘤的辅助治疗

题库

医药大学堂
WWW.YIYAODXT.COM

4. 干扰素具有下列哪些作用（　　　）

    A. 抗肿瘤　　　　　　　　B. 调节免疫　　　　　　　　C. 抑制细胞增殖

    D. 抗真菌　　　　　　　　E. 抗病毒

二、思考题

比较免疫抑制剂和免疫增强剂的药理作用及临床应用。

（徐志立）

Reference answer

Chapter 1

1. D 2. C 3. B 4. E

Chapter 2

1. C 2. D 3. C 4. A 5. B 6. E 7. ABCD 8. BCE 9. ACD

Chapter 3

1. C 2. C 3. C 4. B 5. E 6. A

Chapter 4

1. E 2. A 3. D 4. BDE

Chapter 5

1. B 2. D 3. D 4. A 5. C 6. A 7. ABCD 8. DE

Chapter 6

1. E 2. B 3. C 4. B 5. BDE 6. BCD

Chapter 7

1. D 2. B 3. D 4. A 5. A 6. B 7. AE

Chapter 8

1. A 2. A 3. D 4. C 5. AC 6. CDE

Chapter 9

1. A 2. B 3. B 4. D 5. ABCDE 6. ABCDE

Chapter 10

1. D 2. C 3. B 4. B 5. ABCE

Chapter 11

1. B 2. C 3. B 4. D 5. C 6. C

Chapter 12

1. C 2. A 3. A

Chapter 13

1. C 2. C 3. A 4. D 5. C 6. D

Chapter 14

1. A 2. E 3. C 4. D 5. BCDE 6. ABDE 7. ABD

Chapter 15

1. A 2. E 3. B 4. E 5. A 6. ABCDE 7. ABC

Chapter 16

1. A 2. D 3. D 4. C 5. B 6. A 7. E 8. E 9. E 10. A 11. ABCE 12. ABDE

Chapter 17

1. C 2. B 3. A 4. B 5. C 6. BCD 7. ACDE

Chapter 18

1. E 2. B 3. C 4. A 5. CD 6. ABCDE 7. ABC 8. ABCD

Chapter 19

1. D 2. A 3. C 4. D 5. D 6. B 7. D 8. ABCD 9. ACDE

Chapter 20

1. C 2. A 3. D 4. A 5. C 6. AB

Chapter 21

1. A 2. E 3. E 4. A 5. D 6. ABCDE 7. CDE 8. ABCDE 9. ABCE

Chapter 22

1. A 2. E 3. C 4. E 5. C 6. ABCDE 7. AE

Chapter 23

1. C 2. A 3. C 4. A 5. C 6. A 7. E 8. ABC 9. CD

Chapter 24

1. C 2. D 3. C 4. A 5. D 6. ABCE 7. ABCDE

Chapter 25

1. C 2. E 3. B 4. D 5. B 6. C 7. B 8. BCD 9. ABCD

Chapter 26

1. D 2. A 3. B 4. B 5. ABC

Chapter 27

1. D 2. C 3. B 4. A 5. B 6. AC 7. BDE

Chapter 28

1. A 2. E 3. C 4. D 5. AB

Chapter 29

A

Chapter 30

1. A 2. E 3. C 4. ABC

Chapter 31

1. B 2. D 3. D 4. A

Chapter 32

1. B 2. C 3. B 4. A 5. B 6. ABCDE 7. ABCD

Chapter 33

1. B 2. D 3. C 4. D 5. A 6. ABCE 7. ABE

Chapter 34

1. E 2. B 3. D 4. D 5. ABD 6. BD

Chapter 35

1. D 2. A 3. A 4. D 5. ABCE 6. ABC

Chapter 36

1. C 2. D 3. B 4. C 5. C 6. D 7. BDE 8. ABD 9. ABCDE

Chapter 37

1. E 2. C 3. D 4. B 5. ABC

Chapter 38

1. E 2. C 3. C 4. B 5. ABCD

Chapter 39

1. E   2. D   3. B

Chapter 40

1. D   2. B   3. B   4. A   5. C   6. ABCE   7. ABC   8. ACD

Chapter 41

1. A   2. B   3. E   4. ABDE

Chapter 42

1. C   2. C   3. C   4. B   5. E   6. A   7. CD   8. ABCDE   9. BD

Chapter 43

1. B   2. E   3. ACDE   4. ABCE

References

[1] 廖端芳，周玖瑶. 药理学 [M]. 3版. 北京：人民卫生出版社，2016.

[2] 杨宝峰，陈建国. 药理学 [M]. 9版. 北京：人民卫生出版社，2018.

[3] 娄建石. 药理学（英文版）[M]. 北京：清华大学出版社，2015.

[4] 周宏灏. 药理学 [M]. 北京：科学出版社，2006.

[5] 孙建宁. 药理学 [M]. 北京：中国中医药出版社，2016.

[6] R. A.Harvey.Lippincott's illustrated reviews Pharmacology.5th ed.Lippincott Williams & Wilkins.2012.

[7] Joel G Hardman, Lee E Limbird, Alfred G Gilman.Goodman & Gilman's the Pharmacological Basis of Therapeutics.13th ed. McGraw-Hill Professional.2018.

[8] Humphrey P. Rang,Maureen M. Dale,James M. Ritter, et al. Rang and Dale's Pharmacology. Elsevier Health Sciences.2007.

[9] Bertram G. Katzung,Anthony J. Trevor,Susan B. Masters.Basic and Clinical Pharmacology. 12th ed. Mcgraw Hill Digital.2012.